LAW
&
MENTAL
HEALTH
PROFESSIONALS

GEORGIA

LAW & MENTAL HEALTH PROFESSIONALS SERIES

Bruce D. Sales and Michael Owen Miller, Series Editors

ARIZONA: Miller and Sales
CALIFORNIA: Caudill and Pope
FLORIDA: Petrila and Otto
GEORGIA: Remar and Hubert
MASSACHUSETTS: Brant
MINNESOTA: Janus, Mickelsen, and Sanders
NEW JERSEY: Wulach
NEW YORK: Wulach
TEXAS: Shuman
WASHINGTON: Benjamin, Rosenwald, Overcast, and Feldman
WISCONSIN: Kaplan and Miller

LAW & MENTAL HEALTH PROFESSIONALS

GEORGIA

Robert B. Remar
Richard N. Hubert

American Psychological Association
Washington, DC

Published by
American Psychological Association
750 First Street, NE
Washington, DC 20002

Copies may be ordered from
APA Order Department
P.O. Box 2710
Hyattsville, MD 20784

In the UK and Europe, copies may be ordered from
American Psychological Association
3 Henrietta Street
Covent Garden, London
WC2E 8LU England

Typeset in Palatino by General Graphic Services, York, PA
Text and cover designer: Rubin Krassner, Silver Spring, MD
Printer: Quinn-Woodbine, Inc., Woodbine, NJ
Technical/Production Editor: Miria Liliana Riahi

Library of Congress Cataloging-in-Publication Data
Remar, Robert B.
  Law and mental health professionals.   Georgia / Robert B.
  Remar, Richard N. Hubert.
      p.   cm. — (Law & mental health professionals series)
  Includes bibliographical references and index.
  ISBN 1-55798-364-X
      1. Mental health personnel—Legal status, laws, etc.—
  Georgia.   2. Mental health laws—Georgia.   3. Forensic
  psychiatry—Georgia.   I. Hubert, Richard N.   II. Title.
  III. Series.
  KFG326.5.P73R46   1996
  344.758'044—dc20   96-19783
  [347.508444]   CIP

British Library Cataloguing-in-Publication Data
A CIP record is available from the British Library.

Printed in the United States of America
First edition

Contents

Section 4. Adults, Minors, and Families · 151

vi

Editors' Preface

The Need to Know the Law

For years, providers of mental health services (hereinafter mental health professionals, or MHPs) have been directly affected by the law. At one end of the continuum, their practice has been controlled by laws covering such matters as licensure and certification, third-party reimbursement, and professional incorporation. At the other end, they have been courted by the legal system to aid in its administration, providing such services as evaluating the mental status of litigants, providing expert testimony in court, and engaging in therapy with court-referred juveniles and adults. Even when not directly affected, MHPs find themselves indirectly affected by the law because their clients sometimes become involved in legal entanglements that involve mental status issues (e.g., divorce proceedings or termination of parental rights hearings).

Despite this pervasive influence, most professionals do not know about, much less understand, most of the laws that affect their practice, the services they render, and the clients they serve. This state of affairs is particularly troubling for several reasons. First, not knowing about the laws that affect one's practice typically results in the MHP's not gaining the benefits that the law may provide. Consider the law relating to the incorporation of professionals. It confers significant benefit, but only if it is known about and applied. The fact that it has been enacted by the state legislature does not help the MHP, any more than an MHP will be of help to a distressed person who refuses to contact the MHP.

Second, not knowing about the laws that affect the services they render can result in incompetent performance of, and liability for, the MHP either through the civil law (e.g., malpractice law) or through criminal sanctions. A brief example may help underscore this point. When an MHP is asked to evaluate a party to a lawsuit and testify in court, the court (the law's term for the judge) is asking the professional to assess and testify about whether that litigant meets some legal standard. The court is often not concerned with the defendant's mental health per se, although this may be relevant to the MHP's evaluation of the person. Rather, the court wants to know whether the person meets the legal standard as it is set down by the law. Not knowing the legal standard means that the MHP is most likely evaluating the person for the wrong goal and providing the court with irrelevant information, at least from the court's point of view. Regretfully, there are too many cases in which this has occurred.

Third, not knowing the law that affects the clients that MHPs serve may significantly diminish their capability for handling their clients' distress. For example, a client who is undergoing a divorce and child custody dispute may have distorted beliefs about what may happen during the legal proceedings. A basic understanding of the controlling law in this area will allow the therapist to be more sensitive in rendering therapy.

The Problem in Accessing Legal Information

Given the need for this information, why have MHPs not systematically sought it out? Part of the reason lies in the concern over their ability to understand legal doctrines. Indeed, this is a legitimate worry, especially if they had to read original legal materials that were not collected, organized, and described with an MHP audience in mind. This is of particular concern because laws are written in terms and phrases of "art" that do not always share the common law definition or usage, whereas some terms and phrases are left ambiguous and undefined or are used differently for different legal topics. Another part of the reason is that the law affecting MHPs and their clients is not readily available—even to lawyers. There are no compendiums that identify the topics that these laws cover or present an analysis of each topic for easy reference.

To compound the difficulty, the law does not treat the different mental health professional disciplines uniformly or always specify the particular disciplines as being covered by it. Nor does the law emanate from a single legal forum. Each state enacts its own rules and regulations, often resulting in wide variations in the way a topic is handled across the United States. Multiply this confusion times the one hundred or so topics that relate to mental health practice. In addition, the law within a state does not come from one legal source. Rather, there are five primary ones: the state constitution; state legislative enactments (statutes); state agency administrative rules and regulations; rules of court promulgated by the state supreme court; and state and federal court cases that apply, interpret, and construe this existing state law. To know about one of these sources without knowing how its pronouncements on a given topic have been modified by these other sources can result in one's making erroneous conclusions about the operation of the law. Finally, mental health practice also comes under the purview of federal law (constitutional and statutory law, administrative rules and regulations, and case law). Federal law authorizes direct payments to MHPs for their services to some clients, sets standards for delivery of services in federal facilities (e.g., Veterans Administration hospitals), and articulates the law that guides cases that are tried in federal courts under federal law.

Purposes of This Series

What is needed, therefore, is a book for each state, the District of Columbia, and the federal jurisdictions that comprehensively and accurately reviews and integrates all of the law that affects MHPs in that jurisdiction (hereinafter state). To ensure currency, regular supplements to these books will also need to be drafted. These materials should be written so that they are completely understandable to MHPs, as well as to lawyers. To accomplish these goals, the editors have tried to identify every legal topic that affects mental health practice, making each one the subject of a chapter. Each chapter, in turn, describes the legal standards that the MHP will be operating under and the relevant legal process that the MHP will be operating within. If a state does not have relevant law on an issue, then a brief explanation of how this law works in other states will be presented while noting the lack of regulation in this area within the state under consideration.

This type of coverage facilitates other purposes of the series. Although each chapter is written in order to state exactly what is the present state of the law and not argue for or against any particular approach, it is hoped that the comprehensiveness of the coverage will encourage MHPs to question the desirability of their states' approach to each topic. Such information and concern should provide the impetus for initiating legislation and litigation on the part of state mental health associations to ensure that the law reflects the scientific knowledge and professional values to the greatest extent possible.

In some measure, states will initially be hampered in this proactivity because they will not know what legal alternatives are available and how desirable each alternative actually is. When a significant number of books in this series is available, however, it will allow for nationally oriented policy studies to identify the variety of legal approaches that are currently in use and to assess the validity of the behavioral assumptions underlying each variant, and ultimately lead to a conclusion as to the relative desirability of alternate approaches.[1] Thus, two other purposes of this book are to foster comprehensive analyses of the laws affecting

---

1. Sales, B. D. (1983). The legal regulation of psychology: Professional and scientific interactions. In C. J. Scheirer & B. L. Hammonds (Eds.), *The master lecture series: Vol. 2. Psychology and law* (pp. 5–36). Washington, DC: American Psychological Association.

MHPs across all states and of the validity of the behavioral assumptions underlying these laws, and to promote political, legislative, and legal action to change laws that are inappropriate and impede the effective delivery of services. Legal change may be required because of gaps in legal regulation, overregulation, and regulation based on invalid behavioral and social assumptions. We hope this process will increase the rationality of future laws in this area and improve the effectiveness and quality of mental health service delivery nationally.

There are three remaining purposes for this series. First, although it will not replace the need for legal counsel, this series will make the MHP an intelligent consumer of legal services. This ability is gaining importance in an era of increasing professionalization and litigiousness. Second, it will ensure that MHPs are aware of the law's mandates when providing expert services (e.g., evaluation and testimony) within the legal system. Although chapters will not address how to clinically assess for the legal standard, provider competency will increase because providers now will be sure of the goals of their service (e.g., the legal standard that they are to assess for) as well as their roles and responsibilities within the legal system as to the particular topic in issue. Third and finally, each book will make clear that the legal standards that MHPs are asked to assess for by the law have typically not been translated into behavioral correlates. Nor are there discussions of tests, scales, and procedures for MHPs to use in assessing for the behavioral correlates of the legal standards in most cases. This series will provide the impetus for such research and writing.

Content and Organization of Volumes

Each book in this series is organized into eight sections. Section 1 addresses the legal credentialing of MHPs. Section 2 deals with the different business forms for conducting one's practice, insurance reimbursement, and tax deductions that clients can receive for using mental health services. With the business matters covered, the book then turns to the law directly affecting service delivery. Section 3 covers the law that affects the maintenance and privacy of professional information and discusses the law that limits service delivery and sets liability for unethical and illegal behavior as a service provider. Sections 4 through 8 consider each area of law that may require the services of MHPs: adults, minors, and families; other civil matters; topics that apply similarly in both civil and criminal cases; criminal matters; and voluntary and involuntary receipt of state services by the clients of mental health services.

Collectively, the chapters in these sections represent all topics pertaining to the law as it affects MHPs in their practices. Two caveats are in order, however. First, the law changes slowly over time. Thus, a supplement service will update all chapters on a regular basis. Second, as MHPs become more involved in the legal system, new opportunities for involvement are likely to arise. To be responsive to these developments, the supplements will also contain additional chapters reflecting these new roles and responsibilities.

Some final points about the content of this book are in order. The exact terms that the law chooses are used in the book even if they are a poor choice from an MHP's point of view. And where terms are defined by the law, that information is presented. The reader will often be frustrated, however, because, as has already been noted, the law does not always define terms or provide detailed guidance. This does not mean that legal words and phrases can be taken lightly. The law sets the rules that MHPs and their clients must operate by; thus, the chapters must be read carefully. This should not be too arduous a task because chapters are relatively short. On the other hand, such brevity will leave some readers frustrated because chapters appear not to go far enough in answering their questions. Note that all of the law is covered. If there is no law, however, there is no coverage. If a question is not answered in the text, it is because Georgia law has not addressed the issue. Relatedly, if an obligation or benefit is created by a professional regulation (i.e., a rule of a professional organization) but is not directly recognized by the law, it is not covered. Thus, for example, professional credentials are not addressed in these volumes.

Finally, we want to point out that, in some instances, the pronoun "he" is used generically to refer to both genders. Most notably, the pronoun is used when quoting directly from the law. Legal language is generally consistent in its preference for using the masculine form of the pronoun; it is not always feasible to attempt a rewording.

Bruce D. Sales
Michael Owen Miller
Series Editors

Authors' Preface

This book is primarily a treatment of Georgia law applicable to the mental health professions. Because of the extensive interaction between the law and mental health professionals, not every subject can be treated comprehensively. For example, mental health professionals frequently interact with the criminal justice system. Although this book attempts to address the major issues that mental health professionals will confront in dealing with criminal law issues, it is not possible to deal with the entire range of criminal law. The same may be said for other areas such as business relationships, tort law, probate law, and family law. It would be advisable to consult specific treatises or references in those areas if questions arise that are not addressed in this book.

In addition, this book does not attempt to address the numerous areas of federal law that are relevant to the mental health professions. Federal law, both statutory and constitutional, is a major force in defining the rights of patients and of providers. In particular, federal constitutional law has had a significant impact on the commitment and treatment of the mentally ill and on the rights of criminal defendants. Wherever feasible, an attempt has been made to note the importance of federal law. However, there are areas, particularly in practice arrangements, health care delivery, insurance and third-party payors, and regulatory issues, for which other sources must be consulted.

As to Georgia law, the Georgia Constitution is the organic document that establishes the framework for state government, including the relationship between the branches of government and the function of state constitutional officers. It also provides for the protection of specified individual rights. Citations to the Georgia Constitution appear in the following form: Ga. Const. Art. 1, § 1, ¶ 1. This reference indicates that the citation is to the first paragraph of the first section in the first Article of the Georgia Constitution.

State statutory law is enacted by the Georgia General Assembly. Laws are codified in the Official Code of Georgia Annotated (O.C.G.A.). Citations to Georgia law will therefore appear in the following form: O.C.G.A. § 43-39-1. This citation refers to Title 43, Chapter 39, Section 1 of the Georgia Code. In addition, the laws enacted in each session of the Georgia General Assembly are bound in separate volumes by year called session laws. Reference to the session laws is Ga. Law 1993, page 330, section 2. This reference is to the 1993 session laws volume at page 330.

Much of the work of state government is performed by administrative agencies created by the General Assembly or, in some instances, by the Constitution. These agencies are authorized to promulgate rules and regulations to assist in performing the authority delegated to them by the legislature. For example, the State Board of Examiners of Psychologists is authorized to establish a code of conduct and of ethics. Pursuant to that statutory authority, the Board has adopted a detailed set of ethical and conduct standards. Rules of state administrative agencies are published by the Office of Secretary of State in a multi-volume binder type series. The rules are cited as Ga. Comp. R. & Regs. r. 510-1-.01.

Judicial decisions interpret the Constitution, statutes, and administrative regulations, as well as explain the development of judge-made or common law. Cases involving interpretations of the Constitution of the State of Georgia or of the United States and cases involving title to land, equity, wills, *habeas corpus,* divorce and alimony, and capitol felonies are heard by the Supreme Court of Georgia. Most other cases are initially decided by the Georgia Court of Appeals, with a discretionary review by the Georgia Supreme Court. Citations to decisions of the Georgia Supreme Court are as follows: *Chandler Exterminators, Inc. v. Morris,* 262 Ga. 257, 416 S.E.2d 277 (1992). This refers to volume 262, page 257 of the Georgia Reports. The case is also reported at volume 416, page 277 of the Southeastern Reporter, Second Series. Decisions of the Georgia Court of Appeals are reported as *Ridgeview Institute v. Brunson,* 191 Ga. App. 608, 382 S.E.2d 409 (1989). The first reference is to volume 191 of the Georgia Appeals Reports.

The federal courts primarily decide cases involving interpretation of federal law and the federal constitution. The federal courts may also interpret state law in diversity of citizenship cases. Citations to decisions from the United States District Court are contained in the Federal Supplement (F. Supp.), United States Court of Appeals in the Federal Report (F., F. 2d, or F. 3d), and United States Supreme Court in three reporters (U.S., Sup. Ct., or Law Ed.). Federal legislation is codified in the United States Code and is cited as 42 U.S.C. § 1983. Rules of federal agencies are published in the Code of Federal Regulations and are referred to as C.F.R.

The law is continually evolving both through judicial decisions and legislation. Therefore, this work should be considered current as of June 1996. Future supplements will update developments after that date.

Robert B. Remar
Richard N. Hubert

Acknowledgments

Invaluable research assistance was provided in the preparation of this book by Alex Teel, Megan Gideon, Susan Garrett, Mark D. Oldenburg, David P. Thatcher, Patricia Pentecost, Lila Newberry Bradley, Barbara Bradford, and Tift Hubbard. Attorneys Donald Samuel and Jonathan Zimring and psychologist John Paddock graciously lent their time and expertise in reviewing drafts of the manuscript. Special thanks to Eileen Blenk for her work in preparing the manuscript drafts.

Robert B. Remar

Legal
Credentialing

Licensure and Regulation of Psychiatrists

The licensure and regulation of physicians, including psychiatrists, are governed by state law and by rules adopted by the Composite State Board of Medical Examiners (the Board). Georgia law establishes the Board, defines the terms contained within the law, establishes qualifications and procedures for licensure of physicians, defines the practice of medicine, regulates the conduct of physicians, establishes exceptions to licensure, and prescribes criminal sanctions and penalties for violations of the chapter.[1] There is no separate licensure provision pertaining to the practice of psychiatry. The licensing law is a generic one that regulates the practice of medicine without regard to specialty.

(A) Board of Medical Examiners

(A)(1) Composition

The Board of Medical Examiners is charged with the primary responsibility of licensing and regulating physicians and osteopaths, including psychiatrists and other specialists. The Board is composed of 13 members, all of whom must be citizens of the United States and residents of the state of Georgia. Appointments are made by the governor and confirmed by the Georgia State Senate. Twelve of the members must be practicing physicians of integrity and ability who have been duly licensed to practice in Georgia. Ten of the 12 physician members must be graduates of reputable medical schools conferring the MD degree. The other

---

1. O.C.G.A. § 43-34-20 *et seq.*

two physicians must be graduates of reputable osteopathic schools conferring the DO degree. Members of the Medical Examiners Board who are physicians or osteopaths must have practiced medicine for at least 5 years. The 13th member of the Board is appointed from the state at large and must have no connection whatsoever with the practice of medicine.[2] Members serve 4-year terms. There must be a member from at least each congressional district in the state.[3]

(A)(2) Duties

The Medical Examiners Board has the duty to

1. protect the public health and control and regulate the practice of medicine and osteopathy and to conduct investigations, either through the joint secretary to the state examining boards or independently;

2. appoint a Physician's Assistants' Advisory Committee composed of four physicians, at least two of whom are members of the Medical Examiners Board, and four certified physician's assistants who serve for 2-year terms and who examine applicants for physician's assistant certification and propose legislation concerning physician's assistants;

3. examine applicants to test their qualifications to practice medicine;

4. regulate the denial, revocation, renewal, probation, and suspension of licenses, including alien licenses;

5. employ personnel to assist the Medical Examiners Board in carrying out its duties; and

6. pass on the good standing and reputation of medical and osteopathic colleges and establish examinations and qualifications for aliens and out-of-state applicants to become licensed in the state of Georgia.[4]

(A)(3) Licensure

The Medical Examiners Board may grant a license without examination to a licensee of a board of another state that requires equal or higher qualifications for licensure, on the same basis as such state reciprocates with Georgia, if the applicant for a license has resided within the United States for at least 1 year.[5] Likewise, licensed physicians of other states and foreign countries may be permitted to enter Georgia for consultation with any licensed

---

2. O.C.G.A. § 43-34-21.
3. O.C.G.A. § 43-34-22.
4. O.C.G.A. § 43-34-21.
5. O.C.G.A. § 43-34-30.

physician of this state, provided that no physician may establish an office in this state for practice of the profession, either temporary or permanent, and no physician may practice under another physician's license, unless the applicant obtains a license from the Medical Examiners Board. Thus, reciprocity will apply if the standards of medical licensure of the reciprocating state or foreign country equal those of Georgia, provided that the foreign state or country agrees to license physicians of Georgia on a similar basis.[6]

The joint-secretary, with the approval of the president of the Board, may in his discretion issue a temporary license to an applicant, which has the same force and effect as a permanent license, until the next regular meeting of the Board, at which time the temporary license becomes void. Temporary licenses may not be recorded in the clerk's office of the Superior Court in the county in which the licensee resides.[7]

Institutional licenses were formerly granted to individuals who had resided in the United States for at least 1 year and who had graduated from a school accredited and approved by the Board and who were employed in Georgia in any state-operated institution or state medical college. No new institutional licenses have been granted since July 1, 1983. Individuals holding such licenses before 1980 can continue to renew them. Institutional licenses obtained after 1980 expired July 1, 1985.

Institutional licensees must practice under proper medical supervision in accordance with state licensing law for physicians and are subject to biennial renewal. Institutional licenses do not carry with them the right to engage in private practice, although residency requirements of an individual employed by a state institution or medical college who provides medical services as a teacher, as opposed to providing direct patient care, may be waived. Licensees must undertake 1 year of postgraduate work in a postgraduate training internship approved by the American Medical Association (AMA) or the American Osteopathic Association (AOA) or in some other program acceptable to the Board. Institutional license holders are not permitted to apply for Drug Enforcement Agency registration numbers to write prescriptions to be filled outside the institution.[8]

Provisional licenses for medical practitioners may be issued at the discretion of the Medical Examiners Board if the applicant demonstrates to the Board that he or she possesses all the qualifications and meets all the requirements necessary to become a

---

6. O.C.G.A. § 43-34-31.
7. O.C.G.A. § 43-34-32.
8. O.C.G.A. § 43-34-33.

licensed practitioner in Georgia, except for having passed any required examination. In such case, the Board may waive the examination requirements and grant a provisional license that is valid only so long as the applicant practices in the geographic locality specified upon such license. Such a license expires after 12 months and is subject to renewal or extension only in the event that the provisional licensee demonstrates proof that he or she has practiced in the geographic location specified in the license. Special rules are provided for district health directors of county health boards on the basis of unfulfilled needs for medical services in specific localities. If the licensee fails, for the third or any subsequent time, any examination that is required to be passed to become a licensed physician in Georgia, the applicant will not be eligible to retake such examination until the applicant furnishes proof of having completed 1 year of appropriate education and training as approved by the Medical Examiners Board.[9]

Licenses to practice medicine may be issued by the Board to a person who furnishes satisfactory evidence of attainments and qualifications under the law and the rules and regulations of the Medical Examiners Board. Such licenses are to be scrupulously investigated and policed by the joint-secretary, under the direction of the Board.[10]

(B) Disciplinary Actions Against Physicians

The Medical Examiners Board has the authority to refuse to grant a license to an applicant or to discipline a physician licensed in Georgia upon a finding by the Board that the licensee or applicant has[11]

1. failed to demonstrate qualifications or standards as provided by law and the Board's regulations;
2. knowingly made misleading, deceptive, untrue, or fraudulent representations in the practice of medicine or in any document connected therewith, or practiced fraud or deceit or intentionally made any false statement in obtaining the license to practice medicine, or made a false or deceptive biennial registration with the Board;

---

9. O.C.G.A. § 43-34-34.
10. O.C.G.A. § 43-34-35.
11. O.C.G.A. § 43-34-37.

3. been convicted of a felony in any state or federal court or court of another country or territory (as used in this section, *conviction* includes a verdict of guilty, a plea of guilty, or a plea of *nolo contendere* in a criminal proceeding);
4. committed a crime involving moral turpitude;
5. had his or her license to practice medicine revoked, suspended, or annulled by any lawful licensing authority, or had other disciplinary action taken against him or her, or been denied a license;
6. advertised for or solicited patients, obtained a fee or other thing of value on the representation that a manifestly incurable disease can be permanently cured, or made untruthful or improbable statements, or flamboyant or exaggerated claims concerning his or her professional excellence;
7. engaged in any unprofessional, unethical, deceptive, or deleterious conduct or practices harmful to the public, whether or not such practice resulted in actual injury (*unprofessional conduct* includes any departure from or failure to conform to the minimum standards of acceptable and prevailing medical practice);
8. performed, procured, or aided or abetted in performing or procuring a criminal abortion;
9. knowingly maintained a professional connection or association with any person who is in violation of the law, rules, and regulations of the Board;
10. knowingly aided, assisted, procured, or advised any person to practice medicine contrary to the law and violated or attempted to violate a law, rule, or regulation of the state of Georgia, any other state, the Medical Examiners Board, the United States, or any of the lawful authority without regard to whether the violation is criminally punishable;
11. committed any act or omission that is indicative of bad moral character or untrustworthiness;
12. been adjudged to be mentally incompetent by a court of competent jurisdiction within or without the state of Georgia; or
13. become unable to practice medicine with reasonable skill and safety by reason of illness; or the use of alcohol, drugs, narcotics, chemicals, or any other type of material; or as result of any mental or physical condition. The enforcement procedures dealing with illness or drug or alcohol abuse carry with them the right to require a licensee or applicant to submit to a mental and physical examination, the results of which are

admissible in a hearing before the Medical Examiners Board, notwithstanding any claim of privilege. Permission for mental examination and admission of results of the examination are implied and assumed to be with consent by virtue of the applicant's or licensee's engaging in license application or renewal. The Medical Examiners Board is also authorized to obtain and review any and all records relating to the mental or physical condition of the licensee or applicant, including psychiatric records. Such records of the mental and physical condition of the licensee or applicant, however, shall be received *in camera* and shall not be disclosed to the public.

When the Board finds that an individual is unqualified to be granted a license or finds that an individual should be disciplined, the Board may take one or more of the following actions:

1. refuse to grant a license;
2. administer a public or private reprimand;
3. suspend a license for a definite period;
4. limit or restrict a license;
5. revoke a license; or
6. condition the penalty, or withhold formal disposition, on the physician's submission to care, counseling, or treatment by physicians or other professionals and the completion of such care, counseling, or treatment as directed by the Board.

In addition to and in conjunction with other remedies, the Board may make a finding that is adverse to the licensee, but withhold imposition of judgment and penalty, or impose judgment and penalty, but suspend enforcement thereof, and place the physician on probation, which can be revoked for noncompliance with the terms of probation imposed by the Board. Discipline or corrective measures may be imposed at the discretion of the Board.

The joint-secretary of the state examining boards is vested with the power to investigate as he, the Medical Examiners Board, or a district attorney may deem necessary or advisable in the enforcement of the law. Investigators have access to writings, documents, and material as may be deemed necessary or advisable to make a factual determination. The Board is empowered to issue subpoenas, compel access to documents and enforce the same through the Superior Court. Furthermore, at a hearing to determine the licensee's fitness to practice medicine, any record relating to the patient of the licensee or applicant is admissible in evidence regardless of statutory privilege. The patient may not withhold evidence relating to the licensee's fitness to practice medicine on the grounds of privilege or otherwise; such information, documentation, or other writings shall be received *in camera* and not disclosed to the public.[12]

Any individual, or business association, or other entity who reports the acts or omissions of a licensee is immune from civil or criminal liability, if the report is made in good faith.[13]

There is also a requirement for reporting to the Board medical malpractice judgments or settlements of $20,000 or more. Investigations are required for judgments or settlements in excess of $100,000.[14]

(C) Investigation by the Medical Examiners Board

Board proceedings regarding an applicant's right to practice medicine and matters dealing with the termination, suspension, or limitation of a license require notice to the licensee or applicant and an opportunity for a hearing. Such proceedings are considered to be contested cases within the meaning of the Georgia Administrative Procedure Act (GAPA). Neither refusal of a license nor private reprimand is considered to be a contested case within the meaning of the GAPA. The Board also has the power to issue subpoenas and command the appearance of witnesses before it for testimony and for the production of documents. Generally, the MHP–patient privilege does not apply to an investigation conducted by the Board, but such inquiries are to be *in camera*. Records used in such an investigation must be kept confidential, may not be released for any purpose other than a hearing before the Board, and are not subject to subpoena. However, the Georgia Supreme Court has held that information contained in the investigating file must be turned over to the licensee at his or her request for the purpose of preparing for a hearing before the Board.[15]

In a proper case, the Board may not only take action against the licensee, but may refer matters to the attorney general of the state of Georgia or to the district attorney of the appropriate county. The Board may also report any adverse action to the clerk of the superior court in the county in which the physician resides.[16]

---

12. O.C.G.A. § 43-34-37(e) and (f).
13. O.C.G.A. § 43-1-19(i).
14. O.C.G.A. § 43-34-37(i) and § 33-3-27.
15. Wills v. Composite State Board of Medical Examiners, 259 Ga. 549, 384 S.E.2d 636 (1989). *See* O.C.G.A. §§ 43-1-19 (h) and 43-34-37(d).
16. O.C.G.A. § 43-34-39.

1.2

Licensure and Regulation of Psychiatric Nurses

Licensure and regulation of psychiatric nurses are governed by the Georgia Registered Professional Nurse Practice Act (the Nurse Practice Act), which establishes a Board of Nursing, defines terms contained within the Act, establishes qualifications and procedures for licensure of nurses, defines the practice of nursing, establishes exceptions to licensure, and prescribes sanctions for violations of the Registered Nurse Act.[1] The general licensure provision for nursing pertains to all nurses, without regard to specialty.[2] The Nurse Practice Act makes provisions for "advanced nursing practice," which includes clinical nurse specialists in psychiatric or mental health.[3]

(A) Board of Nursing

(A)(1) Composition

The Board of Nursing (Nursing Board) is the primary administrative body that licenses and regulates registered nurses. It consists of eight members who serve for 3-year terms with a limit of two consecutive terms.[4] The Nursing Board is appointed by the governor with the approval of the Georgia State Senate and consists of seven licensed registered professional nurses who have practiced as registered professional nurses for at least 5 years immediately

---

1. O.C.G.A. § 43-26-1 *et seq.*
2. This law also applies to practical nursing, but our discussion is limited to registered professional nursing because psychiatric nurses must have the additional education required by the latter category.
3. O.C.G.A. § 43-26-3(1).
4. O.C.G.A. § 43-26-3(2) and (4).

prior to their appointment; have engaged in full-time or part-time paid employment as clinical, educational, or administrative personnel; and are citizens of the United States and residents of the state of Georgia.[5] The eighth member of the Nursing Board is appointed by the governor from the public-at-large and must be a citizen of the United States and resident of Georgia with no connection whatsoever with the nursing profession.[6]

(A)(2) Duties

The Nursing Board has the power and duty to

1. establish by rule the standards, curricula, and educational requirements to prepare individuals to practice nursing as registered professional nurses;

2. provide for surveys of educational programs preparing students to practice nursing as registered professional nurses;

3. approve educational programs preparing students to practice nursing as registered professional nurses;

4. deny or withdraw approval from educational programs preparing nurses to practice nursing for failure to meet the provisions of law and the rules adopted by the Nursing Board;

5. examine licenses and renew those of duly qualified applicants for licensure to practice nursing as registered professional nurses;

6. conduct hearings on charges calling for discipline and take actions deemed appropriate, including the administration of a public or private reprimand (a private reprimand is not disclosed to anyone except the licensee); and

7. suspend (to a maximum term of 12 months), limit, or restrict licenses; and revoke or refuse to renew licenses.[7]

(B) Licensure

Applicants may be licensed as registered professional nurses in Georgia if they

1. have completed an approved course of study and graduated from an educational program in nursing approved by the Nursing Board or, if outside the state of Georgia, a program that meets the criteria established by the Nursing Board;

---

5. *Id.*
6. *Id.*
7. O.C.G.A. § 43-26-5.

2. pass a written examination administered and approved by the Nursing Board; or

3. have been duly licensed to practice nursing as a registered professional nurse under the laws of another state or territory of the United States for the 5 years immediately preceding application and, in the opinion of the Nursing Board, the qualifications for licensure in the state of Georgia have been met.[8]

(C) Temporary Licenses

The Nursing Board may issue a temporary permit to practice nursing as a registered professional nurse to applicants during the 6-month period required to complete a program of instruction or during the time that the applicant holds a valid license in other territories or states of the United States.

Upon graduation from an approved program of study, a temporary permit to practice nursing as a registered professional nurse may be issued to the applicant for licensure examination. A temporary permit expires on the day after the examinations are graded and licenses are issued to those who passed. Temporary permits may be renewed if the applicant fails or for any reason is unable to take the first or second examination held after receiving the temporary license. A temporary license will not be issued to any applicant who fails or for any reason is unable to take the third examination after the applicant receives a temporary permit. Temporary permits may also be issued to nurses who hold licenses from outside the United States or its territories in accordance with procedures prescribed for obtaining a temporary license.[9]

Applicants for reinstatement who have not been engaged in the active practice of nursing during the 5 years immediately prior to application must successfully complete a program of instruction in nursing, approved by the Nursing Board, not more than 6 months prior to reinstatement. A temporary permit to practice nursing may be issued during the 6-month period.

(D) Exceptions to Licensing

The nursing licensure law does not prohibit

---

8. O.C.G.A. § 43-26-7.
9. O.C.G.A. § 43-26-8.

1. the furnishing of emergency aid;

2. the practice of nursing as a registered professional nurse that is incidental to a program of study by students enrolled in a nursing educational program approved by the Nursing Board;

3. the practice by any legally qualified registered professional nurse licensed in another state who is employed by the United States government or by any division thereof while in the discharge of official duties;

4. the performance of auxiliary services in the caring of patients when such care and activities do not require the knowledge and skill required of a person practicing nursing as a registered professional nurse and such services are being performed under the orders or directions of a licensed physician, dentist, podiatrist, or individual licensed to practice nursing as a professional nurse;

5. gratuitous nursing of the sick by friends and family members; or

6. the practice of nursing as a registered professional in the case of a disaster.[10]

(E) Regulation: Disciplinary Actions Against a Licensed Nurse

A nurse's license may be suspended, revoked, or placed on probation should the Nursing Board find that a licensee or applicant has

1. failed to demonstrate the qualifications and standards for licensure;

2. knowingly made misleading, deceptive, untrue, or fraudulent representations in the practice of nursing or on a document connected therewith; or practiced fraud or intentionally made false statements in obtaining a license or in communicating with the Nursing Board;

3. been convicted in any court of a state or of the United States of a felony or other crime involving moral turpitude;

4. had a license to practice nursing revoked, suspended, or annulled by any licensing authority or had any disciplinary action taken against him or her;

5. engaged in unprofessional, unethical, deceptive, or deleterious conduct deemed unlawful to the public or likely to deceive,

---

10. O.C.G.A. § 43-26-12.

defraud, or harm the public, including the failure to meet minimal standards of acceptable and prevailing nursing practice;

6. violated any law, statute, rule, or regulation of Georgia;

7. been judged mentally incompetent by a court of competent jurisdiction; or

8. become unable to practice nursing with reasonable skill and safety by reason of illness, use of alcohol, drugs, narcotics; or chemicals; or as the result of any mental or physical condition.[11]

(F) Investigations by the Nursing Board

The Nursing Board shall investigate and seek an injunction from a court of competent jurisdiction to enjoin from the practice of nursing any individual who has not been licensed to practice or whose license has been suspended, revoked, or has expired.[12]

(G) Licensure in an Advanced Nursing Practice

The need to regulate advanced practice nursing as defined in O.C.G.A., section 43-26-2(1), has led to the promulgation of rules governing advanced nursing practice. The rules define the title of Clinical Nurse Specialist in Psychiatric/Mental Health, establish criteria for recognition by the Nursing Board, and establish minimal qualifications for the advanced practice of psychiatric and mental health nursing.[13]

The regulation defines a *clinical nurse specialist in psychiatric/ mental health* as a registered nurse who has completed a program of graduate study; has supervised clinical practice; and has demonstrated depth and breadth of knowledge, competence, and skill in the advanced practice of psychiatric and mental health nursing.[14]

---

11. O.C.G.A. § 43-26-11. *See also* O.C.G.A. § 43-1-19. For administration of anesthesia by nurses, *see* O.C.G.A. § 43-26-11.1.
12. O.C.G.A. § 43-26-10.
13. Reg. of Adv. Nurs. Prac. 410-12-.04(1).
14. Reg. of Adv. Nurs. Prac. 410-12-.04(2).

As of January, 1992, to obtain recognition by the Nursing Board as a clinical nurse specialist in psychiatric/mental health, a nurse must

1. be a registered professional nurse under the laws of Georgia[15]; and

2. have earned a master's degree or higher in nursing with a specialization in psychiatric/mental health nursing, or hold current certification from the American Nurses' Association (ANA) as a clinical nurse specialist in adult psychiatric and mental health nursing or child and adolescent psychiatric and mental health nursing.[16]

To obtain recognition by the Nursing Board after fulfilling the requirements listed above, an applicant must submit

1. a copy of a current Georgia registered professional nursing license,

2. a transcript verifying completion of the graduate degree with a specialization in psychiatric and mental health nursing, and

3. documents verifying ANA certification.[17]

(H) Licensed Practical Nurses

Licensure and regulation of practical nurses is governed by the Georgia Licensed Practical Nurse Act (the Practical Nurses Act),[18] which establishes the Georgia Board of Examiners of Licensed Practical Nurses (the LPN Board). Licensed practical nurses may provide care only under the supervision of a physician, a dentist, a podiatrist, or a registered nurse.[19] Applicants for a license must make application to the LPN Board and must be at least 18 years of age with a high school or equivalent diploma, have graduated from an approved vocational nursing education program, and have passed an examination.[20] The LPN Board may issue a license by endorsement without examination to a person licensed as a practical or vocational nurse in another state or territory of the United States, if the LPN Board determines that the licensure requirements of the other jurisdiction equal or exceed those of Georgia.[21] The LPN Board may refuse to grant a license or revoke

---

15. Reg. of Adv. Nurs. Prac. 410-12-.04(3)(a).
16. Reg. of Adv. Nurs. Prac. 410-12-.04(3)(b).
17. Reg. of Adv. Nurs. Prac. 410-12-.04(5)(a) and (b).
18. O.C.G.A. § 43-26-30.
19. O.C.G.A. § 43-26-32(7).
20. O.C.G.A. § 43-26-36.
21. O.C.G.A. § 43-26-38.

a license if the applicant or licensee has (a) been convicted of a felony, a crime involving moral turpitude, or a crime involving controlled substances; (b) had a license revoked or denied previously; (c) engaged in unprofessional conduct; (d) violated a rule, regulation, or order of the LPN Board or the board of another state; or (e) displayed an inability to practice as a professional nurse.[22]

---

22. O.C.G.A. § 43-26-40.

1.3

Licensure and Regulation of Psychologists

The licensure and regulation of psychologists are governed by state law that establishes a Board of Examiners of Psychologists (the Psychology Examining Board); define terms; establish qualifications, terms of office, and requirements for filling vacancies; and outline the duties of the Board. The statute also provides for the election of officers of the Psychology Examining Board and lists the requirements and duties of its members. It empowers the Board to administer oaths, summon witnesses, issue licenses, and enforce its duties through a joint-secretary. The statute provides for the licensure of individuals engaged in the practice of psychology and sets forth the character, education, and experience requirements for licensure. The statute provides for recordation of licenses; biennial review of licenses; revocation, suspension, or reinstatement of licenses; temporary licenses; and continuing education. The law makes provisions for privileged communications between psychologists and their clients and for restrictions on the use of the title of psychologist. Finally, the law provides for the enforcement of the psychology licensing law by injunction and both civil and criminal penalties.[1]

(A) Psychology Licensing Law

(A)(1) Practice Regulation and Title Protection

Georgia law regulates both the practice of psychology and the use of the title of psychologist. Prior to 1993, the law was unclear as to

---

1. O.C.G.A. § 43-39-1 *et seq.*

whether the psychology licensing law was a practice act or merely a title protection act. In 1992, in the case of *Abramson v. Gonzalez*,[2] the U.S. Court of Appeals for the Eleventh Circuit held that a Florida statute prohibiting unlicensed practitioners of psychology from holding themselves out to the public as psychologists placed an unconstitutional burden on commercial speech. The court based its decision on the fact that Florida's licensing law regulated only the use of the title of psychologist and did not regulate the practice of psychology. This decision caused concern among the mental health professions and led to a joint effort to amend the psychology licensing law, as well as the law licensing professional counselors, social workers, and marriage and family therapists. As amended in 1993,[3] the psychology licensing law prohibits anyone not licensed as a psychologist from practicing psychology.

(A)(2) Scope of Practice

The psychology licensing law defines the scope of *practice of psychology* as follows:

> To render or offer to render to individuals, groups, organizations, or the public for a fee or any remuneration, monetary or otherwise, any service involving the application of recognized principles, methods, and procedures of the science and profession of psychology such as, but not limited to, diagnosing and treating mental and nervous disorders and illnesses, rendering opinions concerning diagnoses of mental disorders, including organic brain disorders and brain damage, engaging in neuropsychology, engaging in psychotherapy, interviewing, administering, and interpreting tests of mental abilities, aptitudes, interests, and personality characteristics for such purposes as psychological classification or evaluation, or for education or vocational placement, or for such purposes as psychological counseling, guidance, or readjustment.[4]

The statutory definition specifically provides that it shall not be construed as permitting the administration or prescription of drugs or as infringing on the practice of medicine.

The definition of practice of psychology was specifically amended in 1993 to overrule a 1992 Georgia Supreme Court decision in *Chandler Exterminators, Inc. v. Morris*.[5] In *Chandler*, the Supreme Court of Georgia held that a neuropsychologist was not qualified to render an opinion concerning a diagnosis of a mental disorder when such disorder required a professional opinion as to a physical disorder, in that case organic brain damage. The court's

---

2. 949 F.2d 1567 (11th Cir. 1992).
3. Ga. Laws 1993, p. 355 (SB 48).
4. O.C.G.A. § 43-39-1(3).
5. 262 Ga. 257, 416 S.E.2d 277 (1992).

decision was not only in conflict with prior decisions regarding the scope of expert witness testimony, but it was based on an overly narrow view of mental disorders and psychology practice. The 1993 amendment, in effect, overruled the decision by explicitly providing that the practice of psychology include "diagnosing and treating mental disorders and illnesses, rendering opinions concerning diagnoses of mental disorders, including organic brain disorders and brain damage [and] engaging in neuropsychology."

(B) Board of Examiners of Psychologists

The Psychology Practice Act, first enacted in 1951, was amended in 1969 to provide for a State Board of Examiners of Psychologists, which consists of six members appointed by the governor of Georgia. Under the law, as amended, no member of the Psychology Examining Board shall be liable in a civil action for any acts performed in good faith in the performance of the members' duties. Five members of the six-member Board are required to be licensed psychologists and one member, deemed to be a consumer member, must not be licensed as a psychologist or have any connection whatsoever with the practice or profession of psychology. The Psychology Examining Board members serve for 5 years or until their successors are appointed and qualified. Board members may be removed only after notice and hearing for incompetence, neglect of duty, malfeasance of duty in office, or commission of a crime involving moral turpitude.[6]

The Psychology Examining Board has the authority to issue licenses and enforce the provisions of the law with regard to the practice of psychology. The Board is authorized to administer oaths, to summon witnesses, and to take testimony in all matters relating to its duties. It issues licenses only to those who present satisfactory evidence of meeting the qualifications of the Psychology Practice Act and the rules and regulations of the Psychology Examining Board. The license, once issued, provides for absolute authority to practice psychology in Georgia. It is the duty of the Board's secretary to provide aid to the prosecuting attorney in the enforcement and prosecution of persons charged with any violation of the Psychology Practice Act.[7]

---

6. O.C.G.A. § 43-39-2.
7. O.C.G.A. § 43-39-6.

Applicants seeking to practice psychology in the state of Georgia are required to make application to the Board through the joint-secretary on such form and in such manner as are adopted and prescribed by the Board.

Candidates for license must furnish to the Psychology Examining Board satisfactory evidence of

1. good moral character; and
2. a doctoral degree from a program in psychology including, but not limited to, clinical psychology, counseling psychology, industrial or organizational psychology, or school psychology, from an accredited educational institution recognized by the Board as maintaining satisfactory standards.

Persons who received a doctoral degree in a field closely allied with the field of psychology could previously meet the degree requirements of the paragraph if

1. the degree in the closely allied field was received no later than July 1, 1991 from an educational institution recognized by the Psychology Examining Board as maintaining satisfactory standards;
2. the training requirements for the degree in a closely allied field were determined by the Board to be substantially similar to those required for a doctoral degree from a program in psychology;
3. the applicant completed the experience requirement of the law no later than July 1, 1991; and
4. the applicant passed the required examination no later than July 1, 1993.

This exception was eliminated effective July 1, 1994.[8] The Act was also amended in 1994 to provide that individuals with a doctoral degree in psychology from an accredited institution recognized by the Board are eligible for licensure if they have completed an organized retraining program in applied psychology.

As of July 1, 1991, an applicant must have at least 2 years of experience in psychology of a type considered to be qualifying in nature by the Psychology Examining Board. The competency of the psychologist must be shown by his or her passing an examination, written or oral or both, in accordance with the Board's rules and regulations.

Examination of applicants is made by the Board at least once a year according to the methods and in such subject fields as may be deemed by the Board to be the most practical and expeditious

---

8. SB 512, Act 767 (1994).

to test the applicants' qualifications. The Board may require the examination to be written or oral or both. In any written examination, applicants are designated by a number instead of a name so that the applicants' identities are not disclosed to the members of the Board until the examination papers have been graded. An unsuccessful candidate may, within 14 days of notice of failure of the final examination and by written request to the Psychology Examining Board, appeal to the Board for a review.[9] Licenses issued by the Board are renewable biannually.[10]

(C) Discipline of Psychologists

The Psychology Examining Board has the authority to refuse to grant or renew a license, to suspend or revoke a license, or to discipline a person licensed by the Board based upon any of the following:

1. the use of fraud or deception in applying for a license or in passing the examination provided for in the Psychology Practice Act;

2. conviction of a felony or any crime involving moral turpitude;

3. the practice of psychology under a false or assumed name or the impersonation of another practitioner of a like or different name;

4. habitual intemperance in the use of alcoholic beverages, narcotics, or stimulants to such an extent as to incapacitate the performance of one's duties;

5. immoral or unprofessional conduct deemed to be deleterious to the profession;

6. knowing assistance to an unlicensed person in the practice of psychology;

7. mental incompetence;

8. display of an inability to practice the profession with reasonable skill and safety; or

9. violation of the Board's rules, including the Code of Ethics and Code of Conduct.

The ethical and conduct codes are based substantially on the ethical principles adopted by the American Psychological Association. Any license revoked by the Board is subject to reinstatement at the Board's discretion. The actions of the Board in grant-

---

9. O.C.G.A. § 43-39-9.
10. O.C.G.A. § 43-39-12.

ing or refusing to grant or renew a license or revoking or suspending or refusing to revoke or suspend an existing license are subject to the Georgia Administrative Procedure Act[11] and may be appealed to the superior court. If the findings of the Board are supported by any evidence, then such findings must be accepted by the court.[12]

(D) Reciprocity

The Board may grant a license without a written examination to any individual who, at the time of application, is licensed by a similar psychology examining board in another state having standards that, in the opinion of the Board, are no lower than those required by the state of Georgia. The Board may require an examination as it deems necessary.[13] In addition, an individual licensed in another state may practice in Georgia for no more than 30 days per year without a Georgia license, provided that the licensure requirements in the other state meet or exceed Georgia's.

(E) Penalties

The Psychology Examining Board is authorized to bring actions to enjoin any individual, firm, or corporation that engages in the practice of psychology without a license. Proceedings for an injunction are filed in the county in which the individual resides or in the county in which the firm or corporation maintains a principal office. If the individual, firm, or corporation is practicing psychology without a license, such an individual, firm, or corporation shall be permanently enjoined from practicing psychology in Georgia. To obtain the injunction described in the Psychology Practice Act, it is not necessary for the Board to allege and prove that there is no adequate remedy at law. The law declares that such unlicensed activities are a menace and a nuisance and are dangerous to the public health, safety, and welfare.[14]

Conviction of a violation carries the punishment of a misdemeanor, and the person will be fined not less than $100 nor more

---

11. O.C.G.A. Title 13, Chapter 50.
12. O.C.G.A. § 43-39-13.
13. O.C.G.A. § 43-39-10.
14. O.C.G.A. § 43-39-18.

than $1,000 for such violation and may be imprisoned for up to 1 year.[15]

(F) Temporary Licenses

The Board may issue a temporary license to an applicant for a permanent license. The temporary license has the same force and effect as a permanent license, but expires 12 months from the date of its issuance and is not renewable. Upon a finding by the Board that the applicant has failed either the written or the oral examination, whichever comes first, the Board must revoke the temporary license.[16] The Board may also issue a provisional license to an applicant for a permanent license who has passed the required examinations, but has not completed the required postdoctoral work experience. The license is not renewable and generally expires in 24 months. A provisional licensee may practice only pursuant to the terms of the supervised work experience.

(G) Privileged Communications

Relations and communications between a psychologist and a client are considered on the same basis as those provided by law between an attorney and a client.[17] Attorneys are charged by law to maintain the confidence and preserve the secrets of their clients,[18] and communications between an attorney and client are not admissible in court.[19] Therefore, psychologists may not disclose confidences, and their client communications are generally not admissible in court. See chapter 3.3.

---

15. O.C.G.A. § 43-39-19.
16. O.C.G.A. § 43-39-14.
17. O.C.G.A. § 43-39-16.
18. O.C.G.A. § 15-19-4(3).
19. O.C.G.A. § 24-9-21.

Practice of Psychology by Subdoctoral and Unlicensed Individuals

As discussed in chapter 1.3, Georgia law regulates both the use of the title of psychologist and the practice of the profession of psychology. However, the psychology licensing law contains a number of exceptions that permit unlicensed individuals to practice psychology in limited circumstances. In addition, the law allows students, trainees, and assistants to engage in activities encompassed within the definition of the practice of psychology so long as such individuals are under the direct responsibility and supervision of a licensed psychologist. The Psychology Examining Board has adopted rules to implement this exception.

(A) Independent Practice by Unlicensed Persons

The psychology licensing law expressly provides that an individual who is not licensed as a psychologist may not practice psychology, may not use the title of psychologist, and shall not imply that he or she is a psychologist.[1] However, the law contains specific exceptions that permit persons who are not licensed as psychologists to engage in independent practice under certain limited circumstances. The exceptions are as follows:

1. An individual who is certified as a school psychologist by the Professional Standards Commission may practice psychology without being licensed while working as an employee of an

---

1. O.C.G.A. § 43-39-7.

educational institution recognized by the State Board of Examiners of Psychologists as meeting satisfactory accreditation standards so long as no fees are charged directly to clients or to a third party.

2. An individual holding a doctoral degree in psychology and working in a research laboratory, college, or university recognized by the Psychology Examining Board as meeting satisfactory accreditation standards may use the title of psychologist in connection with his or her academic or research activities, but may not provide direct psychological services to individuals or groups and may not charge fees directly to clients or through third-party payers.

3. An individual who, prior to July 1, 1996, was engaged in the practice of psychology as an employee of an agency or department of the state government, political subdivisions, or community service boards at an intermediate care or skilled care facility for patients with mental retardation is "grandfathered" and may continue to practice notwithstanding a lack of license. Other governmental or community service board employees are grandfathered if they were practicing psychology at any other facility prior to July 1, 1997. The purpose of this exception is to permit unlicensed persons practicing psychology in the public mental health system on either July 1, 1996 or July 1, 1997 to continue practicing, but to prohibit unlicensed practice by persons employed after that date.

4. Individuals who are in the employ of or serving an "established and recognized religious organization" are permitted to engage in activities and services that may constitute the practice of psychology provided that they do not use the title of psychologist and do not imply that they are psychologists.

In addition, the psychology licensing law specifically states that it does not prohibit an individual from engaging in the lawful practice of medicine, nursing, professional counseling, social work, or marriage and family therapy, provided that such an individual does not use the title of psychologist nor imply that he or she is a psychologist. In this regard, the law recognizes that there may be some overlap between the scope of practice of psychology and the scope of practice of the aforementioned professions. For example, both physicians and psychologists diagnose and treat mental and nervous disorders and illnesses and render opinions concerning diagnoses of mental disorders. Professional counselors and psychologists also administer various types of assessment instruments, although only psychologists may administer psychological tests.[2]

(B) Supervised Practice by Unlicensed Persons

The psychology licensing law contains two exceptions regarding supervised practice by unlicensed persons. First, an individual who holds a doctoral degree in psychology may practice under the supervision of a licensed psychologist to obtain the experience required for licensure. Second, students, trainees, or assistants may engage in activities defined as the practice of psychology if they are under the direct supervision and responsibility of a licensed psychologist and the student, trainee, or assistant does not represent himself or herself to be a psychologist.[3] The State Board of Examiners of Psychologists has developed comprehensive rules concerning both internships and postdoctoral supervised work experiences.[4] Those rules provide qualifications for the supervisor, general standards for internships and internship supervision, and specific standards for internships in clinical psychology and counseling psychology, school psychology, industrial organizational psychology, and the management of mental retardation and other developmental disabilities. The rules also have specific requirements for postdoctoral supervised work experiences, including 2,000 hours of supervised work experience, a written supervision contract, and requirements for regular supervision sessions.

As required by statute, the Psychology Examining Board has also adopted rules regarding the delegation and supervision of psychological services.[5] These rules require, in part, that the psychologist retain full, complete, and ultimate authority and responsibility for the professional acts of his or her supervisee, that the supervisee must be qualified by education and training to provide the services, that the patient or client receiving the services must be fully informed of the supervisee's status, and that regular face-to-face supervision of all services take place.

---

2. O.C.G.A. § 43-10A-22.
3. O.C.G.A. § 43-39-7(7), as amended by SB 512, Act 767 (1994).
4. Ga. Comp. R. & Regs., Chapter 510-2-.05.
5. Ga. Comp. R. & Regs., Chapter 510-5-.06(13).

1.5

Licensure and Regulation of Social Workers

Georgia law, enacted in 1981 and amended in 1990 and 1993, regulates both the practice of social work and the title of social worker by prescribing education and experience requirements for licensure and by outlining the scope of practice of the social work profession. Mental health professionals (MHPs) have to obtain a license to practice social work and to use the title social worker.

(A) Scope of Practice

As discussed in chapter 1.3, in 1993, the law governing professional counselors, social workers, and marriage and family therapists, along with the psychology licensing law, was amended to regulate the practice of those professions, as well as the use of professional titles.[1] As part of the 1993 amendments, the definitions of the scope of practice of each profession were also modified. The *practice of social work* is currently defined as

> that specialty which helps individuals, marriages, families, couples, groups, or communities to enhance or restore their capacity for functioning: by assisting in the obtaining or improving of tangible social and health services; by providing psycho-social evaluations, in-depth analyses and determinations of the nature and status of emotional, cognitive, mental, behavioral, and interpersonal problems or conditions; and by counseling and psychotherapeutic techniques, casework, social work advocacy, psychotherapy, and treatment in a variety of settings which

---

1. Ga. Laws 1993, p. 330 *et seq.*

include but are not limited to mental and physical health facilities, child and family service agencies, or private practice.[2]

A person who is not licensed as a social worker may not practice social work; may not use the title of social worker or advertise as a social worker; nor use any words, letters, titles, or figures indicating or implying that the person is a social worker.[3] However, the law contains numerous exceptions, some of which are applicable just to social work and some of which are applicable to all individuals licensed by the Composite Board of Professional Counselors, Social Workers, and Marriage and Family Therapists (Composite Board). The current exceptions are as follows:

1. individuals licensed to practice medicine or psychology;

2. individuals engaged in the practice of social work as employees of any agency or department of the federal government or any licensed hospital or long-term care facility, but only when engaged in that practice as an employee of such agency, department, hospital, or facility;

3. individuals who engage in the practice of social work as employees of any agency or department of the state of Georgia or any of its political subdivisions, but only when engaged in that practice as employees of such an agency or department and, until 1996, individuals or entities providing social work services under contract to the state or its political subdivisions;[4]

4. students of a recognized educational institution who are preparing to become practitioners of social work, but only if the service they render as practitioners is under supervision and direction and their student status is clearly designated by the title of trainee or intern;

5. individuals who have obtained a master's degree from an accredited program and who are practicing under direction and supervision while preparing to take the master's social work licensing examination, but only for 1 year after receiving their degree;

6. elementary, middle, or secondary school social workers certified by the Professional Standards Commission, but only when practicing within the scope of such certification and only when designated by the title of school social worker;

---

2. O.C.G.A. § 43-10A-3(13).

3. O.C.G.A. § 43-10A-7.

4. The law, with some exceptions, limits the unlicensed practice of professional counseling, and marriage and family therapy for state agencies to those employed prior to July 1, 1997.

7. active members of the clergy, but only when the practice is in the course of their regular service as clergy;

8. members of religious ministries responsible to their established ecclesiastical authority who possess a master's degree or its equivalent in theological studies;

9. individuals engaged in the practice of social work in accordance with biblical doctrine in public or nonpublic agencies or entities or in private practice;

10. individuals engaged in the practice of social work as employees of the Division of Family and Children Services of the Department of Human Resources, but only when engaged in such practice as an employee of that division;

11. individuals with a master's degree from a program accredited by the Council on Social Work Education who are engaged in the practice of community organization, policy, planning, research, or administration;

12. individuals with a bachelor's degree in social work from an accredited program who practice under the direction and supervision of a bachelor's or master's level licensed social worker with 2 years of postdegree practice;

13. rehabilitation counselors employed by an organization accredited by the Commission on Accreditation of Rehabilitation Facilities or the National Accreditation Council for Agencies Serving the Blind and Visually Handicapped; and

14. addiction counselors who have met the certification requirements set by the Georgia Addiction Counselors Association.

The law provides that, unless exempt, a person who is not licensed may not practice social work for any corporation, partnership, association, or other business entity that uses in its corporate, partnership, association, or business name any words, letters, titles, or figures indicating or implying that such entity or any of its employees, officers, or agents are practicing social work.

(B) The Composite Board

The Composite Board issues licenses to practice professional counseling, social work, and marriage and family therapy. The Board consists of 10 members: three professional counselors, three social workers, three marriage and family therapists, and one public member.[5] The Board is divided into three separate

_____
5. O.C.G.A. § 43-10A-4.

standards committees for each respective specialty. Each committee approves, by majority vote, the granting of a license in that specialty, approves the examination and provides for grading the examination in that specialty, and deals with licensing matters relating to its profession.[6] Decisions of the standards committees must be approved by the full Board.[7]

The general eligibility requirements for licensure applicable to the three Composite Board professions are the following:

1. meeting the education, training, and experience requirements for their particular profession;

2. passing the examination established for their profession, except that individuals meeting the requirements of licensure as a marriage and family therapist, pursuant to O.C.G.A. section 43-10A-13, are not required to pass the social work examination; and

3. furnishing two personal references from supervisors, teachers, or any combination thereof and paying the required license fee.

(C) Reciprocity

The Composite Board may issue a license without examination to any applicant licensed in social work under the laws of another jurisdiction having requirements for licensure in social work that are substantially equal to those of the state of Georgia.[8]

(D) The Requirements for Licensure in Social Work

The law recognizes two types of social work licenses: master's social worker and clinical social worker. The education, experience, and training requirements of licensure are as follows:[9]

1. for licensure as a master's social worker, a master's degree in social work from a school accredited by the Council on Social Work Education; and

---

6. O.C.G.A. § 43-10A-6(a).
7. O.C.G.A. § 43-10A-6(b).
8. O.C.G.A. § 43-10A-10.
9. O.C.G.A. § 43-10A-12.

2. for licensure as a clinical social worker:
   a. a master's degree in social work from a school accredited by the Council on Social Work Education; and
   b. 3 years of full-time supervised experience in the practice of social work following granting of the master's degree.

Of the 3 years, only the first 2 must be under ongoing administrative oversight. A doctoral degree in social work, in an allied profession, or in child and family development may substitute for 1 year of such experience. At least 1 year of experience must have taken place within the 2 years immediately preceding the application for licensure as a clinical social worker, or the applicant must have met the continuing education requirements established by the Board for clinical social work during the year immediately preceding the application.

Licensed master's level social workers may render or offer to render to individuals, couples, families, groups, organizations, government units, or the general public, service that is guided by knowledge of social resources, social systems, and human behavior. They may provide evaluation, prevention, and intervention services that include, but are not restricted to, community organization, counseling, and supportive services, such as administration, direction, supervision of bachelor's level social workers, consultation, research, or education. The first 2 years of a master social worker's practice after licensure must take place under direction and supervision. Thereafter, the social worker may engage in private practice, except that those social workers whose practice includes counseling or psychotherapeutic techniques may engage in such practice only under the supervision of a duly qualified supervisor and only for such period of time as is prescribed for qualification to take the clinical social work licensing examination.

Licensed clinical social workers may provide all the services of a master's level social worker and may also provide supervision and direction to other social workers; carry out psychosocial evaluations through data collection and analyses to determine the nature of an individual's mental, cognitive, emotional, behavioral, and interpersonal problems or conditions; offer counseling and psychotherapy to individuals, couples, families, and groups; interpret the psychosocial dynamics of a situation and recommend a course of action to individuals, couples, families, or groups in such settings as private practice, family practice, and counseling agencies, health care facilities, and schools; and provide direct evaluation, casework, social work advocacy, education, training, prevention, and intervention services in situations threatened or affected by social, intrapersonal, or interpersonal stress or health impairment.[10]

(E) Restrictions on Use of Terms in Corporate, Partnership, Association, or Business Names

No corporation, partnership, association, or other business entity may use in its corporate, partnership, association, or business name the term *social work* or any words, letters, titles, or figures indicating or implying that such entity or any of its employees, officers, or agents are practicing social work, unless each person practicing social work in that entity is licensed or exempt from licensure.

Any corporation, partnership, association, or other business entity that violates the law restricting the use of terms in corporate, partnership, association, or business names may be punished for a misdemeanor and, upon conviction thereof, may be fined not less than $500 nor more than $1,000 for each offense.[11]

---

10. O.C.G.A. § 43-10A-12.
11. O.C.G.A. § 43-10A-21.

1.6

Regulation of School Psychologists

The psychology licensing law provides that an individual who is certified as a school psychologist by the state Professional Standards Commission is not required to be licensed while working as an employee in an educational institution recognized by the Psychology Examining Board as meeting satisfactory accreditation standards. In addition, no fees may be charged directly to clients or through a third party.[1]

---

1. O.C.G.A. § 43-39-7(1).

Licensure and Regulation of Professional Counselors

The Composite Board of Professional Counselors, Social Workers, and Marriage and Family Therapists (Composite Board) licenses and regulates the activities of professional counselors, as well as of social workers, and marriage and family therapists. As a result of legislation enacted in 1993 (see chapter 1.3), Georgia law now regulates the use of the title of professional counselor as well as the practice of professional counseling.

(A) Scope of Practice

As part of the 1993 amendments to both the Psychology and Composite Board licensing laws, the definitions of the scope of practice of each profession were modified. The *practice of professional counseling* is currently defined as

> that specialty which utilizes counseling techniques based on principles, methods, and procedures of counseling that assist people in identifying and resolving personal, social, vocational, intrapersonal and interpersonal concerns; utilizes counseling and psychotherapy to evaluate and treat emotional and mental problems and conditions, whether cognitive, behavioral or affective; administers and interprets educational and vocational assessment instruments and other tests which the professional counselor is qualified to employ by virtue of education, training and experience; utilizes information and community resources for personal, social, or vocational development; utilizes individual and group techniques for facilitating problem solving, decision making, and behavior change; utilizes functional assessment and vocational planning and guidance for persons requesting assistance in adjustment to a disability or handicapping condition; utilizes referral for persons who request

counseling services; and utilizes and interprets counseling research.[1]

This broad definition is limited by a statutory restriction that provides that nothing in the Composite Board law authorizes persons licensed under it to practice nursing, occupational therapy, physical therapy, medicine, or psychology, nor are such persons authorized to perform psychological testing.[2]

An individual who is not licensed as a professional counselor may not practice professional counseling, may not use the title of professional counselor or advertise as a professional counselor, nor use any words, letters, titles, or figures indicating or implying that the person is a professional counselor. However, the law contains numerous exceptions, some of which are applicable only to professional counseling and some of which are applicable to all individuals licensed by the Composite Board. The current exceptions are as follows:

1. individuals licensed to practice medicine or psychology;
2. individuals engaged in the practice of professional counseling as employees of any agency, or department of the federal government, or any licensed hospital or long-term care facility;
3. individuals who, prior to July 1, 1997, engaged in the practice of professional counseling as employees of any agency or department of the state or any of its political subdivisions;
4. individuals engaged in the practice of professional counseling as employees of the Department of Corrections, Department of Human Resources, any county board of health, or any community service board, or similar government entity providing services to individuals with disabilities. In addition, individuals or entities who contract to provide professional counseling services with such departments or boards of health are exempt from licensure until January 1, 1996 when engaged in providing professional counseling services pursuant to such contracts;
5. students of a recognized educational institution who are preparing to become professional counselors, but only if they are practicing under supervision and direction and their student status is clearly designated by the title of trainee or intern;
6. individuals who have obtained one of the graduate degrees required for licensure as a professional counselor and who are practicing under supervision and direction to obtain the experience required for licensure;

---

1. O.C.G.A. § 43-10A-3(10), as amended by Ga. Laws 1993, p. 330, § 2.
2. O.C.G.A. § 43-10A-22.

7. elementary, middle, or secondary school counselors certified as such by the Professional Standards Commission, when practicing within the scope of such certification and only when designated by the title of school counselor;

8. individuals registered as rehabilitation suppliers by the Georgia Board of Workers' Compensation, but only when practicing rehabilitation counseling as workers' compensation rehabilitation suppliers;

9. active members of the clergy, but only when the practice of professional counseling is in the course of their service as clergy;

10. members of religious ministries responsible to their established ecclesiastical authority who possess a master's degree or its equivalent in theological studies;

11. individuals engaged in the practice of professional counseling in accordance with biblical doctrine in public or nonprofit agencies or entities or in private practice;

12. individuals practicing professional counseling as employees of the Division of Family and Children Services of the Department of Human Resources;

13. individuals who practice professional counseling, excluding the use of psychotherapy, as employees of organizations that are accredited by the Commission on Accreditation of Rehabilitation Facilities or the National Accreditation Council for Agencies Serving the Blind and the Visually Handicapped; and

14. addiction counselors who have met the certification requirements set by the Georgia Addiction Counselors Association.[3]

(B) The Composite Board

The Composite Board issues licenses to practice professional counseling, social work, and marriage and family therapy. The Board consists of 10 members: three professional counselors, three social workers, three marriage and family therapists, and one member of the public.[4] The Board is divided into three separate standards committees for each respective specialty. Each committee approves, by majority vote, the granting of a license in that specialty, approves the examination and provides for grading the examination in that specialty, and deals with licensing

---

3. O.C.G.A. § 43-10A-7.
4. O.C.G.A. § 43-10A-4.

matters relating to its profession.[5] Decisions of the standards committees must be approved by the full Board.[6]

The general eligibility requirements for licensure applicable to the three Composite Board professions are the following:

1. meeting the education, training, and experience requirements for that particular profession;

2. passing successfully the examination established for their profession; and

3. furnishing two personal references from supervisors, teachers, or any combination thereof and paying the required license fee.

(C) The Requirements for Licensure in Professional Counseling

The law sets forth three methods by which a professional counselor can satisfy the education, experience, and training requirements for licensure. They are

1. a doctoral degree from a recognized educational institution in a program that is primarily counseling in content and that requires at least 1 year of supervised internship in a work setting acceptable to the Board; or

2. a degree in either social work, marriage and family therapy, or professional counseling from a recognized educational institution in a program that is primarily counseling in content with supervised internship or practicum and 2 years of post-master's directed experience under supervision in a setting acceptable to the Board; or

3. a master's degree from a recognized educational institution in a program that is primarily counseling in content with supervised internship or practicum and 4 years of post-master's directed experience under supervision in a setting acceptable to the Board. Up to 1 year of such experience may be in an approved practicum placement as part of the degree program.[7]

The Board may also issue a license without examination to an individual licensed as a professional counselor under the laws of another jurisdiction having requirements for licensure that are substantially equal to the licensure requirements in Georgia.

---

5. O.C.G.A. § 43-10A-6(a).
6. O.C.G.A. § 43-10A-6(b).
7. O.C.G.A. § 43-10A-11.

1.8

Licensure and Regulation of Marriage and Family Therapists

As discussed in chapter 1.3, in 1993, the law governing professional counselors, social workers, and marriage and family therapists, along with the psychology licensing law, was amended to regulate the practice of those professions, as well as the use of professional titles. The Composite Board of Professional Counselors, Social Workers, and Marriage and Family Therapists (Composite Board) issues licenses and regulates the practice of marriage and family therapy.

(A) Scope of Practice

As part of the 1993 amendments to the Composite Board law, the definitions of the scope of practice of the three professions regulated by the Board were modified. The *practice of marriage and family therapy* is currently defined as

> that specialty which evaluates and treats emotional and mental problems and conditions, whether cognitive, affective or behavioral, resolves intrapersonal and interpersonal conflicts, and changes perception, attitudes, and behavior; all within the context of marital and family systems. Marriage and family therapy includes, without being limited to, individual, group, couple, sexual, family, and divorce therapy. Marriage and family therapy involves an applied understanding of the dynamics of marital and family systems, including individual psychodynamics, the use of assessment instruments that evaluate marital and family functioning, and the use of psychotherapy and counseling.[1]

---

1. O.C.G.A. § 43-10A-3(8).

This definition is limited by a statutory provision that marriage and family therapists are not authorized to practice nursing, occupational therapy, physical therapy, medicine, or psychology, nor are they authorized to perform psychological testing.[2]

A person who is not licensed as a marriage and family therapist may not practice marriage and family therapy; may not use the title of marriage and family therapist; nor advertise as a marriage and family therapist; nor use any words, letters, titles, or figures indicating or implying that the person is a marriage and family therapist. However, the law contains numerous exceptions, some of which are applicable only to marriage and family therapists and some of which are applicable to all individuals licensed by the Composite Board. The current exceptions are as follows:

1. individuals licensed to practice medicine or psychology;
2. individuals engaged in the practice of marriage and family therapy as employees of any agency, or department of the federal government, or any licensed hospital, or long-term care facility;
3. individuals who, prior to July 1, 1997, engaged in the practice of marriage and family therapy as employees of any agency or department of the state or any of its political subdivisions, but such individuals may practice only as employees of such agency or department;
4. students of a recognized educational institution who are preparing to become marriage and family therapists, if the services they render are under supervision and direction and their student status is clearly designated by the title of trainee or intern;
5. individuals who have obtained one of the graduate degrees required for licensure as marriage and family therapists and who are practicing under supervision and direction to obtain the experience required for licensure;
6. individuals registered as rehabilitation suppliers by the Georgia Board of Workers' Compensation when practicing rehabilitation counseling for workers' compensation claimants;
7. active members of the clergy, but only when the practice of marriage and family therapy is in the course of their service as clergy;
8. members of religious ministries, responsible to their established ecclesiastical authority, who possess a master's degree or its equivalent in theological studies;

---

2. O.C.G.A. § 43-10A-22.

9. individuals engaged in the practice of marriage and family therapy in accordance with biblical doctrine in public or non-profit agencies or entities, or in private practice;

10. individuals engaged in the practice of marriage and family therapy as employees of the Division of Family and Children Services of the Department of Human Resources; and

11. addiction counselors who have met the certification requirements set by the Georgia Addiction Counselors Association.[3]

(B) The Composite Board

The Composite Board issues licenses to practice professional counseling, social work, and marriage and family therapy. The Board consists of 10 members: three professional counselors, three social workers, three marriage and family therapists, and one member of the public.[4] The Board is divided into three separate standards committees for each respective specialty. Each committee approves, by majority vote, the granting of a license in that specialty, approves the examination and provides for grading the examination in that specialty, and deals with licensing matters relating to its profession.[5] Decisions of the standards committees must be approved by the full Board.[6]

The general eligibility requirements for licensure applicable to the three Composite Board professions are the following:

1. meeting the education, training, and experience requirements for that particular profession;

2. passing successfully the examination established for their profession; and

3. furnishing two personal references from supervisors, teachers, or any combination thereof and paying the required license fee.

---

3. O.C.G.A. § 43-10A-7.
4. O.C.G.A. § 43-10A-4.
5. O.C.G.A. § 43-10A-6(a).
6. O.C.G.A. § 43-10A-6(b).

(C) Requirements for Licensure in Marriage and Family Therapy

The law provides three methods by which individuals may meet the education, experience, and training requirements for licensure as marriage and family therapists. They are

1. a master's degree from a program in professional counseling, social work, or marriage and family therapy; any allied profession, applied child and family development, applied sociology; or any program accredited by the Commission on Accreditation of Marriage and Family Therapy Education, which degree shall have been granted by a recognized educational institution. After July 1, 1987, the degree program must include a course of study in the principles and practice of marriage and family therapy. In addition, the applicant must have 4 years' full-time, post-master's degree experience under direction in the practice of professional counseling, social work, or marriage and family therapy, 1 year of which may have been in an approved internship program before or after the granting of the master's degree and 2 years of which shall have been in the practice of marriage and family therapy. Also, 200 hours of supervision are required, 100 of which shall have been in the practice of marriage and family therapy;

2. a doctoral degree in a program, which degree and program shall meet the requirements stated in the preceding paragraph, 2 years of full-time, post-master's degree experience under direction in the practice of marriage and family therapy, 1 year of which may have been in an approved internship program, and 100 hours of supervision in the practice of marriage and family therapy, 50 hours of which may have been obtained as a student or intern in an accredited doctoral program; or

3. a law degree and specified post-law degree experience in the practice of marriage and family therapy if application for licensure was made prior to July 1, 1989.[7]

The Composite Board may also issue a license without examination to an individual licensed as a marriage and family therapist under the laws of another jurisdiction having licensure requirements that are substantially equal to those in Georgia.

---

7. O.C.G.A. § 43-10A-13.

Certification and Regulation of Hypnotists

Although in some states the law regulates hypnosis and the professional title of hypnotist by prescribing education, experience, and skills requirements, practitioners of the art of hypnosis are not licensed by the state of Georgia. MHPs do not have to obtain certification to use the title of hypnotist and may use the title at their own discretion. The failure to have a licensing law or standards is indicative of the difficulty in formulating appropriate practice standards and measurements of competency in this area.

1.10

Licensure and Regulation of Polygraph Examiners

The basic law governing the licensing and practice of polygraph examiners was repealed in 1992.[1] Prior to its repeal, all polygraph examiners in the state of Georgia were subject to a basic licensing and practice law as set forth in O.C.G.A. section 43-3-61 *et seq.* Although no law governs the licensure and practice now, a recitation and general discussion of the former law may be helpful for any MHP having need to work with or consult a polygraph examiner. However, no statute has ever authorized the introduction into evidence of the results of a polygraph examination in any judicial or administrative proceeding in Georgia.[2] Nevertheless, from the period of 1981 to July 1, 1992, the following laws and provisions applied to polygraph examiners.

(A) Activities Formerly Regulated Under the Polygraph Examiners Law

The General Assembly of Georgia had declared that the state's policy was to restrict the use of a polygraph examination to the measurement of stressful physiological responses by means of devices used for such purposes, to detect deception or verify the truth of statements uttered or to carry out scientific or academic research and experiments. The use of a polygraph or polygraph

---

1. Ga. Laws 1992, p. 3137 § 29, effective July 1, 1992.
2. O.C.G.A. § 51-1-37 authorized a cause of action for the negligent or improper administering of a polygraph examination.

examination intended primarily to frighten or intimidate rather than to measure stressful physiological response was declared improper.

The term *polygraph* means an instrument to measure stressful physiological responses for the purpose of testing or questioning individuals so as to detect deception or verify the truth of a statement. Under former Georgia law, such instruments must, at a minimum, record visually, permanently, and simultaneously a subject's cardiovascular pattern, respiratory pattern, and galvanic skin response. A *polygraph examiner* is a person who measures stressful physiological responses consistent with the definition of polygraph examinations. A *polygraph examiner intern* refers to a person engaged in the study of polygraphy and the administration of polygraph examinations under the personal supervision and control of a polygraph examiner.[3]

(B) Board of Polygraph Examiners

The former Georgia polygraph examiner law created the State Board of Polygraph Examiners, which consisted of seven members. The composition of the polygraph examiners board, since the law has been repealed, no longer merits a discussion.[4]

The Polygraph Examiners Board had the following powers:

1. to determine the qualifications and fitness of the applicants;

2. to issue, renew, deny, suspend, or revoke licenses;

3. to initiate investigations for the purpose of discovering violations;

4. to hold hearings on matters properly brought before the Board, to receive evidence and make necessary determinations, and to enter orders consistent with the Board's findings;

5. to establish continuing education requirements; and

6. to adopt, amend, or repeal all rules necessary to carry out the purposes of the statutes.[5]

(C) Licensing Procedures

Formerly, every person, including an MHP, who administered polygraph examinations had to qualify individually for a license

---

3. O.C.G.A. § 43-36-3 (repealed).
4. O.C.G.A. § 43-36-4 (repealed).
5. O.C.G.A. § 43-36-5 (repealed).

and had to file with the Polygraph Examiners Board a written application to qualify for licensure.[6] Persons pursuing scientific endeavors and academic research were free to use polygraph examinations and devices without licensure, if the sole purpose was for conducting research. However, research and academic endeavors did not include specific employment, law enforcement, or public safety objectives. To qualify for a license, a polygraph examiner was required to

1. be at least 21 years of age;

2. be a citizen of the United States;

3. be a person of good moral character;

4. have a bachelor's degree from a 4-year accredited university or college including at least one course in physical science and one course in psychology, or have completed 2 years of study, or its equivalent, at such a university or college, including at least one course in physical science and one course in psychology and have at least 2 years of experience as an investigator or detective with a municipal, county, state, or federal agency;

5. have completed satisfactorily a formal training course in the use of polygraphs, such training to be of at least 6 weeks' duration at an acceptable polygraph examiner's school;

6. have completed a period of at least 6 weeks of training as a polygraph examiner intern under the supervision of a qualified polygraph examiner in Georgia or have sufficient training and experience in a state, federal, or municipal agency such that the Polygraph Examiners Board, in its discretion, would have recognized the applicant as being properly trained and experienced; and

7. have passed any examination approved by the Polygraph Examiners Board for the purpose of determining qualifications and fitness of applicants for licenses.[7]

Applicants were required to submit to the Polygraph Examiners Board, for its prior approval, the name of a qualified polygraph examiner to supervise the applicant through the intern program. The supervising polygraph examiner had to demonstrate both employment as a polygraph operator and at least 3 years of prior experience. He or she was limited to supervising no more than two interns at one time. The intern had to be personally supervised and controlled by the licensed polygraph examiner on the premises where any testing was conducted, although the Polygraph Examiners Board, in its discretion, could waive the

6. O.C.G.A. § 43-36-8 (repealed).
7. O.C.G.A. § 43-36-6 (repealed).

"on premises" requirements during the internship period in cases of extreme hardship. The supervisor had to be available to the intern for instruction and consultation. The Polygraph Examiners Board's rules limited the number of polygraph examinations that could be taken by an intern during any given period of time and required verification of the examination results. The availability and production of polygraph charts and papers could be required at the Board's discretion before a license was issued.[8]

(D) Issuance of Licenses

Polygraph licenses were issued to those who, pursuant to the application procedure, passed the examination and were deemed morally fit and otherwise qualified. The Polygraph Examiners Board, after satisfying itself that the applicant had met the requirements, delivered to the applicant a license to become a polygraph examiner intern, which was not transferable and could be revoked only by the Polygraph Examiners Board. The intern, after working under the supervision of a licensed polygraph examiner, could then be issued a license as a polygraph examiner. Notwithstanding the other provisions, individuals who were licensed polygraph operators and whose licenses were valid on July 1, 1985, were not required to serve the minimum 6-month polygraph examiner internship under supervision of a polygraph operator or pass an examination.[9]

The statute provided for reciprocity for licensed polygraph operators from states having requirements similar to those of the Georgia licensing law, at the discretion of the Polygraph Examiners Board.[10]

(E) Polygraph Examination Procedures, Testing, and Conditions

Under the former Georgia statute, polygraph examinations were conducted under testing conditions established by the Polygraph Examiners Board, including the following:

1. No chart contained less than 7 nor more than 15 questions.

---

8. O.C.G.A. § 43-36-7 (repealed).
9. O.C.G.A. § 43-36-9 (repealed).
10. O.C.G.A. § 43-36-10 (repealed).

2. Examiners were required to allow a minimum of 10 seconds between questions to allow the subject ample time to respond physiologically to each verbal stimulus.

3. Examiners could not produce a polygraph chart that was not adequately marked to identify, at a minimum, each of the following:

    a. the individual being tested;

    b. the date of the examination;

    c. the time of the chart;

    d. the chart and test number; and

    e. the polygraph examiner's initials.

4. Examiners were required to mark the charts that were produced from instruments that contained electronically enhanced components showing the sensitivity level of the beginning of the chart and any point at which the sensitivity was changed.

5. A polygraph examiner was not permitted to perform more than two examinations per hour nor to exceed 18 polygraph examinations in one 24-hour period; and while the polygraph examination was being administered, no one was to be present in the room other than the polygraph examiner and the examinee, without the knowledge and prior consent of the examinee. No polygraph examination could be monitored with viewing or listening devices without the examinee's knowledge.[11]

Conclusions or opinions of the examiner were required to be in writing and based on analysis of two or more polygraph charts on the examinee covering the same questions. The examiner was allowed to produce only three types of conclusions or opinions. They were (a) deception indicated, (b) no deception indicated, or (c) inconclusive chart analysis.

Upon written request, the conclusions and opinions were required to be provided to the examinee within 15 days of the date of the examination.[12]

---

11. O.C.G.A. § 43-36-12 (repealed).
12. O.C.G.A. § 43-36-13 (repealed).

(F) Areas of Questioning Prohibited During Preemployment or Periodic Employment Examinations

The former statute providing for the proper conduct of a polygraph examination proscribed inquiry into the following areas during preemployment or periodic employment examinations:

1. religious beliefs or affiliations;
2. beliefs or opinions regarding racial matters;
3. political beliefs or affiliations;
4. beliefs, affiliations, or lawful activities regarding unions or labor organizations; or
5. sexual preferences or activities. [13]

(G) The Examinee's Bill of Rights as Relates to Polygraph Procedures

Formerly, each prospective examinee was required to sign a notification, and received a copy of such notification, prior to the beginning of the polygraph examination, which stated that

1. he or she was voluntarily consenting to take the examination;
2. the polygraph examiner could not inquire into any areas dealing with religious beliefs or affiliations, beliefs or opinions regarding racial matters, political beliefs or affiliations, beliefs or affiliations or lawful activities regarding unions or labor organizations; and sexual preferences or activities; and
3. the examinee could terminate the examination at any time.

The examinee, upon written request, had to be provided a written copy of any opinions or conclusions, the name of the polygraph examiner and his license number and business address, the name and address of the Polygraph Examiners Board, and the examinee had the right to file a complaint with the Polygraph Examiners Board if the examinee felt that the examination had been conducted improperly. A form was provided with the exact wording of such notification pursuant to the rules.

---

13. O.C.G.A. § 43-36-14 (repealed).

The law protected the examinee against accusatory interrogation for the purpose of eliciting a confession or admission against interest, coercion or intimidation into signing a confession or confessing to matters released through results of the subject's examination unless the examiner had obtained prior written permission, or conduct of an examination if the examiner knew or had reason to believe the examinee was mentally or physically incapable of undergoing a polygraph examination. The examinee was entitled to tape record an examination on matters directly relating to employment. The examination administered by a polygraph examiner intern or an employee of the licensed polygraph examiner could disclose information acquired from a polygraph only to

1. the examinee or other persons specifically designated in writing by the examinee;
2. the individual, firm or corporation, partnership, business entity, or governmental agency that requested the information; or
3. any person pursuant to and directed by court order.

The rights and procedures provided for the protection of an examinee were not affected by any contract or waiver, and the examiner was prohibited from requesting an examinee to execute such contract or waiver.[14]

The polygraph examination was required to be preserved and kept on file for a minimum of 2 years, and examiners were required to provide professional liability insurance, or a bond or net worth affidavit as an alternative for insurance.[15]

(H) Prohibited Activities

Under the former law, it was unlawful for an employer or prospective employer to charge or require an employee or prospective employee to pay for any polygraph examination as a condition of preemployment or continuing employment.[16]

In 1988, the federal government passed the Employee Polygraph Protection Act (the Federal Polygraph Act).[17] The Federal Polygraph Act prohibits employers from forcing employees to submit to polygraph examinations as a condition of employ-

---

14. O.C.G.A. § 43-36-15 (repealed).
15. O.C.G.A. § 43-36-17 (repealed).
16. O.C.G.A. § 43-36-20 (repealed).
17. 29 U.S.C.A. §§ 2001–2009 (Supp. 1992).

ment,[18] although government agencies[19] and private businesses dealing with security[20] or the distribution or manufacturing of controlled substances[21] are exempt from this prohibition. Furthermore, the Federal Polygraph Act does permit an employer to require an employee to submit to a polygraph examination during the investigation of an act that caused economic injury to the employer.[22]

18. 29 U.S.C.A. § 2002.
19. 29 U.S.C.A. § 2006(a).
20. 29 U.S.C.A. § 2006(e).
21. 29 U.S.C.A. § 2006(f).
22. 29 U.S.C.A. § 2006(d).

1.11

Sunset of Licensing Agencies

O.C.G.A. section 43-2-1 *et seq.* provide for the review of the effectiveness and efficiency of regulatory agencies prior to their termination and the continuation or reestablishment of those agencies. A *regulatory agency* is any board, bureau, or commission of the executive branch of the state government created for the primary purpose of licensing or regulating any profession, business, or trade.[1]

Each regulatory agency will be reviewed by standing committees of both the Senate and House of Representatives, which will conduct a joint public hearing for the purpose of receiving testimony from the public and the officials of such agency. The agency shall have the burden of demonstrating public need. The determination shall take into consideration:

1. whether the absence of regulation would significantly harm, affect, or endanger the public health, safety, or welfare;

2. whether there is a less restrictive method of regulation available that would protect the public adequately;

3. the extent to which the regulatory agency has permitted qualified applicants to serve the public;

4. the extent to which affirmative action requirements of state and federal statutes and constitutions have been complied with by the regulatory agency or the profession, business, or trade that it regulates;

5. the extent to which the regulatory agency has operated in the public interest and the extent to which its operation has been

---

1. O.C.G.A. § 43-2-2.

impeded or enhanced by existing statutes, procedures, practices, and rules and regulations, and any other circumstances, including budgetary, resource, and personnel matters;

6. the extent to which the regulatory agency has recommended statutory changes to the General Assembly, which would benefit the public as opposed to the persons it regulates;

7. the extent to which the regulatory agency has required the persons it regulates to report to it concerning the impact of rules and decisions of the regulatory agency on the public regarding improved service, economy of service, and availability of service;

8. the extent to which persons regulated by the regulatory agency have been required to assess problems in their profession, business, or trade that affect the public;

9. the extent to which the regulatory agency has encouraged participation by the public in making its rules and decisions as opposed to participation solely by the persons it regulates;

10. the efficiency with which formal public complaints filed with the regulatory agency concerning individuals subject to regulation have been processed to completion by the regulatory agency; and

11. the extent to which changes are necessary in the enabling laws of the regulatory agency to comply adequately with the factors listed in the Act.[2]

The state auditor conducts a performance audit for each regulatory agency upon the request of a standing committee to which said agency is assigned. A copy of the audit conducted pursuant to the Act shall be submitted within 15 days of its completion to

1. each member of the House and Senate standing committees to which the regulatory agency has been assigned for review under this chapter;

2. the presiding officers of the Senate and House of Representatives;

3. the governor, the attorney general, and the legislative council;

4. the chairperson of the audited regulatory agency; and

5. the joint-secretary.

Thirty days after the submission of the performance audit, the regulatory agency and the joint-secretary shall each submit a written response to each audit finding in those areas in which the agency or the joint-secretary has been determined to exercise

---

2. O.C.G.A. § 43-2-3.

major responsibilities. The response is required to include the following:

1. whether or not the agency or joint-secretary agrees with the findings and reasons therefor;

2. what steps have been or will be taken to address each issue raised in each finding, whether the steps are regulatory or proposed statutory changes, and the proposed effective date of such regulatory changes; and

3. if no steps have been or will be taken to address any issues raised in the finding, the reason therefor.[3]

The Senate and House committees to which a regulatory agency has been assigned shall issue reports of their findings and recommendations to the governor, to the subject regulatory agency, and to each member of the General Assembly. The reports may be issued separately by the reviewing committees or jointly when a majority of the members of each reviewing committee are in agreement as to the recommendations and findings. The report shall include legislation that must be enacted in order to fulfill the requirements of this Act.[4]

---

3. O.C.G.A. § 43-2-4.
4. O.C.G.A § 43-2-5.

Business Matters

2.1

Sole Proprietorships

MHPs who practice alone and without any formal organization are termed *sole proprietors*. Although professional corporations, partnerships and limited liability companies are subject to direct regulation (see chapters 2.2, 2.3, and 2.4), there is no law regulating sole proprietorships directly. Rather, sole proprietors must abide only by the laws regulating businesses in general.

Professional Corporations[1]

MHPs who do not work for an employer typically organize their business in one of three forms: sole proprietorship (see chapter 2.1), partnership (see chapter 2.3), or professional corporation. The value of the professional corporation form of practice is that it offers many of the tax and practice benefits of regular business corporations. Licensed psychologists, psychiatrists, and registered professional nurses may incorporate under the professional corporation law. Unfortunately, the benefits of professional incorporation are limited to enumerated professions. Professional counselors, marriage and family therapists, and social workers may not avail themselves of the professional corporation form.[2]

(A) Benefits of Incorporation

There are three main benefits to MHPs incorporating their practices. First, certain tax deductions are available only to a corporation (e.g., for the purchase of health insurance, death benefits, and retirement plans). Second, meeting the requisites of corporate law, such as holding shareholder meetings, forces professionals to become more sensitive to the business aspects of their practice. Third, the professional corporate form insulates its shareholders from the business liabilities of the corporation.[3]

---

1. Because the law discussed in this chapter applies to many types of professionals, we attempt only to introduce the reader to the subject rather than to present a comprehensive analysis.
2. O.C.G.A. § 14-7-2; 1977 Op. Att'y Gen. No. 77-14.
3. O.C.G.A. § 14-7-3; see First Bank & Trust Co. v. Zagoria, 250 Ga. 844, 302 S.E.2d 674 (1983).

The insulation from liability afforded to shareholders of a business corporation is not applicable to liability for breach of a professional obligation. The Georgia courts have held that "a profession is a calling which demands adherence to the public interest as the foremost interest of the practitioner,"[4] and therefore a professional corporation will not act as a shield against professional liability.[5]

(B) Incorporation and Operation Procedures

A professional corporation must be organized for the purpose of engaging in only one category of professional service (e.g., provision of psychological services).[6] At least one member of the board of directors and the president of a professional corporation must be licensed to practice the profession for which the corporation is organized.[7] However, the corporation can employ unlicensed individuals in capacities in which they are not rendering professional services to the public in the course of their employment.[8]

In the event that the governing board of a professional corporation includes individuals not licensed in the profession, the corporation must, by the creation of a standing committee of the board or otherwise, vest the responsibility for decisions relating entirely to professional considerations in persons who are so licensed.[9]

(C) Liability and Accountability

The professional corporation is accountable to the board that grants professional licenses to its shareholders (e.g., the State Board of Examiners of Psychologists). The licensing board may establish and enforce standards of practice applicable to the relationship between the person furnishing a professional service and the one receiving such service (e.g., rules regarding confidential communications, ethical standards, and supervision guide-

---

4. *Id.* at 845. The *Zagoria* case involved lawyers, and the court's decision is based, in part, on its power to regulate the legal profession. However, the rationale of the case is equally applicable to other professions.
5. *Id.; see also* Downey v. Bexley, 253 Ga. 125, 317 S.E.2d 523 (1984).
6. O.C.G.A. § 14-7-4(a).
7. O.C.G.A. § 14-7-4(c).
8. O.C.G.A. § 14-7-4(b).
9. O.C.G.A. § 14-7-4(c).
10. O.C.G.A. § 14-7-7.

lines).[12]

(D) Termination of the Professional Corporation

In the event that a professional corporation at any time ceases to have at least one shareholder licensed or otherwise authorized to practice and actually practicing the profession for which the corporation is organized, or if a professional corporation does not redeem, cancel, or transfer the shares of a disqualified, retired, or deceased person in accordance with Georgia law,[13] the professional corporation will cease to exist and must operate as a corporation for profit organized pursuant to Georgia business corporation law[14] for the sole purpose of liquidation. The corporation may, at any time after it ceases to be a professional corporation, change its purpose by amending its articles of incorporation.[15]

---

11. O.C.G.A. § 14-7-5.
12. O.C.G.A. § 14-2-101.
13. O.C.G.A. § 14-7-5(e).

2.3

Partnerships[1]

A *partnership* is a form of doing business whereby two or more individuals, each of whom is a co-owner, enter into a for-profit agreement. It allows the partners to pool their resources to undertake projects that would be financially difficult for one person. The law may find that any joint endeavor is a partnership, regardless of whether or not the individuals labeled it as such. Such a finding could result in a forced sharing of profits and liabilities. Thus, MHPs should be aware of this form of business arrangement whether they form a partnership or merely work in a close business relationship with other persons that could be construed as a partnership.

(A) Formation of a Partnership

A partnership is formed when there is an association of two or more individuals carrying on a business for profit, as co-owners.[2] The intent to share profits is the most important factor in determining whether a partnership exists. For instance, two psychiatrists who work out of a co-owned building under a common name could have partnership status forced upon them if there is an intent to share the profits of their services or if they hold themselves out to the public as being a partnership or a joint practice.

---

1. Because the law discussed in this chapter applies to many types of businesses, we attempt only to introduce the reader to it rather than to present a comprehensive analysis.
2. O.C.G.A. § 14-8-6.

Partners do not have to share equally in profits and losses. Generally, profits and losses are assigned to the partners according to their respective share in the partnership. For example, when a partnership consists of two individuals, one of whom initially contributed $50,000 and the other $100,000, the latter may legitimately claim 66% of the profits. Partners may agree to allocate partnership income and losses in different proportions, although the Internal Revenue Service will not recognize losses in excess of a partner's investment in a partnership.

A mere sharing of debts or employees' salaries does not create partnership status.[3] However, it is not necessary to make a formal declaration or to make a formal filing to create a partnership. Rather, any agreement between the parties that meets the above definition, even an oral one, suffices to initiate a general partnership. (It should be noted that, to form a limited partnership, certain statutory requirements must be met, including filing a certificate of limited partnership in the office of the secretary of the state of Georgia.[4])

(B) Rights and Duties Between Partners

A partnership is more than a business relationship; the law imposes duties on the partners governing their interactions. For instance, the partners have equal rights in the management and conduct of business unless specifically agreed otherwise.[5] Each partner has the right to inspect the partnership books;[6] every partner must account to the partnership for any benefit and hold as trustee for it any profits derived by him or her without the consent of the other partners from any transaction connected with the formation, conduct, or liquidation of the partnership or from any use of partnership property.[7] Each partner shall have the right to a formal accounting as to partnership affairs under certain circumstances,[8] and each partner, who in aid of the partnership makes any payment or advance beyond the amount of capital that he agreed to contribute, must be paid interest from the date of the payment or advance unless specifically agreed otherwise.[9] Other

---

3. O.C.G.A. § 14-8-7(4).
4. O.C.G.A. § 14-9-201.
5. O.C.G.A. § 14-8-18(5).
6. O.C.G.A. § 14-8-19.
7. O.C.G.A. § 14-8-21.
8. O.C.G.A. § 14-8-22.
9. O.C.G.A. § 14-8-18(3).

rights and duties of partners are further set forth by Georgia statute.[10]

The law views each partner as an agent of the partnership. Thus, each partner's acts bind each of the other partners[11] so long as the acts are within the partner's authority. Unless authorized by the other partners or unless they have abandoned the business, one or more but less than all the partners have no authority to

1. assign the partnership property in trust for creditors or on the assignee's promise to pay the debts of the partnership;
2. dispose of the goodwill of the business;
3. perform any other act that would make it impossible to carry on the ordinary business of the partnership;
4. confess a judgment; or
5. submit a partnership claim or liability to arbitration or reference.[12]

Perhaps most important, any wrongful act or omission of any partner acting in the ordinary course of the business of the partnership or with the authority of his partners that results in a loss, injury, or penalty accrues to all of the partners.[13] Therefore, when one partner acting within the scope of his apparent authority receives money or property of a third person and misapplies it; or when the partnership in the course of its business receives money or property of a third person and the money or property so received is misapplied by any partner while it is in the custody of the partnership, the partnership is bound to make good the loss.[14] The partners are jointly and severally liable for all partnership liabilities, which means that a person wronged by the professional negligence of a partner may sue one, several, or all of the partners.[15]

(C) Dissolution of a Partnership

A partnership is dissolved[16]

1. by the termination of the definite term or particular undertaking specified in the agreement;

---

10. O.C.G.A. § 14-8-18.
11. O.C.G.A. § 14-8-9(1).
12. O.C.G.A. § 14-8-9(3).
13. O.C.G.A. § 14-8-13.
14. O.C.G.A. § 14-8-14.
15. O.C.G.A. § 14-8-15.
16. O.C.G.A. § 14-8-31.

2. by the express will or withdrawal of any partner;

3. by the expulsion of any partner from the business in accordance with the terms of the agreement between the partners;

4. by any event that makes it unlawful for the business of the partnership to be carried on or for the members to carry it on in partnership;

5. by the death of any partner, unless there is a written agreement between the partners expressly providing otherwise;

6. by decree of court pursuant to Georgia law;[17] and

7. in other circumstances as provided in the agreement between the partners.

Generally, the dissolution of a partnership terminates the authority of the partners except to wind up the partnership affairs.[18] This does not absolve the partners of whatever liability may have accrued to the partnership prior to dissolution.

17. O.C.G.A. § 14-8-32.
18. O.C.G.A. §§ 14-8-33, 14-8-35, and 14-8-38.

The Georgia Limited Liability Company: A New Option for Structuring the Professional Practice[1]

On March 1, 1994, the Georgia Limited Liability Company Act went into effect. The Act creates a new form for the organization of business entities known as the *Limited Liability Company* (LLC). The advent of the Georgia LLC increases to five the number of organizational structures from which professionals may choose. These include the sole proprietorship, the partnership, the professional corporation, and the professional association.

(A) Sole Proprietorship

The simplest of these structures is the *sole proprietorship*, in which the business is owned entirely by an individual who assumes personal liability for the business's debts, for his own actions, and, under most circumstances, for the acts and omissions of his employees and agents.

(B) Partnership

A *partnership* may arise whenever two or more principals enter into an agreement to share revenues and expenses. The partnership as an entity may be held liable for its business debts and for the wrongful acts of partners, employees, and agents of the part-

---

1. This chapter was authored by Susan M. Garrett, an attorney with the Atlanta law firm of Kirwan, Goger, Chesin & Parks, PC. The chapter originally appeared in the *Georgia Psychologist* (Spring 1994).

nership,[2] but the individual partners remain personally liable, "jointly and severally," for all of the partnership's obligations.[3] This means that a creditor may look to any one partner for full satisfaction of a partnership debt or obligation. Therefore, in partnerships rendering professional services, each partner is potentially liable for the professional negligence of his partners as well as that of the partnership's employees and agents.

Although Georgia's Uniform Partnership Act sets out the formal legal requirements for the formation of a partnership,[4] it is important to note that even in the absence of the legal formalities, a partnership may be inferred when two or more individuals hold themselves out to the public as a partnership.[5] For example, assume that two psychologists are conducting separate practices but operate in a space-sharing arrangement under a common practice name. There is a significant risk that they would be treated as *de facto* partners for liability purposes if members of the public reasonably rely upon the representation that a partnership exists. This risk may be reduced by including a conspicuous disclaimer on letterhead, signs, or wherever the practice name appears. A better solution may be to abandon the use of the practice name or consider organizing as a professional corporation or an LLC.

(C) Professional Corporation

Under the Georgia Professional Corporation Act, a professional corporation (PC) may be formed by an individual or group of individuals licensed to practice a profession in Georgia.[6] The owners of the PC are its shareholders, who practice their profession as employees of the corporate entity. A PC may practice only one profession, and every shareholder must be a licensed member of that profession.[7] This restriction prevents, for example, a licensed psychologist and a licensed physician from forming a professional corporation. However, a professional corporation owned by psychologists could employ physicians and other professionals.

The advantage of this organizational structure is that, unlike the partners in a partnership, the shareholders in a PC are

---

2. O.C.G.A. § 14-8-13.
3. O.C.G.A. § 14-8-16.
4. O.C.G.A. § 14-8-1 *et seq.*
5. O.C.G.A. § 14-8-16(a); Kaplan v. Gibson, 192 Ga. App. 466, 385 S.E.2d 103 (1989).
6. O.C.G.A. § 14-7-1 *et seq.*
7. O.C.G.A. §§ 14-7-5, 14-7-6.

shielded from personal liability for the business debts of the corporation. However, this liability shield does not extend to professional malpractice. A shareholder in a professional corporation remains liable not only for his own professional misdeeds but for those of the other shareholders in the corporation.[8]

(D) Professional Association

Georgia law also permits two or more licensed members of the same profession to organize as an unincorporated professional association (PA). The PA is distinct from the partnership only in that its members cannot be held liable for the business debts of the association unless they personally participated in the transaction from which the claim arose. However, as in professional corporations, this limited liability shield does not extend to claims for professional negligence.[9] The PA form of organization provides few, if any, advantages over other forms of organization.

(E) The Limited Liability Company

The new Limited Liability Company Act provides that an LLC may be organized "for any lawful purpose." The Act also expressly states that limited liability companies may be organized for the purpose of providing professional services. Ownership of the LLC is vested in its members, whereas the business affairs of the company may be managed either by the members or by managers, if the articles of organization or written operating agreement so provide. Although the Act's provisions have not yet been interpreted by the courts, the LLC structure presents a number of potential advantages over other organizational structures that may be of particular interest to health care professionals.

(F) Liability Issues

One advantage of the Limited Liability Company Act is its extremely broad limitation on personal liability to third parties:[10]

An individual who is a member, manager, agent, or employee of a limited liability company is not liable, solely by reason of

---

8. First Bank & Trust Co. v. Zagoria, 250 Ga. 844, 302 S.E.2d 674 (1983).
9. O.C.G.A. § 14-10-7.
10. O.C.G.A. § 14-11-303.

being a member, manager, agent, or employee of the limited liability company, under a judgment, decree, or order of a court, or in any other manner, for a debt, obligation, or liability of the limited liability company, whether arising in contract, tort, or otherwise, or for the acts or omissions of any other member, manager, agent, or employee of the limited liability company, whether arising in tort, contract, or otherwise.

This provision appears to expand upon the liability shield available to shareholders of professional corporations by protecting members of the LLC from liability not only for business debts of the company but also from liability for the acts or omissions of fellow members. However, it may not be assumed that members of an LLC will be shielded from liability for each other's professional malpractice.

On the one hand, the Act provides that "the laws of this state relating to establishment and regulation of professional services are amended and superseded to the extent such laws are inconsistent with [the formation of limited liability companies] and are deemed amended to permit the provision of professional services within this state by limited liability companies."[11] On the other hand, the Act provides that it "does not alter any law applicable to the relationship between a person rendering professional services and a person receiving those services, including liability arising out of those professional services."[12] The Act also provides that it is not intended to restrict the authority of any regulatory or licensing bodies to license individuals or to regulate the practice of professions.[13] This resembles the professional corporation statute that has been judicially interpreted to permit shareholders in a professional corporation to be held liable for the professional misdeeds of other shareholders.[14] Although no court has had an opportunity to interpret these provisions of the Limited Liability Company Act, the most prudent approach is to assume that members of the LLC must share the risk of professional liability just as shareholders in a professional corporation do. This risk can be reduced through the purchase of appropriate professional liability insurance.

(G) Structure

A second attractive feature of the Limited Liability Company Act is that it appears to permit ownership by members of different

---

11. O.C.G.A. § 14-11-1107.
12. O.C.G.A. § 14-11-314.
13. O.C.G.A. § 14-11-117.
14. *See* Note 8, *supra*.

professions, because it does not contain the express prohibitions found in the statutes governing professional associations and professional corporations.[15] This would permit licensed members of different professions, such as psychologists and physicians, to practice together as members of an LLC. It remains to be seen, however, whether this restriction may be engrafted onto the Act through judicial interpretation.

A third advantage of the LLC, at least as compared with the professional corporation, is the relative simplicity of formation and structure. Instead of being shareholders in a corporation, owners of the LLC possess an undivided interest in the company which more closely resembles a partnership interest. Instead of a separate board of directors, the management of the company is vested in the members, unless they choose to designate managers for this purpose. The LLC counterparts to the articles of incorporation and bylaws are the articles of organization and an optional operating agreement. However, the statute contains detailed default provisions for the operation and management of the LLC which apply unless there is a provision to the contrary in the articles or operating agreement. Moreover, the Act contains a streamlined procedure through which existing corporations or partnerships may elect to reorganize as limited liability companies.[16]

Whether they practice solo or in groups, MHPs should give careful consideration to the type of business entity under which they will practice their profession. The scope of potential personal liability is an important issue, but by no means the only factor to be considered. MHPs should consult with an attorney and financial advisor to select the organizational structure best suited to their needs.

---

15. The Professional Corporation Code provides that shares may be owned only by persons licensed to practice the profession for which the corporation is organized; see O.C.G.A. § 14-7-5(a). For example, a non-physician cannot be a shareholder in a medical professional corporation; see Sherrer v. Hale, 248 Ga. 793, 285 S.E.2d 714 (1982).
16. O.C.G.A. § 14-11-21.

2.5

Health Maintenance Organizations

Generally, a health maintenance organization (HMO) provides health care services to an enrollee who individually or as part of a group pays a single, usually annual, fee. Under Georgia law, a public or private HMO must provide, or arrange for, health care services that are more than mere indemnification against the cost of such services.[1]

(A) Establishing an HMO

Operation of an HMO in Georgia requires the application to the Insurance Commissioner for a certificate of authority.[2] A certificate of authority is predicated on a showing of willingness and potential ability to ensure availability and accessibility of adequate personnel and facilities. In addition, arrangements for an ongoing quality assurance program, program of statistical compilation, and out-of-area emergency services program must be made.[3] The standard of health care that any HMO is required to maintain is set forth in rules and regulations of the Department of Human Resources.[4]

---

1. O.C.G.A. § 33-21-1.
2. O.C.G.A. § 33-21-2.
3. O.C.G.A. § 33-21-3.
4. These rules are set forth in the Rules of the Department of Human Resources, Public Health, Chapter 290-5-37.

(B) Benefits for Mental Health Services

Georgia law[5] provides that to maintain a valid certificate of authority to operate, an HMO must provide, or arrange for, *basic health care services*. These services are defined generally as services that might reasonably be required in order to maintain good health.[6] More specifically, they include emergency and preventive care, usual physician services, laboratory, X-ray, inpatient hospital care, outpatient medical services, and out-of-area coverage.[7]

The Rules of the Department of Human Resources[8] require that as a part of its basic health care services, the HMO shall provide:

1. outpatient evaluative and crisis intervention mental health services. These basic mental health services may be provided through lesser or longer time periods if enrollees are equitably assured the equivalency of 20 full 50–55 minute session visits per enrollee per year;

2. diagnosis and medical treatment for the abuse of or addiction to alcohol and drugs, including detoxification on either an outpatient or inpatient basis, whichever is medically determined to be appropriate, in addition to the treatment for other medical conditions; and

3. alcohol and drug referral services for either medical or for nonmedical services. Medical services shall be a part of basic health services; nonmedical ancillary services need not be a part of basic health services.

With regard to the personnel of an HMO, the rules[9] provide that "all HMO personnel and providers of service shall be currently licensed to perform the service they provide, when such services require licensure or registration under applicable state law."

The only other relevant regulations require an HMO to provide continuing education to its staff or providers of care and to maintain a personnel folder on each person. An MHP may, therefore, provide services as an employee of the HMO or on a fee-for-service basis if the HMO complies with the above rules.

---

5. O.C.G.A. § 33-21-5.
6. O.C.G.A. § 33-21-1.
7. O.C.G.A. § 31-6-2.
8. Chapter 290-5-37.03.
9. Chapter 290-5-37.07.

2.6

Preferred Provider Arrangements

The Georgia Preferred Provider Arrangements Act regulates the formation, organization, and operation of preferred provider arrangements and became effective July 1, 1988.[1] The Act seeks to establish minimum standards for preferred provider arrangements and health benefit plans associated with those arrangements. A *health benefit plan* is defined as the health insurance policy or subscriber agreement setting forth the covered services and benefit levels between the covered person, as the policy holder, and the health care insurer.[2]

A *preferred provider* is a health care provider or group of providers that contract with employers, unions, or third-party payers (such as an insurance company) to provide services to employees, members, or insureds under an arrangement that may provide incentives for covered persons to use health care services.[3] Preferred providers render services that include, but are not limited to, hospital, medical, surgical, dental, vision, chiropractic, psychological, and pharmaceutical services.[4]

In addition to proposing to ensure "fair, reasonable and equitable mechanisms for assignment and payment of benefits to nonpreferred providers," the Act undertakes to minimize the cost of the health care plan and to control the use of health care services. The Act also seeks to ensure that preferred provider arrangements have procedures for determining whether health care services are medically necessary.

---

1. O.C.G.A. § 33-30-21.
2. O.C.G.A. § 33-30-2(2).
3. O.C.G.A. § 33-30-22(6).
4. O.C.G.A. § 33-30-22(5).

The Act prohibits arrangements that unfairly deny health benefits, have differences in benefit levels that unfairly deny benefits for covered services, have differences in co-insurance percentages applicable to benefit levels for services provided by preferred and nonpreferred providers that differ by more than 30%, or have co-insurance percentages applicable to benefit levels for services provided by nonpreferred providers that exceed 40% of the benefit levels under the policy for services.[5]

Entities not licensed as health care insurers are required to file with the State Insurance Commissioner a description of the contract that they use with health care providers. Employers that enter into such contracts with health care providers for the exclusive benefit of their employees and dependents are exempt from this filing requirement.[6]

Incentive policy provisions for covered persons to use preferred providers are required to contain provisions for emergency care when a preferred provider is not available. Policy holders must be reimbursed at parity with the usual, customary, and reasonable charges applicable to preferred providers and be shown specifically the differences in benefit levels for preferred provider and nonpreferred providers.[7]

Although limits may be placed on the number or classes of preferred providers, the statute prohibits discrimination on the basis of religion, race, color, national origin, age, sex, marital, or corporate status. The Act provides that qualified providers in the service area shall be given an opportunity to apply to become preferred providers without discrimination.[8]

---

5. O.C.G.A. § 33-30-23(b).
6. O.C.G.A. § 33-30-23(d).
7. O.C.G.A. § 33-30-24.
8. O.C.G.A. § 33-30-25.

2.7

Individual Practice Associations

An *individual practice association (IPA)* is a group of health care providers that contract to provide services for an organization that provides a prepaid health plan, frequently an HMO.[1] The members of the IPA practice in their own offices, but are compensated by the organization on a fee-for-service or fee-per-patient basis.

There is no Georgia law regulating the formation or operation of IPAs, other than basic contract law.

---

1. An IPA is a new form of health care organization, and an exact definition has yet to be widely adopted.

2.8

Hospital, Administrative, and Staff Privileges

Hospital staff privileges and administration in Georgia are governed by the rules and regulations of the Department of Human Resources (DHR).[1]

The DHR is charged[2] with governing, the licensing, and regulating of health care institutions.[3] The rules and regulations of the DHR concerning hospitals are based on a classification of the type of institution involved.[4] The three types of hospitals are general, institutional, and specialized.

Each type of hospital is under the control of a governing body.[5] This body appoints a licensed professional staff to perform the professional services for patients and establishes policy to ensure professional staff judgment in all matters that are necessary for the safety and health of patients. All of a hospital's services must be under the supervision of professional staff members.

---

1. Public Health Chapter 290-5-6.
2. O.C.G.A. § 31-7-2.1.
3. Health care institutions include community mental health and mental retardation facilities, hospitals, nursing homes, personal care homes, abortion clinics, health testing facilities, emergency care clinics, or birthing centers (O.C.G.A. § 31-7-1).
4. O.C.G.A. § 31-7-2; Public Health Chapter 290-5-6.03.
5. Public Health Chapter 290-5-6.01.

Historically, the professional hospital staff has been restricted to physicians, dentists, or osteopathic physicians.[6] However, recent changes in Georgia law provide that licensed psychologists are eligible to serve on hospital staffs with full privileges consistent with their scope of practice.

Under Georgia law and the Joint Commission on Accreditation of Healthcare Organizations (JCAHO) standards, psychologists may serve on hospital medical staffs and may provide inpatient psychological services to the full extent of their licensure.[7] In addition, recently enacted legislation has expanded the role of psychologists in the admission, treatment, and discharge of patients under the Georgia Mental Health Code.[8]

The exercise of staff or administrative privileges in any medical facility or institution is subject to the rules, regulations, and procedures of the institution. As such, privileges may be limited, restricted, or revoked when such rules are violated. Georgia law specifies, however, that staff privileges may not be restricted for violation of a rule unless the particular rule has been applied, in good faith, in a nondiscriminatory manner to all practitioners on staff at the institution.[9]

Furthermore, the Georgia legislature, in enacting the Health Service Provider Psychologist Act[10] stated:

> The General Assembly finds and declares that the treatment of psychological problems of persons residing within the community would in some cases be advanced by temporary hospitalization. The interests of the people of this State demand that all appropriate resources, including inpatient facilities, be available to assist in the diagnosis, prevention, treatment, and amelioration of psychological problems and emotional and mental disorders. The General Assembly recognizes that psychology is

---

6. *See* O.C.G.A. § 31-7-7. A physician licensed to practice in Georgia does not have an absolute right to be on staff at a hospital. Staff decisions are under the total control of the governing board so long as the board is reasonable and nondiscriminatory in its decisions; *see* Yeargin v. Hamilton Memorial Hospital, 225 Ga. 661 (1969). The governing body is created by the Hospital Authority Act (Act 1964, pp. 499, 598), the Board of Trustees, the partnership, the corporation, the association, the person or group of persons who maintain and control the hospital.

7. O.C.G.A. § 31-7-160 defines a *health service provider psychologist* as a licensed psychologist who is trained and experienced in direct, preventive assessment and therapeutic intervention services. O.C.G.A. § 31-7-161 states that "[a] medical facility or institution may provide for the appointment of health service provider psychologists on such terms and conditions as the medical facility or institution shall establish. Psychologists shall be eligible to hold membership and serve on committees of the medical or professional staff and may possess clinical privileges and carry professional responsibilities consistent with the scope of their licensure and their competence, subject to the reasonable rules of the medical facility or institution."

8. O.C.G.A. Title 37, Chapters 3, 4, and 7.

9. O.C.G.A. § 31-7-164.

10. O.C.G.A. § 31-7-160 *et seq.*

an independent health profession as set forth and proscribed by the State Board of Examiners of Psychologists and Chapter 39 of Title 43 of the Official Code of Georgia Annotated. It is therefore the intent of the General Assembly in enacting this act, to authorize medical facilities and institutions, on local determination, to make psychological services available in an inpatient setting.[11]

The Georgia legislature's intent to permit psychologists to play a full and active role in the hospital setting is further evidenced by amendments made to the Hospital Practice Act in 1990.[12] The Hospital Practice Act addresses, in part, the refusal or revocation of staff privileges. The 1990 amendment prohibits discrimination against psychologists in the granting of hospital staff privileges. The statute, as amended, provides in relevant part:

> The provisions of this Code Section [refusal or revocation by public hospital staff of staff privileges] shall not be construed to mandate such hospital to grant or to prohibit such hospital from granting staff privileges to other licensed practitioners of the healing arts who are otherwise qualified for staff privileges pursuant to the bylaws of the governing body of the hospital and, in addition, shall not be construed to modify or restrict the rights of health service provider psychologists to be treated in a nondiscriminatory manner as provided in Code Sections 31-7-161 and 31-7-164.[13]

Legislation enacted at the 1992 session of the Georgia General Assembly further enhances the psychologists' role in the hospital setting. House Bill 408[14] substantially expands the role of psychologists in the examination, commitment, and treatment of patients under the Georgia Mental Health Code. The changes made by the legislation include the following:

1. The chief medical officer of a facility may designate a treating psychologist to make discharge decisions (section 2);

2. A psychologist may execute a certificate (commonly known as the 1014 certificate) that authorizes a patient to be detained in a facility for purposes of evaluation for up to 5 days (section 3);

3. A psychologist, along with a physician, may execute a certificate (commonly known as the 1021 certificate) authorizing a patient to be detained for purposes of civil commitment (section 6);

4. A provision that all patients in a mental health facility shall be treated by either a physician or a psychologist (section 12); and

---

11. Ga. Laws, 1983, § 1, p. 1426.
12. O.C.G.A. Title 31, Chapter 7.
13. O.C.G.A. § 31-7-7(c).
14. Ga. Laws 1992, p. 1902.

5. Numerous changes expanded psychologists' roles in the out-patient setting.

Comparable changes were also made in Chapter 7 of Title 37 dealing with the treatment of alcohol- and drug-dependent individuals.

In addition, at the 1991 session of the General Assembly the patient's rights provision of the Mental Health Code[15] was amended to provide as follows:

> If a patient hospitalized under this chapter is able to secure the services of a private physician or psychologist, he shall be allowed to see his physician or psychologist at any reasonable time. The chief medical officer is authorized and directed to establish regulations designed to facilitate examination and treatment which a patient may request from such private physician or psychologist.[16]

Both House Bill 408 and House Bill 889, although dealing with patients hospitalized under the Mental Health Code, reinforce existing Georgia law that psychologists are eligible to serve on a hospital's medical staff and to possess clinical privileges and responsibilities consistent with the scope of their licensure. Under these amendments to the Mental Health Code, facilities designated by the DHR as either emergency receiving, evaluating, or treating facilities may use psychologists to admit, treat, and discharge patients. This is in addition to prior law that specifically provides that psychologists are eligible to hold full clinical privileges and responsibilities consistent with the scope of their licensure.[17]

---

15. O.C.G.A. § 37-3-162(d).
16. House Bill 889, Ga. Laws 1991, p. 1059.
17. O.C.G.A. § 31-7-161.

2.9

Zoning

State and local governments guide the rate and type of community growth through zoning regulations. The goal of such zoning regulations is to promote the "long-range requirements of the public health, safety, and welfare."[1] Georgia law delegates zoning authority to local government, but local zoning process is subject to state law.[2] In some areas, zoning laws have been used to exclude from particular communities or areas classes of people who are thought to be undesirable. Community homes for the mentally different are often considered "undesirable," and zoning laws may be used in an attempt to discriminate against them. The Georgia Supreme Court has held that group homes may be established in areas zoned residential as long as the definition of the zoned area permits groups of nonmarried, unrelated individuals living together.[3]

---

1. O.C.G.A. § 36-67-2.
2. O.C.G.A. § 36-67-3 *et seq*.
3. Macon Association for Retarded Citizens v. Macon-Bibb County Planning and Zoning Commission, 252 Ga. 484 (1984); Douglas County Resources, Inc. v. Daniel, 247 Ga. 785 (1981).

Insurance Reimbursement for Services

Typically, accident and sickness insurance carriers (insurers) provide reimbursement, to some degree, for mental health services. Georgia law requires that insurers in Georgia make available to the insured coverage for the treatment of mental disorders.[1] The Georgia code does not specify the particular health care provider whose services are covered. If the policy in question provides coverage for services that are within the lawful scope of practice of a psychologist[2] licensed to practice in Georgia, however, then such services are entitled to reimbursement regardless of whether they are rendered by a doctor of medicine or a duly licensed psychologist.[3] Given this limit, it would be possible for an insurance plan to meet the required coverage, but not cover services performed by MHPs other than physicians or psychologists.

(A) Types of Insurance Affected

The types of accident and sickness insurance benefit plan, policy, or contract covered by the code include

1. individual accident and sickness insurance policy or contract;

2. group and blanket accident and sickness insurance policy or contract;

---

1. O.C.G.A. § 33-24-28.1.
2. The term *psychologist* means that the person is duly licensed, has a doctoral degree and 1 year of experience, meets continuing education requirements, and adheres to the American Psychological Association's ethical standards; *see* O.C.G.A. § 33-24-27(a).
3. O.C.G.A. § 33-24-27(b).

3. group contract issued by a nonprofit hospital service corporation;

4. group contract issued by a health care plan;

5. group contract issued by a nonprofit medical service corporation;

6. group contract issued by HMOs; and

7. any similar accident and sickness benefit plan, policy, or contract.[4]

(B) Required Provision for Coverage

Under the code, the phrase *mental disorder* has the same meaning as it does under *The Diagnostic and Statistical Manual of Mental Disorders* (American Psychiatric Association), *The International Classification of Diseases* (World Health Organization), or the Insurance Commission rules and regulations.[5]

Covered insurers must "make [mental health coverage] available" as a part of, or as an optional endorsement to, all policies that provide major medical coverage (after January 1, 1982).[6] This coverage must be at least as extensive as like coverage of physical illnesses in the policy and must cover the spouse and dependents of the insured. The law further specifies that the mental disorder

---

4. O.C.G.A. § 33-24-28.1.

5. *Id.*

6. "Every insurer authorized to issue accident and sickness insurance benefit plans, policies, or contracts shall be required to make available, either as a part of or as an optional endorsement to all such policies providing major medical insurance coverage which are issued, delivered, issued for delivery, or renewed on or after July 1, 1984, coverage for the treatment of mental disorders, which coverage shall be at least as extensive and provide at least the same degree of coverage as that provided by the respective plan, policy, or contract for the treatment of other types of physical illnesses. Such an optional endorsement shall also provide that the coverage required to be made available pursuant to this Code section shall also cover the spouse and the dependents of the insured if the insured's spouse and dependents are covered under such benefit plan, policy, or contract. In no event shall such an insurer be required to cover inpatient treatment of more than a maximum of 30 days per policy year or outpatient treatment for more than a maximum of 48 visits per policy year under individual policies or to cover inpatient treatment for more than a maximum of 60 days per policy year or outpatient treatment for more than a maximum of 50 visits per policy year under group policies." O.C.G.A. § 33-24-28.1(b).

coverage provided cannot be limited by a provision that is not a general limitation on all similar benefits.[7]

It is noteworthy, however, that the law loses much of its potential benefit because it can be satisfied by coverage made available to a master policyholder even if the availability is not passed on to the insured.[8]

(C) Coverage for Spouse and Dependents

Coverage for a spouse may not be automatically terminated because of the death of the insured or the divorce of the insured and the spouse. The insurer must offer a similar policy to the surviving or divorced spouse, upon application made to the company within 31 days following the entry of the divorce decree and upon payment of the appropriate premium. The surviving or divorced spouse need not offer evidence of insurability. Any probationary or waiting periods are deemed waived.[9] However, these requirements do not apply to credit accident and sickness insurance.

(D) Continuation of Coverage: Georgia Law

Continuation of coverage is also required under the code for employees covered by group policies.[10] Group members are not entitled to have coverage continued if they are terminated for

---

7. "The optional endorsement required to be made available under subsection (b) of this Code section shall not contain any exclusions, reductions, or other limitations as to coverages, deductibles, or coinsurance provisions which apply to the treatment of mental disorders unless such provisions apply generally to other similar benefits provided or paid for under the accident and sickness insurance benefit plan, policy, or contract." O.C.G.A. § 33-24-28.1(c).
8. "The requirements of this Code section with respect to a group or blanket accident and sickness insurance benefit plan, policy, or contract shall be satisfied if the coverage specified in subsections (b) and (c) of this Code section is made available to the master policyholder of such plan, policy, or contract. Nothing in this Code section shall be construed to require the group insurer, nonprofit corporation, health care plan, health maintenance organization, or master policyholder to provide or to make available such coverage to any insured under such group to blanket plan, policy, or contract." O.C.G.A. § 33-24-28(e).
9. O.C.G.A. §§ 33-24-20 (individual policies) and 33-24-21 (group policies).
10. O.C.G.A. § 33-24-21.1.

cause, if they fail to pay required contributions, or if group coverage is terminated in its entirety or replaced by similar group coverage. If terminated for other reasons, they are entitled to continued coverage for 3 policy months upon payment in advance of the premium.

A recent change in Georgia law expands continuation of coverage for any employee who has reached the age of 60 years and whose employment terminates for health reasons, or for the surviving or divorced spouse of such an employee.[11] After the period set forth in O.C.G.A. section 33-24-21.1 expires, an employee 60 years or older may continue coverage indefinitely. A cap on the premium is also set by the new legislation.

(E) Waiver of Copayment

An MHP may be asked by a patient to waive the copayment normally paid by the patient and to provide services for the portion of the fee reimbursed by the insurer. This practice may constitute insurance fraud, which is a crime. O.C.G.A. section 33-1-9 states:

> Any natural person who knowingly or willfully: (1) makes or aids in the making of any false or fraudulent statement or representation of any material fact or thing in any written statement or certificate, . . . for the purpose of procuring or attempting to procure the payment of any false or fraudulent claim by an insurer . . . commits the crime of insurance fraud.

The penalty for insurance fraud when the money or benefit received exceeds $500 is imprisonment from 1 to 5 years and/or a fine of not more than $5,000.

The waiver of the copayment constitutes insurance fraud because the MHP is misrepresenting to the insurer the actual fee charged for services. The insurer reimburses based on the fee charged and if the practitioner represents that the fee is $100 per hour, when in fact he or she has agreed to accept $80 per hour (20% typically being the copayment required), the claim submission constitutes a false and fraudulent statement. The Attorney General of Georgia has rendered an official opinion that a dentist who waived the copayment without full disclosure to the insurer may have violated the insurance fraud statute and was subject to disciplinary action.[12]

---

11. *See* House Bill 1202 (1992), which will be enacted into law as O.C.G.A. § 33-24-21.2.
12. Op. Att'y Gen. 83-25.

MHPs may also be subject to having their license revoked because of this practice. Grounds for revoking licenses include "knowingly [making] misleading, deceptive, untrue, or fraudulent representations in the practice of a business or profession."[13] This general section is also incorporated in the specific grounds for revocation of a psychologist's license.[14]

An additional dilemma for the MHP who waives copayment and accepts only the reimbursed portion of a fee is that the insurer may decide that the reduced fee (the 80%, for example) is the proper amount upon which to base payment. The insurer may then refuse to reimburse more than 80% of the reduced amount. For example, if the fee charged is $100 per hour and the psychologist has waived copayment of 20% and seeks reimbursement from the insurer of $80, the insurer may decide to reimburse only 80% of $80, or $64. The insurer may also determine that the psychologist's usual and customary fee is only 80% of the amount billed and may pay only that amount on other claims submitted by the MHP.

---

13. O.C.G.A. § 43-1-19(a)(2).
14. O.C.G.A. § 43-39-13.

2.11

Mental Health Benefits in State Insurance Plans

In some states, the law mandates that any health insurance plan provided for state government employees must include certain mental health benefits. Georgia law, however, does not specify which health benefits must be offered to state employees.

Tax Deductions for Services

An individual may deduct the medical care expenses paid for self, spouse, or dependents if they itemize their personal deductions. These expenses are deductible only to the extent that they exceed 7½% (before 1987, 5%) of adjusted gross income. In addition, expenses must be reduced by any reimbursement from an insurer.[1]

(A) Mental Health Services as a Medical Deduction

Deductible medical expenses under federal tax law cover much more ground than most people realize. They encompass not only professional services related to treatment of mental or emotional disorders, but also professional diagnostic services, transportation to get medical care, and prescribed drugs.

Obviously, services performed by a psychiatrist are eligible for deduction. In addition,

> amounts paid psychologists who are qualified and authorized under State law to practice psychology for services rendered by them in connection with the diagnosis, cure, mitigation, treatment, or prevention of disease, or for the purpose of affecting any structure or function of the body, constitute expenses paid for medical care within the meaning of section 23(x) of the Internal Revenue Code and may be deducted in computing net

---

1. I.R.C. § 213.

income for Federal income tax purposes, to the extent provided therein.[2]

Even payment to an unlicensed practitioner can be deductible:

> Accordingly, it is held that amounts paid for medical services rendered by practitioners, such as chiropractors, psychotherapists, and others rendering similar type services, constitute expenses for "medical care" within the provisions of section 213 of the Code, even though the practitioners who perform the services are not required by law to be, or are not (even though required by law) licensed, certified, or otherwise qualified to perform such services.[3]

Some specific examples of tax treatment for mental health care costs are as follows:

1. Costs of psychiatric therapy of sexual inadequacy and incompatibility at a hospital are deductible.[4]

2. Costs of inpatient treatment at a therapeutic center for alcoholism, and expenses for meals and lodging furnished as necessary incident to treatment, are deductible.[5]

3. Costs of marriage counseling that is not for the alleviation of a mental defect or illness, but rather to help improve the taxpayer's marriage, are not deductible.[6]

4. Cost of maintaining a person at a therapeutic center that helps patients adjust from life in a mental hospital to life in the community, upon recommended and continued supervision of a psychiatrist, is deductible.[7]

Georgia income tax laws follow the federal rules in that a taxpayer is allowed "the sum of all itemized non business deductions if the taxpayer used itemized non business deductions in computing federal income tax."[8] Therefore, the federal allowable deductions provided by an MHP provider described would also be deductible for Georgia income tax purposes.

---

2. Rev. Rule 143, 1953-2 C.B. 129.
3. Rev. Rule 91, 1963-1 C.B. 54.
4. Rev. Rul. 75-187, 1975-1 C.B. 92.
5. Rev. Rul. 73-325, 1973-2 C.B. 75.
6. Rev. Rul. 75-319, 1975-2 C.B. 88.
7. Ltr. Rul. 7714016, 1977.
8. O.C.G.A. § 48-7-27.

(B) Mental Health Services as a Business Deduction

Section 162(a) of the Internal Revenue Code provides that "[t]here shall be allowed as a deduction all the ordinary and necessary expenses paid or incurred during the taxable year in carrying on any trade or business."[9] The key factors in this definition are not only that there be a "trade or business," but also that the expense be both ordinary and necessary. *Ordinary* is determined by examining the transaction out of which the obligation arose and its normalcy in the particular business.[10] Compliance with the requirement that an expense be "necessary" would appear to be less of a problem than the "ordinary" requirement. Generally, an expense is "necessary" if it is "appropriate and helpful."[11]

---

9. 26 U.S.C. § 162(a).
10. Deputy v. Dupont, 308 U.S. 488, *rev'd*, 188 F.2d 269, which had affirmed 14 T.C. 1066.
11. Welch v. Helvering, 290 U.S. 11 (1933).

Privacy of Professional Information

3.1

Informed Consent for Services

Georgia law makes a distinction between the concepts of consent to surgical or medical treatment and informed consent for specific surgical or diagnostic procedures. The Georgia medical consent law differentiates between surgical and medical treatment generally, in which only the treatment or course of treatment has to be disclosed, and specifically defined invasive procedures, in which the risks, benefits, and alternatives must be disclosed. The general Georgia medical consent law provides that

> [a] consent to surgical or medical treatment which discloses in general terms the treatment or course of treatment in connection with which it is given and which is duly evidenced in writing and signed by the patient or other person or persons authorized to consent pursuant to the terms of this chapter shall be conclusively presumed to be a valid consent in the absence of fraudulent misrepresentations of material facts in obtaining the same.[1]

In interpreting this code section, the Georgia courts have consistently held that the duty of disclosure does not include disclosure of the risks of treatment and that the doctrine of "informed consent" is not a viable principle of law in Georgia.[2] The courts have held, however, that a physician has a duty to respond honestly when questioned about the risks of the procedure.[3] Therefore, a physician's duty in dealing with a noninvasive treatment is merely to disclose in general terms the treatment or course of treatment and to obtain the consent of the patient. The

---

1. O.C.G.A. § 31-9-6.
2. McMullin v. Vaughn, 138 Ga. App. 718, 227 S.E.2d 440 (1976). As discussed *infra*, the General Assembly has made the concept of informed consent applicable to specific invasive procedures.
3. Spikes v. Heath, 175 Ga. App. 187, 332 S.E.2d 889 (1985).

failure to do so will give rise to a claim for battery. Unless the physician fraudulently misrepresents a material fact in obtaining the consent, the consent will be deemed valid.

In 1989, in reaction to public dissatisfaction regarding the lack of informed consent in Georgia, the General Assembly amended the medical consent law to provide for the disclosure of certain information to individuals undergoing specific surgical or invasive diagnostic procedures.[4] Any individual who undergoes a surgical procedure under general anesthesia, spinal anesthesia, or major regional anesthesia, or any individual who undergoes an amniocentesis procedure or a diagnostic procedure involving the intravenous or intraductal injection of a contrast material not only must consent to the procedure but also must be informed in general terms of the following:

1. a diagnosis of the patient's condition requiring the proposed surgical or diagnostic procedure;

2. the nature and purpose of the proposed procedure;

3. the material risks generally recognized and accepted by reasonably prudent physicians that, if disclosed to a reasonably prudent person in the patient's position, could reasonably be expected to cause the person to decline the procedure;[5]

4. the likelihood of success;

5. the generally recognized and accepted practical alternatives; and

6. the prognosis if the procedure is rejected.

It is the responsibility of the physician to ensure that the information is disclosed and that proper consent is obtained. The required information may be provided through the use of videotapes, audiotapes, pamphlets, or booklets, or through communications with allied health professionals, such as nurses, physicians, and counselors.

The law further provides that the failure to comply with the informed consent procedures does not give rise to a separate legal claim for relief, but may give rise to an action for medical malpractice if the patient suffered an injury that was proximately caused by the procedure, the information concerning the injury suffered was not disclosed, and a reasonably prudent person would have refused the procedure or would have chosen an alternative if the information had been disclosed. In addition to

---

4. O.C.G.A. § 31-9-6.1.

5. The risks are specifically identified as infection, allergic reaction, severe loss of blood or loss of function of any limb or organ, paralysis or partial paralysis, paraplegia or quadriplegia, disfiguring scar, brain damage, cardiac arrest, or death.

the general requirements in any medical malpractice action that an expert witness affidavit be attached to the complaint, the affidavit must also state that the patient suffered an injury that was proximately caused by the procedure and that such injury was a material risk required to be disclosed.[6]

The disclosure of information and consent are not required in an emergency. An *emergency* is defined as a situation in which the treatment or procedure is reasonably necessary, a person authorized to consent is not available, and a delay in treatment could reasonably be expected to jeopardize the life or the health of the individual affected or could result in disfigurement or impaired faculties.[7]

The individuals authorized to consent to surgical or medical treatment are also set forth in the statute. They are

1. an adult, either directly or by living will;
2. an individual authorized to give consent for an adult under a durable power of attorney;
3. in the absence or unavailability of a living spouse, any parent, whether an adult or a minor, for his minor child;
4. any married person, whether an adult or a minor, for himself and his spouse;
5. an individual standing temporarily in the place of a parent, whether formally serving or not, for a minor under his care;
6. any guardian for a ward;
7. any woman, regardless of age or marital status, for herself when given in connection with pregnancy, pregnancy prevention, or childbirth; and
8. upon the inability of an adult to consent for himself and in the absence of any other individual authorized to consent, then in priority order, an adult child for a parent, a parent for an adult child, an adult for a brother or sister, or a grandparent for a grandchild.

The medical consent law specifically applies to the care and treatment of patients in facilities for the mentally ill.[8] In addition, the Georgia Mental Health Code specifically provides that, unless disclosure to the patient is determined by the chief medical officer, by the treating physician, or by a psychologist to be detrimental to the physical or mental health of the patient, the patient shall have the right to review his medical file, to be told the nature of his diagnosis, to be consulted on the treatment recommendations

---

6. O.C.G.A. § 31-9-6.1(d).
7. O.C.G.A. § 31-9-3(a).
8. O.C.G.A. § 31-9-4.

and to be fully informed concerning medication, including its side effects and available treatment alternatives.[9]

By its terms, the medical consent law applies only to procedures that are performed or prescribed by a physician. Although not governed by the terms of the medical consent law, any health care provider who performs services that involve any physical contact with a patient should obtain consent to the treatment. Otherwise, the patient would have a claim for battery. Moreover, good professional care dictates providing the patient with information concerning the diagnosis, course of treatment, risks of treatment, alternatives to treatment, and prognosis. For example, both the Rules of the State Board of Examiners of Psychologists and the *Ethical Principles of Psychologists* require that informed consent to therapy be obtained.

---

9. O.C.G.A. § 37-3-162(b).

Extensiveness, Ownership, and Maintenance of and Access to Records

Georgia law distinguishes between mental health records and other types of health records. O.C.G.A. Title 31, Chapter 33, which governs the disclosure of health records in general, specifically excludes psychiatric, psychological, and other mental health records.[1] In general, mental health records are protected as products of the confidential and privileged communications between MHPs and their patients.[2] Prior to July 1, 1995, only communications between psychiatrists and psychologists and their patients were regarded as being privileged. As a result of legislation enacted in 1995, the privilege was extended to communications between a patient and a licensed clinical social worker, clinical nurse specialist in psychiatric mental health care, licensed marriage and family therapist, and licensed professional counselor during the psychotherapeutic relationship.[3]

The Georgia Mental Health Code regulates the maintenance, confidentiality, and release of clinical mental health records.[4] The code applies to state facilities, community mental health centers, U.S. Veterans Administration hospitals, and private hospitals designated by the Department of Human Resources as receiving, evaluating, or treating facilities. The record-keeping provisions of the Mental Health Code do not apply to MHPs in independent, private practice settings.[5] The code provides that clinical mental health records maintained by these institutions are not public records, are not subject to public disclosure under the Open Rec-

---

1. O.C.G.A. § 31-33-4.
2. O.C.G.A. §§ 24-9-21(5), (6), (7) and (8), and 43-39-16.
3. Ga. Laws 1995, p. 858.
4. O.C.G.A. § 37-3-166.
5. O.C.G.A. § 37-3-1(7).

ords Act, and may be released only under certain narrowly defined circumstances.[6] The statutory provisions do not, however, delineate the record-keeping responsibilities of different categories of mental health professionals within those facilities.

Records of drug-dependent individuals who seek treatment or counseling from any program licensed under the Drug Abuse Treatment and Education Act must also be maintained and shall be confidential.[7] Federal law also restricts the disclosure of records maintained by a facility for the treatment of drug and alcohol abuse if the facility receives federal financial assistance.[8]

(A) Ownership

Georgia law does not specifically address the question of the ownership of mental health records. Because the law is silent on this matter, it can be presumed that in the private practice sector, the MHP owns the record.[9] However, because the MHP–patient relationship is essentially a contractual one, and because the record is being maintained in connection with that relationship, the patient arguably has a contractual right of access to the record.[10] In addition, the MHP may owe a duty of care to the patient to make the patient's records available to other MHPs when the records would be useful in the care and treatment of the patient. Psychologists should also be aware that under standards adopted by the American Psychological Association, psychologists may

---

6. In Southeastern Legal Foundation, Inc. v. Ledbetter, 400 S.E.2d 630 (1991), the Georgia Supreme Court held that clinical records maintained under the Mental Health Code are not public records and are not subject to disclosure under the Open Records Act.
7. O.C.G.A. § 26-5-17.
8. 42 U.S.C. §§ 290dd-3 and 290ee-3; 42 C.F.R. Part II.
9. For psychiatrists, the American Medical Association (AMA) states that the records are the personal property of the physician. AMA Opinion, Section 7.02, provides in pertinent part that "[n]otes made in treating a patient are primarily for the physician's own use and constitute his personal property."
10. In contrast, O.C.G.A. § 31-33-2 requires a health care professional to furnish the patient with a complete copy of the record upon written request and payment of copying charges. Mental health records are specifically exempted.

not withhold records imminently needed for a patient's treatment solely because payment has not been received.[11]

Under the Mental Health Code, each facility, through its chief medical officer, retains ultimate responsibility for and authority over the release of patient records. The exercise of this authority is subject only to the MHP–patient privilege, the subpoena power of the courts, the limited right of the patient to review the records, and, under some circumstances, the patient's consent to release the records to third parties.[12]

The rules and regulations governing intensive residential treatment programs for children and adolescents state that the clinical record required to be maintained by those treatment programs is the property of the facility and is maintained for the benefit of the patient, staff, and the facility.[13] The rules governing other types of programs or facilities do not specifically discuss ownership of the records.

An opinion from the Georgia Court of Appeals suggests, however, that at least in the private sector, the mental health facility is the owner of the records.[14] In that case, the victim of a shooting sought access to the deceased perpetrator's records from a private mental health facility. Although the deceased patient's estate had consented to the release of the records, the court determined that, even assuming that the facility was authorized to release the records, it was still under no legal obligation to do so unless ordered to release the records by a court. Implicit in the decision was the suggestion that the hospital owned the records and that because the patient was dead, the hospital was under no obligation to make its property available to third parties. However, a 1994 amendment to the Mental Health Code provides that a copy of the record may be released to the legal representative of a deceased patient's estate, except in the case of privileged matters.[15]

The failure of a hospital, physician, or other health care provider to furnish medical records upon proper request may result in the tolling of the statute of limitations for bringing a

---

11. American Psychological Association (APA), *Ethical Principles of Psychologists*, Standard 5.11 (1981). Standard 5.10 is ambiguous on the issue of ownership of records. As to access by patient, *see* APA, *General Guidelines for Providers of Psychological Services*, Section 2.3.7 (1987); APA, *Specialty Guidelines for the Delivery of Services*, Guideline 2.3.5 (1981). The principles of medical ethics that have been adopted by the American Psychiatric Association are silent as to the right of a patient to access his records (American Psychiatric Association, *The Principles of Medical Ethics with Annotations Especially Applicable to Psychiatry*, Section 4, 1989).
12. O.C.G.A. § 37-3-166(a).
13. Ga. Comp. R. & Regs. r. 290-4-4-.06(j)(6)(ii).
14. Ridgeview Institute, Inc. *v*. Brunson, 191 Ga. App. 608, 382 S.E.2d 409 (1989).
15. O.C.G.A. § 37-3-166(a)(8.1), as amended by House Bill 1405, Act 1160 (1994).

medical malpractice action for up to 90 days. If records are not furnished within 85 days after the request, the patient may petition the court for an order requiring delivery of the records.[16]

(B) Content

Georgia law does not contain any requirements for the content and maintenance of mental health records in the private practice setting, other than the Mental Health Code requirements governing private facilities licensed by the Department of Human Resources. However, the Composite State Board of Medical Examiners and the State Board of Examiners of Psychologists do have specific record-keeping requirements.[17]

The Medical Board generally requires physicians to maintain records that "furnish documentary evidence of the course of the patient's medical evaluation, treatment and response."[18] Whenever Schedule II drugs are prescribed, the physician must maintain appropriate records that must contain, at a minimum, the patient's name, drug quantity, and diagnosis for all Schedule II prescriptions, and the patient's history.[19]

The Psychology Board requires psychologists to maintain records that include

1. the presenting problem(s) or purpose of diagnosis;
2. the fee arrangement;
3. the date and substance of each billed contact or service;
4. test results and basic test data;
5. formal consults with other providers; and
6. copies of all reports prepared.

The record shall be maintained for at least 5 years.[20] In addition, generally accepted professional standards require that written records be kept even in the absence of a licensing board rule. See, for example, American Psychological Association, *General Guidelines for Providers of Psychological Services* (1987) requiring that "[a]ccurate, current, and pertinent records of essential psy-

---

16. O.C.G.A. § 9-3-97.1.
17. The Rules of the State Board of Examiners of Psychologists provide that psychologists must function in accordance with the *Ethical Principles of Psychologists* (APA, 1981), which would include Principle 5 governing patient records. *See* Note 11, *supra.*
18. Rules of the Composite State Board of Medical Examiners; Ga. Comp. R. & Regs. r. 360-2-.09(f)(3).
19. Ga. Comp. R. & Regs. r. 360-2-.09(d).
20. Rules of the State Board of Examiners of Psychologists; Ga. Comp. R. & Regs. r. 510-5-.03(7).

chological services [be] maintained" and that "[a]t a minimum, records kept of psychological services should include identifying data, dates of services, types of services, and where appropriate, . . . a record of significant actions taken."[21] Courts may very well consider such standards in determining whether an MHP has exercised due care in treating a patient. Some courts have also considered the lack of adequate treatment records in determining an MHP's liability for professional malpractice.[22]

As to MHPs governed by the Mental Health Code, the code defines the clinical record as follows:

> *Clinical record* means a written record pertaining to an individual patient and shall include all medical records, progress notes, charts, admission and discharge data, and all other information which is recorded by a facility or other entities responsible for a patient's care and treatment under this chapter and which pertains to thepatient's hospitalization and treatment. Such other information as may be required by the rules and regulations of the board shall also be included.[23]

The Rules of the Georgia Department of Human Resources also address the content and maintenance of patient records in several specific contexts. There are sets of rules for

1. drug abuse treatment programs licensed by the state;[24]

2. community mental health, mental retardation, or substance abuse programs operated or funded by the state;[25]

3. intensive residential treatment facilities for children and youths;[26] and

4. all other facilities, including hospitals owned, operated, or licensed by the state.[27]

Drug abuse treatment records are required to contain a complete Management Information System (MIS) form; a complete medical examination form, including results of laboratory tests; a signed consent to treatment form; medical notes; a urine report form; counselor notes; including notes of failure to keep appoint-

---

21. *See also* American Psychological Association, *Specialty Guidelines for the Delivery of Services*, Guidelines 2.3.3–2.3.5 (1981). Unfortunately, there is apparently no clear understanding among Georgia psychologists as to required record-keeping practices. See Record-Keeping Practices of Psychologists–Psychotherapists, *Georgia Psychologist* (July 1989).

22. *See, e.g.,* Abille v. United States, 482 F. Supp. 703 (N.D. Cal. 1980); Donaldson v. O'Connory, 493 F.2d 507 (5th Cir. 1974), 422 U.S. 563 (1975); Whitree v. State, 290 N.Y.S.2d 486 (1968). *See also* Klein, *Legal Issues in the Private Practice of Psychiatry* (American Psychiatric Press, 1984), pp. 50–55.

23. O.C.G.A. § 37-3-1(2).

24. Ga. Comp. & R. Regs. r. 290-4-2-.05(6).

25. Ga. Comp. & R. Regs. r. 290-4-9-.05.

26. Ga. Comp. & R. Regs. r. 290-4-4-.01 *et seq.*

27. Ga. Comp. & R. Regs. r. 290-4-6-.05.

ments; medication records; treatment notes; a client treatment plan form; and a discharge summary.[28] Copies of the drug abuse treatment records may be required to be furnished to the director of the Division of Mental Health from time to time.[29]

Community mental health, mental retardation, and substance abuse programs are required to maintain a service record for each client that includes data pertaining to admission and "such other information as may be required under regulations and standards of the Department."[30] This reference to "other information" obliges community mental health centers to keep records at least in accordance with the definition of "clinical record," that is, all medical records, progress notes, charts, and admission and discharge data. Service records for alcohol and drug abuse clients must also be maintained in accordance with federal regulations.[31] Because clinical records play an essential role both in safeguarding the patient's well-being and in shielding the mental health care provider from liability, private facilities and MHPs should establish and adhere to a prudent record retention policy.[32]

It is important for MHPs to maintain a complete set of all patient records in the event a malpractice action is threatened or filed. There is an ultimate statute of limitations of 5 years for all medical malpractice actions.[33] However, a damages claim for alleged improper health care may be brought as an action for breach of contract. The statute of limitations for breach of a simple contract in writing is 6 years.[34] It would, therefore, be prudent for MHPs and health care facilities to maintain a complete set of patient records for at least 7 years after the last patient contact.

There are particularly stringent rules regulating the control of records in drug abuse treatment programs.[35] All materials must be kept in a secure area and stored in locked cabinets marked "Confidential Client Information." Charts are to be centrally filed and removed and returned to the locked file on a daily basis. No

---

28. Ga. Comp. & R. Regs. r. 290-4-2-.05(6).
29. Ga. Comp. & R. Regs. r. 290-4-2-.03(9).
30. Ga. Comp. & R. Regs. r. 290-4-9-.05(1).
31. Among the boards regulating physicians, psychologists, professional counselors, marriage and family therapists, and social workers, only the Psychology Board has a specific rule regarding maintenance of records. Psychologists must maintain the complete record for a minimum of 5 years. *See* Ga. Comp. R. & Regs. r. 510-5-.03(7)(b).
32. O.C.G.A. § 9-3-71. *Medical malpractice* is defined as any claim for damages arising out of the provision of health, medical, dental, or surgical services or services rendered by a hospital, nursing home, clinic, facility, or institution.
33. O.C.G.A. § 9-3-24. *See* Ballard v. Rappaport, 168 Ga. App. 671, 310 S.E.2d 4 (1983).
34. Ga. Comp. & R. Regs. r. 290-4-2-.05.
35. O.C.G.A. § 37-3-167(a) (mentally ill); O.C.G.A. § 37-4-126(a) (mentally retarded); and O.C.G.A. § 37-7-167(a) (substance abuser).

list of names may be posted in an area visible to outsiders. A client may not carry his file from one center to another: transport must be by mail, the alcohol and drug abuse services section delivery vehicle, or an authorized staff person. The weekly Management Information System (MIS) computer output is to be destroyed by shredding or incineration.

(C) Access by the Client

Under the Mental Health Code, every patient has the right to examine all medical records kept in his name by the department or facility in which he was hospitalized or treated.[36] In addition, the "patients' rights" provisions found in the rules and regulations of the Department of Human Resources also permit client access to mental health records in state-owned or state-operated hospitals or similar facilities and community mental health centers.[37] A patient's access to his own records may be limited only when "the disclosure to the patient is determined by the chief medical officer or the patient's treating physician to be detrimental to the physical or mental health of a patient" and a notation to that effect is placed in the patient's record.[38] A patient's right of access to his own records includes the right to request that any inaccurate information be corrected.[39]

(D) Access by Others

Under the Mental Health Code, the patient may consent to the disclosure of his records to third parties. These third parties include his attorney,[40] those present at a hearing,[41] or any other individual or entity designated by the patient.[42] The chief medical officer may deem the release of the records essential for continued treatment and may release them to other physicians without the patient's consent in state-owned or state-operated hospitals or similar facilities, but only with the patient's consent in the case of records maintained in community health centers.[43] Records may

---

36. Ga. Comp. & R. Regs. r. 290-4-6-.05(3); 290-4-9-.02(1)(c).
37. O.C.G.A. § 37-3-162(b) (mentally ill); O.C.G.A. § 37-4-122(c) (mentally retarded); and O.C.G.A. § 37-7-162(b) (substance abuser).
38. O.C.G.A. § 37-3-167(b); Ga. Comp. & R. Regs. r. 290-4-6.05(4).
39. Ga. Comp. & R. Regs. r. 290-4-6-.05(2)(a)5 and r. 290-4-9-.05(1)(f).
40. Ga. Comp. & R. Regs. r. 290-4-6-.05(2)(a)7 and r. 290-4-9-.05(1)(h).
41. Ga. Comp. & R. Regs. r. 290-4-6-.05(2)(a)2 and r. 290-4-9-.05(1)(c).
42. Ga. Comp. & R. Regs. r. 290-4-6-.05(2)(a)1 and r. 290-4-9-.05(1)(b).
43. Ga. Comp. & R. Regs. r. 290-4-6-.05(2)(a)3 and r. 290-4-9-.05(1)(d).

also be released to another admitting facility[44] and to any employee in a facility when necessary for proper treatment.[45] The records may also be released without consent in a bona fide medical emergency.[46] A law enforcement officer may be informed, in the course of a criminal investigation, whether a person is or has been a patient and the patient's current address.[47] The fact that information has been released under any of the foregoing situations does not relieve the MHP or the facility from the continuing obligations to maintain the confidentiality of the records as to other third parties.

An institution for the treatment of drug and alcohol abuse that receives federal financial assistance is restricted in the disclosure of patient records. Absent written patient consent, disclosure is permitted only in cases of medical emergency, for research or program evaluations, or by court order upon a showing of good cause.[48] In determining good cause, the court must weigh the public interest and the need for disclosure against the injury to the patient, to the MHP–patient relationship, and to the treatment services.[49] The Georgia courts have concluded that this "good cause" showing is satisfied as to nonprivileged portions of records if the patient has put his treatment in issue in a civil case. However, those portions of the records that contain privileged MHP–patient communications may not be disclosed (see chapter 3.3).[50]

---

44. Ga. Comp. & R. Regs. r. 290-4-6-.05(2)(a)4 and r. 290-4-9-.05(1)(e).
45. Ga. Comp. & R. Regs. r. 290-4-6-.05(2)(a)6 and r. 290-4-9-.05(1)(g).
46. Ga. Comp. & R. Regs. r. 290-4-6-.05(2)(a)9.
47. 42 U.S.C. §§ 290dd-3(b) and 290ee-3(b).
48. 42 U.S.C. §§ 290dd-3(b)(2)(C) and 290ee-3(b)(2)(C).
49. Aetna Casualty and Surety Co. v. Ridgeview Institute, 194 Ga. App. 805, 392 S.E.2d 286 (1990).
50. *Id.*

3.3

Confidential Relations and Communications

Under Georgia law, communications between a patient and an MHP are considered to be both confidential and, if with statutorily specified MHPs, privileged. Confidential and privileged are two distinct legal concepts. Confidential means that the communications occur in the context of the therapist–patient relationship and with an expectation that they will be kept secret. The MHP has a duty to maintain the secrecy of confidential communications. Breach of that duty may give rise to a damages action by the patient for invasion of privacy. It may also constitute an ethical violation.

Communications between a patient and statutorily specified MHPs are also deemed privileged. That is, neither the patient nor the MHP may be compelled to disclose the privileged communications except in certain narrow circumstances. However, the federal courts in Georgia do not recognize the MHP–patient privilege. In the absence of other statutes, such as a drug abuse confidentiality statute, an MHP can be compelled to testify in federal court to communications that are privileged under state law.[1]

The concepts of both confidential and privileged communications arise from the generally recognized understanding that effective treatment cannot occur unless the patient has assurances that what he says in the course of therapy will remain inviolate. However, the law permits disclosure of confidential and privi-

---

1. United States v. Corona, 849 F.2d 562 (11th Cir. 1988); Hancock v. Hobbs, No. 90-9067 (11th Cir. July 14, 1992). The U. S. Supreme Court is expected to rule on the applicability of the privilege in federal courts during the term that ends June 1996.

leged communication in certain limited circumstances when disclosure is required to protect countervailing interests.[2]

(A) Privilege for Psychologists

Georgia law provides the following privilege for communications between a patient and a licensed psychologist:

> The confidential relations and communications between a licensed psychologist and client are placed upon the same basis as those provided by law between attorney and client; and nothing in this chapter shall be construed to require any such privileged communication to be disclosed.[3]

The statute, by its terms, applies only to licensed psychologists and treats the communications the same as communications between an attorney and his client. The statutes governing the attorney–client privilege state:

> Communications to any attorney or to his employee to be transmitted to the attorney pending his employment or in anticipation thereof shall never be heard by the court. The attorney shall not disclose the advice or counsel he may give to his client, nor produce or deliver up title deeds or other papers, except evidences of debt left in his possession by his client. This Code section shall not exclude the attorney as a witness to any facts which may transpire in connection with his employment.[4]

> No attorney shall be competent or compellable to testify for or against his client to any matter or thing, the knowledge of which he may have acquired from his client by virtue of his employment as attorney or by reason of the anticipated employment of him as attorney. However, an attorney shall be both competent and compellable to testify for or against his client as to any matter or thing, the knowledge of which he may have acquired in any other manner.[5]

---

2. Ethical standards governing the behavior of psychologists, psychiatrists, professional counselors, social workers, and marriage and family therapists also require that communications between patient and therapist be kept confidential. *See* American Psychological Association (APA), *Ethical Principles of Psychologists*, Standard 5 (Rule 510-5-.07 of the Rules of the State Board of Examiners of Psychologists, 1982); APA, *General Guidelines for Providers of Psychological Services*, Guidelines 2.3.7 and 2.3.8 (1987); APA, *Specialty Guidelines for the Delivery of Services*, Guideline 2.3.5 (1981); American Psychiatric Association, *The Principles of Medical Ethics With Annotations Especially Applicable to Psychiatry*, Section 4 (1989); Rule 135-7-.03 of the Rules of the Composite Board of Professional Counselors, Social Workers, and Marriage and Family Therapists.
3. O.C.G.A. § 43-39-16. In 1995, the psychologist privilege was added to the Georgia evidence code along with privileges for psychiatrists and other MHPs. *See* O.C.G.A. § 24-9-21(b); Ga. Laws 1995, p. 858.
4. O.C.G.A. § 24-9-24.
5. O.C.G.A. § 24-9-25.

These statutes make clear that any information communicated by a client to a psychologist, or to the psychologist's employee for transmission to the psychologist, shall not be divulged. However, if the information comes from an outside source and not directly from the patient, it may not be privileged.

(B) Privilege for Psychiatrists

Georgia law provides that communications between a psychiatrist and his patient are privileged on the grounds of public policy.[6] The privilege is contained in the same code section that protects attorney–client communications. Thus, the scope of the psychologist–patient and psychiatrist–patient privileges are the same.

Georgia law does not contain a statutory definition of the term "psychiatrist," and there is no licensing designation for psychiatrists. The meaning of the term "psychiatrist" has, therefore, been left to the courts. In *Wiles v. Wiles*, the Georgia Supreme Court held that "the psychiatrist–patient privilege extends to a person authorized to practice medicine who devotes a substantial portion of his or her time in the diagnosis or treatment of a mental or emotional condition, including alcohol and drug addiction."[7] *Wiles* was a child custody dispute in which the husband sought the medical records of a patient of his wife, a licensed medical doctor. (The court did not address how the patient's records could possibly be relevant to a custody dispute between Mr. and Dr. Wiles as the issue was not raised on appeal.) Dr. Wiles testified that she treated one third of her patients for mental problems, that providing counseling was part of her practice, and that she had treated this particular patient for a mental condition. The court concluded that Dr. Wiles was a physician who spent a substantial portion of her time treating mental and emotional problems and that the privilege was applicable.

The court found that its definition was necessary to protect people who need psychiatric treatment, but live in areas of the state where there are no physicians with postgraduate training in psychiatry. The court also noted that its definition acknowledges the absence of a general physician–patient privilege by restricting the privilege to only those physicians who spend a significant time diagnosing and treating mental illness.

The broad scope of the psychiatrist–patient privilege is further demonstrated by the "physician shield" statute. This statute

6. O.C.G.A. § 24-9-21.
7. Wiles v. Wiles, 264 Ga. 594, 448 S.E.2d 681 (1994).

protects medical doctors from liability for releasing confidential information under court order or subpoena or pursuant to a waiver from the patient, but specifically does not apply to psychiatrists or to hospitals in which a patient has been treated solely for mental illness.[8] This is because under Georgia law, while communications between a medical doctor and patient are confidential, they are not privileged and may be disclosed as provided in the statute. However, communications between psychiatrist and patient are confidential and privileged. Thus, the exclusion of psychiatrists and hospitals treating mental illness in the "physician shield" statute demonstrates that disclosure of communications made to a psychiatrist or contained in the records of a mental health facility is prohibited.[9]

(C) Other Mental Health Professionals

Prior to July 1, 1995, communications to MHPs other than psychologists and psychiatrists were not privileged under Georgia law. Efforts to expand the privilege by court decisions were rebuffed. One case recognized that although communications to other MHPs should arguably be covered as a matter of public

---

8. The text of the physician shield statute is as follows: "[n]o physician licensed under Chapter 34 of Title 43 and no hospital or health care facility, including those operated by an agency or bureau of the state or other governmental unit, shall be required to release any medical information concerning a patient except to the Department of Human Resources, its divisions, agents, or successors when required in the administration of public health programs pursuant to Code Section 31-12-2 and where authorized or required by law, statute, or lawful regulation; or on written authorization or other waiver by the patient, or by his or her parents or duly appointed guardian ad litem in the case of a minor, or on appropriate court order or subpoena; provided, however, that any physician, hospital, or health care facility releasing information under written authorization or other waiver by the patient, or by his or her parents or guardian ad litem in the case of a minor, or pursuant to law, statute, or lawful regulation, or under court order or subpoena shall be liable to the patient or any other person; provided, further, that the privilege shall be waived to the extent that the patient places his care and treatment or the nature and extent of his injuries at issue in any civil or criminal proceeding. This code section shall not apply to psychiatrists or to hospitals in which the patient is being or has been treated solely for mental illness." O.C.G.A. § 24-9-40.

9. Although the psychologist–patient and psychiatrist–patient privileges are coextensive, the physician shield statute exempts only psychiatrists. In Jarallah v. Schwartz, 413 S.E.2d 210 (Ga. App. 1991), the Court of Appeals *in dicta* suggested that psychologists were included in the statutory coverage. This conclusion was unnecessary to the decision, as it was clear that the communications were not privileged since treatment was neither given nor contemplated.

policy, the courts should not expand the scope of the privilege in the absence of specific legislation to that effect.[10]

At its 1995 session, the General Assembly passed legislation extending the privilege to communications between patient and licensed clinical social workers, clinical nurse specialists in psychiatric/mental health care, licensed marriage and family therapists, and licensed professional counselors during the "psychotherapeutic relationship."[11] The term "psychotherapeutic relationship" is defined as the relationship that arises between a patient and the specified MHP using "psychotherapeutic techniques."[12] Although seemingly circular, the language was intended to limit the privilege to communications that are made in the context of psychotherapy. To that extent, the scope of the privilege is probably somewhat narrower than the psychologist/psychiatrist–patient privilege.

In addition, the evidence code was amended at the same time to protect communications between MHPs regarding a patient's privileged communications.[13] This amendment was designed to overrule cases in which the court had held that the privilege did not extend to communications made to a nurse unless the nurse was the agent of the attending psychiatrist.[14] The amendment is designed to protect communications among specified members of the treatment team regarding a plaintiff's privileged communications. As of July 1, 1995, the following are privileged:

> Communications between or among any psychiatrist, psychologist, licensed clinical social worker, clinical nurse specialist in psychiatric/mental health, licensed marriage and family therapist, and licensed professional counselor who are rendering psychotherapy or have rendered psychotherapy to a patient, regarding that patient's communications which are otherwise privileged. . . .[15]

The 1995 amendments also add the psychologist–patient privilege to the evidence code, in addition to its existing location in the Psychology Practice Act.[16] Thus, all MHP–patient privi-

---

10. Lipsey v. State, 170 Ga. App. 770, 318 S.E.2d 184 (1984) (no privilege for communications to intake counselor or behavior specialist). See also White v. State, 180 Ga. App. 185, 348 S.E.2d 728 (1986). The privilege did not extend to nurses or attendants unless they were the agents of the attending psychologist; Annandale at Suwanee v. Weatherly, 194 Ga. App. 803, 503 S.E.2d 27 (1990).
11. O.C.G.A. § 24-9-21(7); Ga. Laws 1995, p. 858.
12. O.C.G.A. § 24-9-21.
13. O.C.G.A. § 24-9-21(8).
14. Meyers v. State, 251 Ga. 883, 310 S.E.2d 504 (1984), in which the nurse was held to be an agent of the hospital, not of the psychiatrist; therefore, statements made to her were not privileged. See also Weksler v. Weksler, 173 Ga. App. 250, 325 S.E.2d 874 (1985).
15. O.C.G.A. § 24-9-21(8).
16. O.C.G.A. § 24-9-21(6).

leges are now listed in one Code section.

(D) Basis for the Privilege

The rationale behind the protection accorded communications between patient and MHP is that "most psychiatric analysis and treatment must come from the mind of the patient whereas much information useful to a physician in treating a patient comes from empirical data."[17] To ensure proper treatment, the MHP must obtain all necessary information from the patient. Patients would necessarily be reluctant to disclose their private thoughts and secrets if such information would be disclosed by their therapist. Because the privilege is designed to foster the MHP–patient relationship, it applies only if treatment is given or contemplated. Therefore, if an individual sees an MHP for purposes of obtaining testimony in a court proceeding, or if the visit is pursuant to a court-ordered evaluation, no privilege attaches because the patient is not seeking treatment and no treatment is given or contemplated.[18]

In addition, psychiatrists and psychologists are specifically permitted to give evidence, including evidence as to communications that would normally be privileged, at hearings held under the Mental Health Code for involuntary hospitalization or involuntary outpatient treatment.[19]

(E) Hospitals and Other Mental Health Facilities

As noted earlier, hospitals in which patients are being or have been treated solely for mental illness are specifically excluded from the physician shield statute. Even if such facilities release confidential information pursuant to a subpoena or notice to produce, they may still be held liable. This is because records main-

---

17. Gilmore v. State, 175 Ga. App. 376, 333 S.E.2d 210, 211 (1985).
18. Fullbright v. State, 194 Ga. App. 827, 392 S.E.2d 298 (1990); *In re*: R.M.C.C. and I.M., 194 Ga. App. 888, 392 S.E.2d 13 (1990); Rachals v. State, 184 Ga. App. 420, 361 S.E.2d 671 (1987), *aff'd*, 258 Ga. 48, 364 S.E.2d 867 (1988); Massey v. State, 226 Ga. 703, 177 S.E.2d 79 (1970); Payne v. Sherrer, 458 S.E.2d (1995) (employer-mandated evaluation).
19. "In connection with any hearing held under this chapter, any physician, including any psychiatrist, who is treating or who has treated the patient shall be authorized to give evidence as to any matter concerning the patient, including evidence as to communications otherwise privileged under Code Section 24-9-40." O.C.G.A. § 37-3-166(b), 1974 Op. Att'y Gen. 474–486.

tained by a mental hospital frequently contain privileged communications, whereas records maintained by a general hospital do not. Mental health records should be released only pursuant to valid consent or court order. In addition, the statute refers only to hospitals, and no case has decided whether it applies to other mental health facilities such as clinics. One case has held that a private psychiatric hospital, Ridgeview Institute, was authorized, but not required, to release mental health records because the patient's estate had consented.[20]

(F) Assertion and Waiver of the Privilege

Before the privilege will attach to communications, the court must be convinced that the requisite relationship between the patient and the MHP exists.[21] The person asserting the privilege must first establish that the communications were, in fact, made to a licensed MHP or to an agent of the MHP while treating the patient,[22] or to members of the treatment team specified in O.C.G.A. section 24-9-21(8). This can be done by producing a certificate of licensure or through testimony.

Second, the existence of the MHP–patient relationship must be established. Under Georgia law, the relationship is created when an individual seeks mental health care and receives treatment. Merely having a conversation with an MHP does not create the relationship.[23] Seeking out the assistance of a psychologist/hypnotist to have one's memory of an event "improved" through age regression does not constitute the type of relationship that gives rise to the privilege, as treatment is not the primary focus of the relationship.[24]

---

20. Ridgeview Institute, Inc. v. Brunson, 191 Ga. App. 608, 382 S.E.2d 409 (1989).
21. Donalson v. State, 192 Ga. App. 37, 383 S.E.2d 588 (1989), in which defendant argued that use of a subpoena *duces tecum* to secure medical records regarding his hospitalization for psychiatric treatment was improper, but defendant failed to establish that the information "originated as communications from appellant to an attending psychiatrist or his agent," *quoting* Johnson v. State, 254 Ga. 591, 597, 331 S.E.2d 578 (1985).
22. White v. State, 180 Ga. App. 185, 348 S.E.2d 728 (1986).
23. Rachals v. State, 184 Ga. App. 420, 361 S.E.2d 671 (1987), *aff'd*, 258 Ga. 48, 364 S.E.2d 867 (1988), *cert. denied*, 108 S.Ct. 2909 (nurse convicted of aggravated assault of patient, who threatened to commit suicide on night of arrest and voluntarily agreed to be admitted into psychiatric ward for one night to avoid going to jail, but who received no real treatment, could not assert privilege).
24. Emmett v. Ricketts, 397 F. Supp. 1025 (N.D. Ga. 1975).

If an individual is required to undergo an evaluation, the communications are not protected.[25] For example, if a court appoints a psychiatrist or psychologist to conduct a court-ordered evaluation of a criminal defendant, no treatment is contemplated and no psychiatrist/psychologist–patient relationship exists. The communications are, therefore, not privileged.[26] In fact, a court-appointed psychiatrist was permitted to testify concerning statements made by the defendant describing his participation in a murder in which the statements were relied on by the psychiatrist to formulate his opinions that the defendant was sane at the time of the crime. In addition, a defendant who raises a defense of insanity in a criminal trial and who seeks to present expert testimony on the issue is deemed to have waived the privilege.[27]

A patient may waive the privilege in a number of ways. Waiver may occur if a third party is present who is not an agent of the MHP to whom the privilege extends. There is no waiver of the privilege, however, when persons consult an MHP jointly and the presence of both is "necessary and customary." Thus, if a husband and wife attend joint counseling sessions, one spouse may not waive the privilege for the other spouse.[28]

No waiver of the MHP–patient privilege occurs when a patient places his mental state in issue, for example, by claiming damages for mental pain and suffering in a civil lawsuit.[29] If a patient sues his MHP for alleged malpractice, however, the privilege is waived to the extent disclosure is necessary to defend the case.

In the criminal context, a defendant's right to confront and cross-examine the witness against him may result in the loss of the privilege claimed by the witness. Before abrogating the privilege, the defendant must establish that the information sought is

25. Bobo v. State, 256 Ga. 357, 349 S.E.2d 690 (1986), *citing* Kimble v. Kimble, 240 Ga. 100, 101, 239 S.E.2d 676 (1977).
26. Plummer v. State, 229 Ga. 749, 194 S.E.2d 419 (1972); Massey v. State, 226 Ga. 703, 177 S.E.2d 79, *cert. denied*, 401 U.S. 964 (1970). *See* chapters 7.5 and 7.9, this volume *infra*.
27. Harris v. State, 256 Ga. 350, 349 S.E.2d 374 (even though defendant waived the psychologist–patient privilege by using an insanity defense, the court must consider whether the use of statements made to a psychologist admitting the commission of a murder violates the privilege against self-incrimination). *Cf.* Isley v. Dugger, 877 F.2d 47 (11th Cir. 1989) (psychiatrists permitted to repeat defendant's statements because they formed the basis for opinion on insanity). *Also see* Bright v. State, 455 S.E.2d 37 (1995).
28. Sims v. State, 251 Ga. 877, 311 S.E.2d 161 (1984). *Also see* Mrozinski v. Pogue, 205 Ga. App. 731, 423 S.E.2d 405, 408 (1992).
29. Wilson v. Bonner, 166 Ga. App. 9, 303 S.E.2d 134 (1983); *see also* Aetna Casualty and Surety Co. v. Ridgeview Institute, 194 Ga. App. 805, 392 S.E.2d 286 (1990); Plunkett v. Ginsburg, 465 S.E.2d 595 (1995).

"critical to his defense and that substantially similar evidence is otherwise unavailable."[30]

The privilege survives the death of the communicant, so even if the patient has died, the MHP should assert the privilege on behalf of his client and maintain the confidentiality of the communuications.[31]

(G) Limitations on the Scope of the Privilege

Not every communication between patient and MHP is protected. The mere fact that one has consulted an MHP or has sought admission to a psychiatric hospital is not privileged nor are the dates of treatment.[32]

Another limitation on the scope of both the privilege and confidential communications is the requirement that MHPs report child abuse. Georgia law[33] requires that health professionals, including licensed psychologists, physicians, nurses, professional counselors, social workers, and marriage and family therapists report child abuse. An unlicensed psychologist or other professional not listed in the statute cannot be held criminally responsible for failing to report child abuse.[34]

Georgia law permits a physician who learns that a patient is infected with human immunodeficiency virus (HIV, the AIDS virus) and who reasonably believes that the spouse, sexual partner, or child of the patient is at risk of being infected with HIV by that patient to reveal to the spouse, sexual partner, or child that the patient is infected after notifying the patient that the disclosure is going to be made.[35]

Furthermore, health care providers, the definition of which includes psychologists, professional counselors, social workers, and marriage and family therapists,[36] may disclose AIDS confidential information to other health care providers or health care facilities that have provided, are providing, or will provide treatment to a patient infected with HIV if the disclosure is reasonably necessary to protect personnel or other patients or if the facility

---

30. Bobo v. State, 256 Ga. 357, 349 S.E.2d 690 (1986).
31. Sims v. State, *supra* note 28 at 165.
32. National Stop Smoking Clinic–Atlanta, Inc. v. Dean et al., 190 Ga. App. 289, 378 S.E.2d 901 (1989); Johnson v. State, 254 Ga. App. 591, 331 S.E.2d 578 (1985); Cranford v. Cranford, 120 Ga. App. 470, 170 S.E.2d 844 (1969).
33. O.C.G.A. § 19-7-5.
34. Gladson v. State, 258 Ga. 885, 376 S.E.2d 362 (1989).
35. O.C.G.A. § 24-9-47(g).
36. O.C.G.A. § 31-22-9.1(g).

has a legitimate need for the information.[37] The Department of Human Resources has the authority to determine whether mandatory, nonanonymous reporting of positive HIV tests is reasonably necessary and to require health care providers to report this information to the Department of Human Resources.[38] The department has not yet made such a determination.

The duty to warn a third party of possible harm from a patient may also outweigh the privileged and confidential nature of communications between patient and therapist. In *Bradley Center, Inc. v. Wessner,*[39] the Supreme Court of Georgia found that because of the special relationship between the mental health facility and the patient, the Bradley Center was under a duty to exercise reasonable care to control the patient to prevent him from doing bodily harm to a third person.[40] Although the *Bradley Center* case actually involves the duty to control a potentially dangerous patient as opposed to the duty to warn, the legal theory used by the court could also be used to establish a duty to warn. This is because the court held that a duty to prevent harm to others may arise from the special nature of the therapist–patient relationship.

In *Jacobs v. Taylor*, the Georgia Court of Appeals declined "to impose a blanket liability on ... doctors for failing to warn members of the general public ... of the risk posed by ... a patient with a history of violence who made generalized threats."[41] The court further found that there was no duty to warn when the victim had knowledge of the patient's violent tendencies. Although it did not directly address the question of whether there is a duty to warn, the court impliedly recognized the obligation under Georgia law. Thus, if a reasonably prudent MHP believes that a patient presents a risk of imminent harm to identifiable third parties, the privilege will be overcome by the obligation to warn of the patient's potential risk of violence.

(H) Liability for Violation

There is no criminal liability for violating the MHP–patient privilege or for disclosing confidential information, only civil liabil-

---

37. O.C.G.A. § 24-9-47(i).
38. O.C.G.A. § 24-9-47(2).
39. 287 S.E.2d 716, *aff'd*, 250 Ga. 199, 296 S.E.2d 693 (1982). *Also see* Ermutlu v. McCorkle, 416 S.E.2d 792 (Ga. App. 1992).
40. Bradley Center, Inc. v. Wessner, 296 S.E.2d at 696, *citing* Restatement (Second) of Torts, Section 319.
41. Jacobs et al. v. Taylor et al., 190 Ga. App. 520, 379 S.E.2d 563 (1989); *cf.* Swofford v. Cooper, 184 Ga. App. 50, 360 S.E.2d 624, *aff'd*, 258 Ga. 143, 368 S.E.2d 518 (1988).

ity.[42] The civil liability flowing from the wrongful disclosure of privileged information is generally framed in terms of the tort of invasion of privacy.[43] However, there is no liability when the MHP is acting out of a countervailing duty imposed by law, such as the duty to warn. In those instances, the law classifies the communication to third parties as *legally privileged*, that is, not subject to an action for defamation or invasion of privacy.

For example, one unreported decision permitted a psychiatrist to reveal to the supervisor of a nurse whom he was treating that the nurse had psychiatric problems that could adversely affect the welfare of her patients.[44] Because the psychiatrist was acting out of a "legal or moral private duty"[45] and without malice, his communications were deemed to be privileged and, therefore, not tortious. In addition to civil liability, psychologists, professional counselors, social workers, and marriage and family therapists are subject to license revocation for revealing client confidences in violation of licensing board rules.[46] Psychiatrists are also subject to admonishment, reprimand, suspension, or expulsion from the American Psychiatric Association for breach of the ethical duty to maintain confidentiality.[47]

---

42. Cranford v. Cranford, 170 S.E.2d at 848.
43. Mrozinski v. Pogue, 205 Ga. App. 731, 423 S.E.2d 405 (1992).
44. Baawo et al. v. Thorneloe (Ga. Ct. of Appeals No. 74206, April 16, 1987).
45. O.C.G.A. § 51-5-7.
46. Ga. Comp. R. & Regs. r. 510-5 of the Rules of State Board of Examiners of Psychology; O.C.G.A. § 43-39-13; Ga. Comp. R. & Regs. r. 135-7 of the Rules of the Composite Board of Professional Counselors, and so on.
47. American Psychiatric Association, *The Principles of Medical Ethics With Annotations Especially Applicable to Psychiatry*, Section 4 (1989).

3.4

Privileged Communications

For specific professionals, Georgia law handles confidential communications and privileged communications together (see chapter 3.3).

3.5

Search, Seizure, Subpoena, and Production of Records

A warrant for the search and seizure of evidence and a subpoena for testimony or the production of documents or tangible things are two ways in which a court might require information from an MHP. In addition, under the Georgia Civil Practice Act, any party to a lawsuit can serve a request for the production of documents, including mental health records. Search and seizure occurs in the context of a criminal investigation in which a court has probable cause to believe that evidence of criminal activity can be found in a certain location. A subpoena may be issued in the course of either a criminal or civil proceeding. In addition to requiring the appearance of an MHP in court, a civil subpoena may also command the MHP to appear for the taking of a deposition. A deposition is the taking of testimony under oath before a court reporter and occurs outside the courtroom, generally without judicial supervision. A subpoena may also require the production of records either in court or at a deposition.

(A) Search and Seizure

Various constitutional protections[1] prevent the government from searching and seizing things in which individuals have a reasonable expectation of privacy. Searches may occur with or without a warrant. Searches without a warrant are generally limited to emergency situations incident to an arrest, such as seizing the fruits of a crime, or searching for weapons to ensure the officer's

---

1. U.S. Const. amend. IV; Ga. Const., art. 1, § 1, par. 13.

safety.[2] Warrantless searches are unlikely to be an issue for MHPs.

Warrants are typically issued by magistrates and permit a law enforcement officer to search a specific place for specific items, generally evidence of a crime.[3] There are statutes governing the execution of the search warrant,[4] the scope of the search warrant,[5] and the personnel authorized to execute the search warrant.[6] The officer is required to make a written list of all items seized by filing an inventory with the judicial officer named in the warrant. If requested, the judicial officer shall furnish a copy of the inventory of seized items to the person from whom the items were seized.[7]

(B) Subpoena for the Production of Records

In civil cases, there are two methods by which parties may seek to compel the pretrial disclosure of mental health records: by subpoena for the taking of a deposition or by the service of a request for production of documents.[8] A subpoena is legal process issued by the clerk of the court upon the request of a party. Subpoenas are generally issued in blank and filled out by the party or the party's attorney. Subpoenas can compel a witness's attendance at a deposition and can also direct the individual to produce for inspection and copying documents, including mental health records. A subpoena may be served by any person over the age of 18 or by registered or certified mail. In order to compel the appearance of a witness who resides out of the county where the testimony is to be given, the subpoena must be accompanied by a $10 witness fee and mileage at the rate of 20 cents per mile for travel expenses for going from and returning to the witness's place of residence. As to deposition subpoenas, a person can be compelled to attend a deposition only in the county in which the individual resides, is employed, or transacts business; in the county in which he is served with the subpoena; or in any place that is not more than 30 miles from the county seat in which the person resides, is employed, or transacts business.

---

2. O.C.G.A. § 17-5-1.
3. O.C.G.A. § 17-5-21.
4. O.C.G.A. § 17-5-25.
5. O.C.G.A. § 17-5-23.
6. O.C.G.A. § 17-5-24.
7. O.C.G.A. § 17-5-29.
8. In the federal courts, a notice to produce is not available against a nonparty to the proceedings.

An MHP who receives a subpoena should immediately notify the patient or the patient's attorney. If the patient executes a written authorization for release of the information, the MHP may produce the records. If the MHP is unable to obtain the patient's express authorization, then the MHP should, within 10 days after the service of the subpoena or on or before the time specified in the subpoena for compliance if such time is less than 10 days after service, deliver to the attorney designated in the subpoena a written objection to inspection or copying of the records.[9] MHPs who are covered by the privilege provisions of the evidence code should assert the MHP–patient privilege. Other MHPs should assert the confidentiality of the records (see chapter 3.3). Once objection is made, the party serving the subpoena is not entitled to inspect and copy the materials except pursuant to an order of the court.

(C) Request for Production of Documents

An alternative method by which parties to civil litigation may obtain mental health records in Georgia courts is by serving a request for production of documents, sometimes called a notice to produce, on the MHP. The request is issued without court approval and directs the MHP to produce for inspection and copying all or part of the record. The request is supposed to be served upon all parties of record in the case. Although the patient will generally be a party to the case, it is possible that the patient may not be a party and, therefore, may not have notice of the request. The applicable code section provides that the MHP or any party may file an objection with the court to the furnishing of the requested materials. If no objection is filed within 10 days of the request, the MHP must then decide whether to comply with the request.

The disclosure by psychiatrists of otherwise privileged information pursuant to requests for production of documents has resulted in a number of lawsuits. Most recently, the Georgia Court of Appeals decided the case of *Jones v. Able*,[10] in which Dr. Able, a psychiatrist, was served with a request for production of documents. On the 15th day after receipt of the request, Dr. Able, having received no response from the patient, forwarded a sub-

---

9. In federal courts, the time period is 14 days. The rules regarding fees and geographic enforceability are also different.
10. 434 S.E.2d 822 (1993).

stantial portion of the medical record, including notes of his conferences with the patient, to the attorney for an individual who was suing the patient. The patient later filed an objection to the production, believing that he had 30 days in which to object. In fact, his objection was untimely because an objection must be filed within 10 days of a request directed to a health care practitioner, whereas in all other cases, there are 30 days in which to object. The patient then sued Dr. Able for disclosure of privileged materials.

At trial, Dr. Davis, another psychiatrist, testified that it was the standard of care in the psychiatric profession to wait 13 days after receipt of the request and, if no objection was received from the patient, to forward the records to the requesting attorney. The jury returned a verdict in favor of Dr. Able. The Court of Appeals affirmed, finding that Dr. Able had not violated the standard of care on the basis of Dr. Davis's testimony that the standard of care required production of the records notwithstanding their privileged nature because no objection had been filed by the patient. Three judges of the Court of Appeals vigorously dissented, concluding that there had been no waiver of the privilege and that the psychiatrist was obligated to assert the privilege on the patient's behalf by objecting to the request for production of documents. The *Jones v. Able* decision is potentially at odds with other Georgia cases that have narrowly construed waivers of the privilege.[11]

Another case involving a request for production of documents is *Jones v. Thornton*,[12] in which a nonparty physician received a request to produce the medical records of one of his patients. The very next day the physician mailed copies of the records to the requesting attorney. The patient sued the physician for invasion of privacy and libel on the basis of his compliance with the discovery request. The court ruled that on the particular facts presented, the physician was not liable for invasion of privacy because of the failure of the patient's lawyer to object. However, the court cautioned that the physician placed himself at risk by complying immediately and thereby denying the patient the opportunity to object to the request and obtain a court ruling.

Given the current confusion in the law as to an MHP's obligations, it would be prudent for an MHP who receives a request for production of documents and who does not have the patient's written authorization to file with the court an objection to producing the records on the basis of either privilege, if applicable, or confidentiality. Although the code section is not explicit as to the time in which the MHP, as opposed to the patient, must

---

11. *See, for example,* Mrozinski v. Pogue, 205 Ga. App. 731, 423 S.E.2d 405 (1992).
12. 172 Ga. App. 412, 323 S.E.2d 217 (1984).

file the objection, it would be prudent to do so within 10 days of the request. The objection need only set forth the caption of the case and a statement that the MHP is asserting privilege or confidentiality, as the case may be, on behalf of the patient. The issue will then be decided by the court.

(D) Subpoenas for Appearance in Court

An MHP may be subpoenaed to appear in court and to testify and to produce the patient's record. The subpoena may direct the MHP's attendance at a civil or criminal proceeding or before a grand jury. The subpoena may be served by any person over the age of 18 years or by registered or certified mail. A subpoena may compel an MHP's attendance anywhere in the state of Georgia, but to be effective outside the county of the witness's residence or place of business, it must be accompanied by the witness fee for one day's attendance and appropriate mileage.[13]

If the MHP obtains the client's written authorization, then the MHP may produce the records and testify. However, if no written authorization is obtained, then the MHP must assert privilege and confidentiality on the patient's behalf. This may be done by retaining counsel who can file a motion to quash the subpoena and possibly obtain a ruling prior to the date of the MHP's appearance. Otherwise, the MHP should advise the attorney requesting the information that the MHP will be required to assert privilege or confidentiality and should request that the attorney release the MHP from the subpoena. If the MHP does not obtain a written confirmation of release from the subpoena from the party who issued it, the MHP should not disclose any of the records nor testify as to any privileged communications, except by direction of the court. If called as a witness, the MHP should explain the circumstances, assert the privilege, and await the court's ruling.[14] If the court orders the MHP to testify or to produce the records, then the MHP should do so.

---

13. Criminal defendants and state agencies are not required to tender witness fees; see O.C.G.A. § 24-10-24.
14. For example, in Freeman v. State, 196 Ga. App. 343, 396 S.E.2d 69 (1990), the court refused to permit the witness's psychologist to testify without a written waiver or oral testimony under oath that the patient waived the privilege.

3.6

Georgia Freedom of Information Act (Georgia Open Records Act)

Georgia law permits inspection of public records by any citizen who makes a request.[1] Specifically exempted from public disclosure are medical records, "the disclosure of which would be an invasion of personal privacy."[2] Furthermore, the definition of *clinical record* set out in the Mental Health Code states that the clinical records "shall not be a public record." Thus, clinical records maintained pursuant to the Mental Health Code are not subject to inspection under the Open Records Act.[3]

---

1. O.C.G.A. § 50-18-70.
2. O.C.G.A. § 50-18-72.
3. O.C.G.A. § 37-3-166(a); Southeastern Legal Foundation, Inc. v. Ledbetter, 400 S.E.2d 630 (1991).

Right to Refuse Treatment

Georgia statutorily recognizes the right of an adult over 18 years of age to refuse to consent to medical treatment.[1] The Georgia Supreme Court has also held that the constitutional right of privacy prevents the state from forcing medical treatment and food on a mentally competent prisoner.[2] The right to refuse treatment does not, however, act as a bar to the involuntary commitment of mentally ill persons (see chapters 4.19 and 8.4). A patient in a mental health facility has certain limited rights to refuse medication and object to treatment, although a physician, with the concurrence of a second physician, may overrule the patient's objections.[3] With limited exceptions, minors, even those who may be mature enough to make their own decisions, do not have the right to refuse treatment.[4]

(A) Georgia Living Will

Georgia law provides for the execution of a living will that authorizes the withdrawal of life-sustaining procedures in the event of terminal illness or imminent death.[5] The living will is similar to a durable health care power of attorney and is applicable in the event that the declarant does not have a health care power of attorney or the named agent under the health care

---

1. O.C.G.A. § 31-9-7; Kirby v. Spivey, 167 Ga. App. 751, 307 S.E.2d 538 (1983).
2. Zant v. Prevatte, 248 Ga. 832, 286 S.E.2d 715 (1982).
3. O.C.G.A. § 37-3-163.
4. Novak v. Cobb County Kennestone Hospital Authority, 849 F. Supp. 1559 (N.D. Ga. 1994).
5. O.C.G.A. § 31-32-1.

power of attorney fails to or is unable to make the health care decision on the declarant's behalf. In fact, Georgia law provides that a living will is inoperative as long as a health care agent is available and is authorized under the health care power of attorney to deal with the subject of life-sustaining or death-delaying procedures on the declarant's behalf.[6]

As with the health care power of attorney, there are moral, ethical, and legal implications to the signing of the living will, including the declarant's designation as to whether to have certain life-sustaining procedures withdrawn or withheld. The person executing the living will must specify, within the document itself, exactly what procedures should be withheld or withdrawn. For example, the declarant must specifically choose whether nourishment and/or hydration will be withheld.

The living will must be signed by the declarant in the presence of two witnesses. If the declarant signs the living will while in a hospital or skilled nursing facility, the declarant's signature must be witnessed by a staff member, physician, or hospital designee not participating in the care of the patient.[7]

A living will executed on or after March 28, 1986 is effective until revoked; a living will signed prior to that date is effective for a period of 7 years unless the termination clause is stricken from the document and initialed by the declarant.[8]

(B) Durable Health Care Power of Attorney

Another means provided by law for the refusal of medical treatment is that of a durable health care power of attorney.[9] This power of attorney can give broad and comprehensive authority to a designated person (the attorney-in-fact) to make decisions for the principal concerning the principal's personal care, medical treatment, hospitalization, and health care, including the withholding or withdrawal of any life-sustaining or death-delaying treatment (including termination of nourishment and hydration). The power of attorney gives the attorney-in-fact access to the principal's medical records and the right to disclose the contents to others.[10] The attorney-in-fact also has full power to make a disposition of any part or all of the principal's body for medical

---

6. O.C.G.A. § 31-36-11.
7. O.C.G.A. § 31-36-3.
8. O.C.G.A. § 31-32-6.
9. O.C.G.A. § 31-36-1 *et seq.*
10. O.C.G.A. § 31-36-5.

purposes, authorize an autopsy of the body, and direct the disposition of the principal's remains.[11] The health care power of attorney applies exclusively to a principal's health care and does not provide any powers over non–health care matters, such as bank accounts and personal assets. The principal may revoke a signed health care power of attorney at any time.

The principal is allowed to specify within the power of attorney itself exactly the types of health care treatment that the agent may or may not control. The durable power of attorney describes the circumstances under which health care treatment may be withheld or withdrawn.

The principal is required to designate the date or event on which the power of attorney becomes legally effective. The principal can designate, for example, that the power of attorney becomes effective only when the principal is determined by a court to be disabled or incapacitated. If a specific date or event is not provided, the power of attorney becomes effective immediately upon the signature of the principal with regard to all powers specified in the documents, even though the principal may be in perfect mental and physical health at the time of the signing.

The principal also designates in the power of attorney when, if ever, the document terminates. If the principal fails to set forth the termination date, the document is effective indefinitely or until it is revoked.

(C) Mental Health Facilities

Patients in mental health facilities, whether voluntarily or involuntarily, are afforded the protections of the Georgia medical consent law,[12] with two exceptions. First, a patient may refuse medication except in emergency cases in which a physician determines that refusal would be unsafe to the patient or to others. If the patient continues to refuse medication after the initial emergency treatment, then medication may be continued if a second physician concurs.[13]

Second, if immediate surgical or other intervention is necessary to prevent serious physical harm or death and delay in obtaining consent would create a grave risk of harm, then, on the authorization of two physicians, essential surgery or treatment may be administered without obtaining consent. This provision is expressly limited to the situation of an individual who cannot

---

11. O.C.G.A. § 31-36-4.
12. O.C.G.A. § 37-3-163(d); O.C.G.A. § 31-9-4. *See* chapter 3.1, this volume *infra*.
13. O.C.G.A. § 37-3-163(b).

understand the consequences of withholding consent because of advanced age, impaired thinking, or other disability.[14] A patient who objects to the administering of a treatment has the right to seek a protective order from the court.[15]

14. O.C.G.A. § 37-3-163(e).
15. O.C.G.A. § 37-3-163(c).

3.8

Regulation of Aversive and Avoidance Conditioning

There is no specific statute that regulates the use of behavioral therapies using aversive stimuli. Although the law does not prohibit the use of aversive stimuli, MHPs who use these methods should be aware of the possibility of certain common law and ethical restraints on the use of such treatment methods (and of the statutory requirement that a mental health patient's "dignity as an individual" be respected at all times).[1] In particular, aversive therapies should be not experimental and generally recognized. Proper informed consent must also be obtained.

Georgia law provides by statute that a patient's dignity as an individual is to be respected at all times, including any occasions during which he or she is taken into custody, detained, or transported. There is to be no distinction between medical patients and mental health patients or those suspected of being mentally ill. Except when required under the most extraordinary cases of extreme urgency, procedures, facilities, and restraining devices normally used for criminals or persons accused of a crime are not to be used in connection with the mentally ill.[2]

The law further mandates that each patient receiving services for mental illness shall receive care and treatment that is suited to the person's needs and is the least restrictive appropriate care and treatment. Any treatment is to be administered skillfully, humanely, and with respect for the patient's dignity and personal integrity. Patients have the right to participate in their care and treatment, and they shall have reasonable access to their medical files unless disclosure would be harmful, in which event a

---

1. O.C.G.A. § 37-3-160.
2. *Id.*

notation to that effect must be made a part of the medical record. Patients have the right to be told the diagnosis and treatment recommendation and to be fully informed as to medication being prescribed, including its side effects, and available treatment alternatives.

All treatments administered to patients must be suitable for their condition and must conform to recognized standards of psychiatric treatment. No nonstandard treatments may be administered without the written consent of the patient or guardian. If consent is given by someone other than the patient or guardian, court approval must be obtained.

To the extent that aversive therapies require the use of physical restraints, they may not be used in mental health facilities. Physical restraints may be used only when absolutely necessary to prevent patients from injuring themselves or others. Restraints may not be used for treatment purposes.[3]

---

3. O.C.G.A. §§ 37-3-165(b) and 37-4-124(b).

Quality Assurance for Hospital Care

Under Georgia law, a medical review committee may be formed in health care facilities "to evaluate and improve the quality of health care rendered by providers of health services or to determine that health services rendered were professionally indicated or were performed in compliance with the applicable standard of care."[1] The medical review committee may also inquire into the cost of the services rendered to assess whether they are reasonable under the standards that exist for health care professionals in the area. The committee may consist of members of a state or local professional authority, or of a medical staff of a licensed hospital, nursing home, or medical foundation, provided that the medical staff operates pursuant to written bylaws that have been approved by the governing board of the hospital or nursing home.

Georgia law provides that there will be no monetary liability on the part of, and no cause of action for damages against, any member of the duly appointed medical review committee for any act or undertaking within the scope of the functions of such committee, unless there is malice or fraud.[2] Such immunity, of course, does not bar a tort or contract claim brought by patients or their successors or assigns against the treating health care professional.[3] Additionally, committee proceedings and records are immune from discovery and may not be used as evidence in any legal proceedings. Proceedings conducted and records generated in connection with such reviews are deemed to be confidential. However, information, documents, or records otherwise avail-

---

1. O.C.G.A. § 31-7-140.
2. O.C.G.A. § 31-7-141.
3. O.C.G.A. § 31-7-142.

able from original sources are subject to discovery and may be used in any civil action, notwithstanding the fact that they were presented during the proceedings of such committee.[4] Furthermore, a witness who testifies at a committee proceeding will not be prevented from testifying at trial about the same matters, but may not be questioned about any appearance before the committee or any testimony presented there. The Georgia Supreme Court has held that the statute forbidding discovery of information produced in a committee review applies to any cause of action brought against the committee, including allegations of fraud and conspiracy.[5]

Georgia law also provides for the review of the quality of a health care professional's services by a group of his or her professional peers.[6] The proceedings of the peer review committee are also confidential, and members of the committee are protected from liability for their good faith actions.[7]

4. Cobb County Kennestone Hospital v. Martin, 208 Ga. App. 326 (1993).
5. Emory Clinic v. Houston, 258 Ga. 434 (1988).
6. O.C.G.A. § 31-7-130 et seq.
7. O.C.G.A. §§ 31-7-132 and 133.

3.10

Malpractice Liability

Malpractice is professional negligence. A *malpractice suit* is a civil action for money damages in which the plaintiff claims that he or she was injured as a result of the failure of a professional to exercise the degree of skill and care required of such professional generally in like or similar circumstances. MHPs, as individuals providing health care, are subject to malpractice suits. Although malpractice is a form of negligence, there are specific rules regarding the filing and presentation of malpractice suits.

(A) Elements of a Malpractice Claim

Georgia law provides that a "person professing to practice surgery or the administering of medicine for compensation must bring to the exercise of his profession a reasonable degree of care and skill. Any injury resulting from a want of such care and skill shall be a tort for which a recovery may be had."[1] Although this statute applies only to physicians, including psychiatrists, it sets forth the standard that is generally applicable to health care professionals and that has been adopted by the courts in establishing the duty of care that health professionals owe to their patients.

There are three essential elements that must be proved by the plaintiff in order to recover in a professional negligence case. They are

---

1. O.C.G.A. § 51-1-27.

1. the existence of a duty of care imposed by the professional–patient relationship;
2. the breach of that duty by the failure of the professional to exercise the requisite degree of skill and care in the situation; and
3. an injury sustained as a result of that breach of duty.[2]

Likewise, an action for malpractice against a hospital or other health care facility requires the establishment of the duty of the hospital to the patient; the breach of that duty by the failure of hospital employees to exercise the requisite degree of skill and care; and proof that the failure to exercise such care was the proximate cause of the injury.[3]

When the negligence relates to a matter of professional judgment on the part of a physician or MHP who is an independent contractor and not an employee of the hospital, and when the employer does not exercise or have the right to exercise control in the diagnosis or treatment of the patient, then the hospital cannot be liable for the professional's alleged negligence.[4]

The liability of hospitals for the acts of employed professionals is confused under Georgia law. Generally, a hospital will be liable for the negligence of its employed professionals. A hospital may also be liable for the negligent acts of its employees in carrying out a physician's instructions in performing administrative or clerical acts requiring no medical judgment. However, if a physician or other professional gives orders to hospital employees or exercises personal supervision over these employees, then the physician will be deemed liable for their conduct as well.[5]

(B) Duty of Care

The first element of any professional negligence claim is to establish the existence of a duty of care owed by the professional to the plaintiff. In general, before a plaintiff may recover on the basis that he or she received negligent treatment from a physician or other MHP, the plaintiff must show that an MHP–patient rela-

---

2. Cogin v. Goldman, 209 Ga. App. 251, 433 S.E.2d 85 (1993); Hawkins v. Greenberg, 166 Ga. App. 574, 304 S.E.2d 922 (1983).
3. McClure v. Clayton County Hospital Authority, 176 Ga. App. 414, 336 S.E.2d 268 (1985).
4. Moore v. Carrington, 155 Ga. App. 12, 270 S.E.2d 222 (1980); Stewart v. Midani, 525 F. Supp. 843 (N.D. Ga. 1981).
5. Swindell v. St. Joseph's Hospital, 161 Ga. App. 290 (1982); Miller v. Atkins, 142 Ga. App. 618 (1977); Ross v. Chatham County Hospital Authority, 258 Ga. 234, 367 S.E.2d 793 (1988); Gray v. Vaughn, P.C., 460 S.E.2d 86 (1995).

tionship existed between them. The existence of an MHP–patient relationship creates a duty of care from the MHP to the patient.[6]

There are, however, occasions when an MHP may owe a legal duty to a third party. In the seminal case of *Tarasoff v. Regents of University of California*,[7] the California Supreme Court found that therapists owe a duty of care to third parties who may be endangered by the conduct of their patients, including a duty to control and to warn others of such conduct in appropriate circumstances. In *Bradley Center, Inc. v. Wessner*, the Georgia Supreme Court held that a private mental health facility could be held civilly liable for a murder committed by a patient over whom the hospital could exercise control. The court identified the legal duty as follows:

> Where the course of treatment of a mental patient involves an exercise of "control"over him by a physician who knows or should know that the patient is likely to cause bodily harm to others, an independent duty arises from that relationship and falls upon the physician to exercise that control with such reasonable care as to prevent harm to others at the hands of the patient.[8]

The Georgia courts have also held that the duty of care, at least in the hospital setting, extends to taking reasonable precautions to prevent a patient from committing suicide. In *Brandvain v. Ridgeview Institute, Inc.*, a wrongful death action was filed against Ridgeview Institute based upon the suicide of a patient in the impaired professionals treatment program. The Georgia Supreme Court articulated the standard of care as follows:

> A private hospital in which patients are placed for treatment by their physicians, and which undertakes to care for the patients and supervise and look after them, is under the duty to exercise such reasonable care in looking after and protecting a patient as the patient's condition, which is known to the hospital through its agents and servants charged with the duty of looking after and supervising the patient, may require. This duty extends to safeguarding and protecting the patient from any known or reasonably apprehended danger from himself which may be due to his mental incapacity, and to use ordinary and reasonable care to prevent it.[9]

The court further noted that the fact that the death occurred at the patient's own hand was not an intervening circumstance that would relieve the hospital from liability. Rather, if the defen-

---

6. Bradley Center, Inc. v. Wessner, 250 Ga. 199, 296 S.E.2d 693 (1982).
7. 511 P.2d 334 (1976).
8. 296 S.E.2d at 695-696. *Also see* Swofford v. Cooper, 184 Ga. App. 50, 360 S.E.2d 624 (1987), *aff'd*, 258 Ga. 143, 368 S.E.2d 518 (1988).
9. Brandvain v. Ridgeview Institute, Inc., 188 Ga. App. 106, 372 S.E.2d 265, 271, *aff'd*, 259 Ga. 376, 382 S.E.2d 597 (1989), *quoting* Emory University v. Shadburn, 47 Ga. App. 643 (1933).

dant's suicide was foreseeable, then the hospital would be liable if it failed to take reasonable steps to protect the patient from his own conduct.

(C) Standard of Care

The general rule in Georgia is that a health care professional, including an MHP, is required to exercise that degree of care and skill ordinarily exercised by members of the profession generally under similar conditions and circumstances.[10] The standard is of the profession generally and not in the particular locality in which the professional practices.[11]

It is necessary for the plaintiff to establish, through expert testimony, the standard of care applicable in the particular situation. There is a presumption that an MHP has performed pursuant to the standard of care, and the plaintiff must produce expert testimony to overcome the presumption. It is necessary to present testimony from an expert in the same specialty as the defendant, unless the specialties are substantially similar.

The Georgia Civil Practice Act establishes a heightened pleading requirement in professional malpractice actions. In any such action, the plaintiff must file, with the complaint, an affidavit of an expert competent to testify, which affidavit must set forth specifically at least one negligent act or omission and the factual basis for the claim.[12] The term *professional* in the malpractice affidavit section has been defined as an individual who is required to be licensed pursuant to Title 43 of the Georgia Code.[13] This includes physicians, nurses, psychologists, professional counselors, marriage and family therapists, and social workers. Although a pharmacist is clearly a professional, an affidavit is not required in a malpractice action against a pharmacist because pharmacists are licensed under a different statute.

Georgia law also provides that, in any action for medical malpractice in which damages in excess of $10,000 are sought, the demand for judgment in the complaint must state that the plaintiff "demands judgment in excess of $10,000 and no further monetary amount shall be stated."[14] A medical malpractice action includes any claim arising from health, medical, dental, or surgical care and treatment.

---

10. Emory University v. Porubiansky, 248 Ga. 391, 282 S.E.2d 903 (1981); Williams v. Ricks, 152 Ga. App. 555, 263 S.E.2d 457 (1979).
11. Sullivan v. Henry, 160 Ga. App. 791, 287 S.E.2d 652 (1982).
12. O.C.G.A. § 9-11-9.1.
13. Harold v. Lusk, 263 Ga. 895, 439 S.E.2d 896 (1994).
14. O.C.G.A. § 9-11-8(a)(1).

(D) Statute of Limitations

Georgia law provides that an action for medical malpractice must be brought within 2 years after the date on which an injury or death arising from a negligent or wrongful act or omission occurred. An action for medical malpractice is defined as any claim for damages resulting from death or injury arising out of health, medical, dental or surgical services, diagnosis, prescription, treatment or care, as well as care or service rendered by any hospital, nursing home, clinic, facility, or institution.[15]

In interpreting the statute, the Georgia courts have adopted the discovery rule in medical malpractice cases. Under the discovery rule, the statute of limitations does not begin to run until the plaintiff, through the exercise of reasonable diligence, discovers the injury and the causal connection between the injury and the professional's conduct.[16] However, the Georgia statute provides for an ultimate 5-year statute of repose and abrogation.[17] This means that no action for medical malpractice may be brought more than 5 years after the date on which the negligent act or omission occurred, even if the injury is discovered more than 5 years after the negligent act.

Although the discovery rule does not operate to toll (suspend) the 5-year statute of ultimate repose, the statute will be tolled if the defendant fraudulently conceals his negligent or wrongful acts or omissions from the patient.[18] However, in *Hickey v. Akren*,[19] a case involving alleged sexual abuse by a psychotherapist, the court rejected the theory that the limitations period was tolled by the defendant's fraud based on evidence that the patient had not been deterred by the defendant from seeking treatment elsewhere. The court found that the patient was aware of her injuries and of their causal connection with the therapist's misconduct during the 2-year statute of limitations. However, in a case in which a therapist engages in improper conduct and affirmatively advises the patient that this conduct is proper and not harmful, and the patient is not aware that damage is being inflicted, it is likely that the statute of limitations would be tolled on a fraud theory.

The Georgia statute of limitations further provides that individuals who are legally incompetent because of mental retardation or mental illness are not exempt from the limitations periods.

---

15. O.C.G.A. § 9-3-70.
16. Whitaker v. Zerkle, 188 Ga. App. 706, 374 S.E.2d 106 (1988); Vitner v. Miller, 208 Ga. App. 306, 430 S.E.2d 671 (1993).
17. O.C.G.A. § 9-3-71(c).
18. Hill v. Fordam, 186 Ga. App. 354, 367 S.E.2d 128 (1988).
19. 98 Ga. App. 718, 403 S.E.2d 229 (1991).

Likewise, minors are subject to the 2-year statute of limitations and of the 5-year ultimate statute of repose. A minor who has not attained the age of 5 years shall have 2 years from the date of the minor's fifth birthday within which to bring a malpractice action if the claim arose before the minor attained the age of 5 years. In such cases, the statute of repose bars claims brought after the tenth birthday if the child was under 5 years of age at the time the negligent act occurred or 5 years from the date on which the negligent act or omission occurred if the minor was 5 years or older on such date.

The periods of limitations for bringing an action for medical malpractice may be tolled based on a request for provision of the injured person's medical records. The statute of limitations may be tolled for up to 90 days while the custodian of the medical records responds to the request.[20]

---

20. O.C.G.A. § 9-3-97.1.

3.11

Other Forms of Professional Liability

Most claims brought against MHPs are for malpractice and assert that the professional failed to conform to the requisite standard of care. However, other legal theories may be used to bring claims against MHPs. Although such claims are frequently asserted as part of malpractice actions, they may also be asserted separately to avoid the particular rules applicable in malpractice actions. For example, other claims may be used to avoid the malpractice statute of limitations or the requirement of expert testimony in a medical malpractice action.

(A) Breach of Contract

The MHP–patient relationship is, at its simplest, a contract. That is, the MHP agrees, for consideration, to render care and treatment to the patient. No written or express contract is required to create the contractual relationship. In a professional setting, the contract contains an implied term that the professional will possess and exercise ordinary care and skill in rendering the services. Thus, the failure of the MHP to conform to the applicable standard of care may constitute a breach of contract, as well as the tort of malpractice. In some instances, a breach of contract claim may be brought even though the statute of limitations has expired on the malpractice claim. Actions for breach of simple contracts in writing must be brought within 6 years after the breach. All other actions upon contracts, whether express or implied, must be brought within 4 years after the right of action accrues.[1]

---

1. O.C.G.A. §§ 9-3-24 and 9-3-26.

(B) Sexual Misconduct

Engaging in sexual conduct with a patient during the course of treatment is a crime in Georgia, violates ethical and licensing standards, and may constitute malpractice. It may also give rise to a separate and independent claim for sexual assault. Such a claim would subject the defendant to a claim for punitive damages, damages that are not generally available in malpractice actions.

The question of whether conduct can be characterized as malpractice or sexual misconduct may be particularly important on the issue of insurance coverage. In *St. Paul Fire & Marine Insurance Company v. Mitchell*,[2] the issue was whether a psychiatrist's conduct in engaging in sexual relations with a patient constituted malpractice for purposes of insurance coverage. The court held that the psychiatrist's alleged negligence in mishandling the transference phenomenon during therapy, which resulted in the psychiatrist having sexual relations with the patient, could constitute the failure to exercise proper professional care, which would be covered under the policy of insurance. However, in *St. Paul Fire & Marine Insurance Company v. Alderman*,[3] the court granted summary judgment to the same insurance carrier on the basis that the physician's conduct did not involve medical treatment, but was designed purely to satisfy the physician's own sexual interests. The physician, an internist, engaged in sexual physical touching with the patient during the course of a physical examination. The court held that the physician's conduct did not involve medical treatment or the application of medical skills and, therefore, did not constitute a professional service covered under the physician's malpractice insurance policy. In *American Home Assurance Company v. Smith*,[4] the Georgia Court of Appeals upheld a provision in a psychologist's professional liability policy that limited recovery to $25,000 for claims arising out of actual or alleged erotic physical conduct.

(C) Assault and Battery

Assault and battery is an intentional tort that involves unconsented physical contact between the patient and the MHP. If treatment is to involve any type of physical touching, then specific consent must be obtained. In addition, informed consent must be obtained

---

2. 164 Ga. App. 215, 296 S.E.2d 126 (1982).
3. 216 Ga. App. 777, 455 S.E.2d 852 (1995) .
4. 426 S.E.2d 441 (1995).

in which certain invasive procedures are performed. (See chapter 3.1, this volume.)

(D) False Imprisonment

False imprisonment consists of an unlawful restraint on an individual's liberty. Therefore, involuntarily committing an individual without complying with the procedures in the Mental Health Code may give rise to a claim for false imprisonment.[5] If the procedures of the Mental Health Code are followed, then the MHP is immune from liability unless there is a showing of bad faith.[6]

(E) Abandonment

The tort of *abandonment* occurs when an MHP withdraws care and treatment from a patient in a manner that causes injury to the patient. A physician or other MHP who agrees to treat a patient may not refuse to continue treatment at a critical stage when to do so would cause harm to the patient.[7] An MHP who seeks to withdraw from the treatment of a patient should do so at the appropriate time, should make an appropriate referral, and should advise the patient of the consequences of not seeking further treatment.

(F) Invasion of Privacy

As discussed in chapter 3.3, the unauthorized disclosure of patient records or communications may give rise to a claim of invasion of privacy.

---

5. Kendrick v. Metropolitan Psychiatric Center, Inc., 158 Ga. App. 839, 282 S.E.2d 361 (1981).
6. O.C.G.A. § 37-3-4.
7. Norton v. Hamilton, 92 Ga. App. 727, 89 S.E.2d 809 (1955); Kenney v. Piedmont Hospital, 136 Ga. App. 660, 222 S.E.2d 162 (1975).

3.12

Criminal Liability

(A) Sexual Assault

Under Georgia law, it is a felony for an MHP to engage in sexual contact with a patient or to use the treatment or counseling relationship to facilitate sexual contact. The law provides that

> [a] person commits sexual assault when, as an actual or purported practitioner of psychotherapy, he or she engages in sexual contact with another person who the actor knew or should have known is the subject of the actor's actual or purported treatment or counseling, or, if the treatment or counseling relationship was used to facilitate sexual contact between the actor and said person.[1]

Psychotherapy is defined as the professional treatment or counseling of a mental or emotional illness, symptom, or condition. *Sexual contact* is broadly defined as any contact for the purpose of sexual gratification with the "intimate parts" of the patient.

The law makes it a crime both to have sexual contact with a person currently in treatment and to have sexual contact with a former patient if the treatment or counseling relationship is used to facilitate the sexual contact. Consent of the victim is not a defense. There are, to date, no Georgia cases defining the circumstances under which treatment or counseling could be deemed to facilitate the sexual contact.

---

1. O.C.G.A. § 16-6-5.1(c)(2).

(B) Battery

An individual commits the crime of battery by intentionally, knowingly, or recklessly causing physical injury or an unwanted touching upon another person with the intent to insult, provoke, or injure the person.[2] Therefore, an MHP who touches a patient without consent in a manner that causes physical injury or in a manner that would naturally cause harm may be guilty of simple battery.

(C) Assisted Suicide

Georgia law makes it a felony to assist in the commission of suicide. Under the law, a person who publicly advertises, offers, or holds himself out as offering that he will actively assist a person in the commission of suicide and who commits an overt act to further the suicide is guilty of a felony. Likewise, any person who knowingly and willfully commits any act designed to destroy the volition of another or who exercises undue influence on another thereby intentionally causing the person to commit suicide shall be guilty of a felony.[3]

---

2. O.C.G.A. § 16-5-20.
3. O.C.G.A. § 16-5-5.

Liability of Licensing Boards

The issue of sovereign and official immunity is a complicated one in Georgia. Sovereign immunity derives from the common law concept that the "king can do no wrong." Thus, the state of Georgia, as the "sovereign," is immune from suit unless it consents. The Georgia Constitution provides that the General Assembly may waive the state's sovereign immunity from suit by enacting a State Tort Claims Act.[1]

Official immunity is a doctrine under which officers and employees of the state may not be sued for their negligent conduct. The Georgia Constitution provides that, except as provided by the General Assembly in a State Tort Claims Act, all officers and employees of the state and its departments may be subject to suit for damages caused by the negligent performance of their ministerial functions and may be liable for injuries if they act with actual malice or intent to cause injury. A *ministerial function* is generally defined as one that does not involve the exercise of discretion and that the officer is required to perform by law.

In 1992, the Georgia General Assembly enacted a State Tort Claims Act pursuant to a constitutional amendment. Members of state licensing boards are specifically considered to be officers or employees of the state for purposes of the State Tort Claims Act.[2] The Act states that it constitutes the exclusive remedy for any tort committed by a state officer or employee. A state officer or employee who commits a tort while acting within the scope of official duties is not subject to suit. A person who brings an action based on the tortious conduct of a state officer or employee may

---

1. Ga. Const. art. 1, § 2, ¶9.
2. O.C.G.A. § 50-21-22(7).

not name the individual directly, but must name the governmental entity for which the officer was acting.[3] Therefore, a member of a state licensing board has immunity from suit for torts committed by the member in the course of official duties as a licensing board member.

However, if the licensing board member is acting outside the scope of official duties, then there is no immunity from suit. Actions taken by licensing board members at board meetings or in furtherance of board business will clearly be immunized from suit. It is only if the board member acts outside the scope of official responsibilities that liability may be imposed. For example, a board member who is involved in a board investigation of unprofessional conduct or who votes to revoke a license will clearly be acting within the scope of official duties.

The State Tort Claims Act further provides that the state has no liability for quasi-judicial or prosecutorial action or inaction. Therefore, the actions of a state licensing board and its members in investigating complaints against licensees and adjudicating those complaints will not subject the state or the board members to liability.

The state has created an insurance fund managed by the State Department of Administrative Services to defend and pay claims made against state officers, including licensing board members. The attorney general's office will provide a defense to a board member who is sued for actions taken in connection with his or her status as a board member.

It should also be noted that Georgia law provides good faith immunity from suit for individuals who report violations to licensing boards and who testify or engage in peer review for licensing boards. The law provides immunity from civil and criminal liability for reporting or investigating the acts or omissions of a licensee or applicant if such report is made or the investigation is taken in good faith without fraud or malice. Any individual who testifies or who makes a recommendation to a state examining board in the nature of peer review, in good faith and without fraud or malice, is also immune from civil and criminal liability.[4]

---

3. O.C.G.A. § 50-21-25.
4. O.C.G.A. § 43-1-19(i). *Also see* O.C.G.A. § 43-39-20, which provides for immunity for psychologists who testify in good faith as to an applicant's fitness to practice psychology or who make a report or recommendation to the Psychology Board in the nature of peer review.

3.14

Antitrust Limitations to Practice

Antitrust laws were enacted to prevent the formation of monopolies and abuses of economic power. Health care providers and provider organizations have increasingly become targets of antitrust litigation. Activities that are generally prohibited under the antitrust laws include *price fixing*, an agreement among competitors to establish a common price or a system for setting prices; *division of markets*, an agreement among competitors to allocate certain markets to certain participants who would otherwise be competitors; *a group boycott*, an agreement among competitors to patronize only certain businesses; and *tying arrangements*, by which a party agrees to sell a certain product or service only on condition that the buyer also purchase a different product. All of these activities fall within the general prohibitions against restraints of trade.

The vast majority of antitrust litigation is brought in federal court under federal law. Litigation may be brought by the federal government, by competitors, and by individuals who claim to have suffered an antitrust injury. Health care providers have attempted, generally unsuccessfully, to use the antitrust laws as a remedy for denial or removal of staff privileges.

To recover under the federal antitrust laws, a plaintiff must prove that two or more distinct entities agreed to take concerted action against the plaintiff and that it had an anticompetitive effect on the market and an effect on interstate commerce. The plaintiff must also demonstrate that he or she suffered damages of the type that the antitrust laws were intended to prevent.[1]

Georgia law also prohibits certain anticompetitive activities. The Georgia Constitution provides that "[t]he General Assembly shall not have the power to authorize any contract or agreement which may have the effect of or which is intended to have the effect of defeating or lessening competition, or encouraging a monopoly, which are hereby declared to be unlawful and void."[2] Georgia also provides that contracts that are in restraint of trade are against public policy and cannot be enforced.[3] These provisions provide not only a mechanism to render such agreements unenforceable, but also provide a common law tort action in favor of third parties who are injured by a conspiracy in restraint of trade.[4]

Georgia law also provides a claim for relief for tortious interference with the business relationships between a plaintiff and its customers or suppliers. To be held liable, the defendant

> must have (1) acted improperly and without privilege, (2) purposely and with malice with the intent to injure, (3) induced a third party or parties not to enter into or continue a business relationship with the plaintiff, and (4) [caused] plaintiff [to] suffer some financial injury.[5]

Of particular interest to health care providers is the question of the enforceability of restrictive covenants. Such agreements are frequently used in the employment context, as well as between partners or shareholders in a professional venture. Noncompetition contracts restrict an individual from engaging in a business or professional activity that is competitive with the employer or person with whom the agreement is made. A customer nonsolicitation agreement prohibits the solicitation of business from the employer's customers or prospective customers. Nonsolicitation agreements may also prohibit a former employee or partner or shareholder from luring away the employees or personnel of the employer or practice. Agreements may also attempt to restrict the use of confidential or trade secret information acquired during the course of employment.

---

1. *See generally*, Todorov v. D.C.H. Health Care Authority, 921 F.2d 1438 (11th Cir. 1991); Robles v. Humana Hospital-Cartersville, 758 F. Supp. 989 (N.D. Ga. 1992); Bolt v. Halifax Hospital Medical Center, 891 F.2d 810 (11th Cir. 1990); Boczar v. Manatee Hospitals and Health Systems, Inc., 993 F.2d 1514 (11th Cir. 1993).
2. Ga. Const., art. III, § 6, ¶5(c).
3. O.C.G.A. § 13-8-2.
4. U.S. Anchor Manufacturing, Inc. v. Rule Industries, Inc., 7 F.3d 986 (11th Cir. 1993).
5. *Id.* at 1003, *citing* DeLong Equipment Company v. Washington Mills Abrasive Company, 887 F.2d 1499, 518 (11th Cir. 1989).

The Georgia courts have severely restricted the use of restrictive covenants ancillary to employment contracts. In *Jackson & Coker, Inc. v. Hart*, the Georgia Supreme Court held unconstitutional a statute that authorized contracts containing broad postemployment covenants not to compete.[6] Generally, to be enforceable, covenants not to compete must be reasonable and specific regarding geographic scope, nature of restriction, and time. Postemployment customer nonsolicitation provisions are analyzed under the same standards. However, a nonsolicitation provision may be enforceable without regard to territorial limitation if it applies only to customers with whom the employee had contact while employed.[7]

The Georgia Trade Secrets Act also prohibits the misappropriation of trade secrets. Under the Act, a contractual duty to maintain or limit the use of a trade secret is not void or unenforceable because of lack of a durational or geographic limitation.[8]

---

6. Jackson & Coker, Inc. v. Hart, 261 Ga. 371, 405 S.E.2d 253 (1991), *addressing* O.C.G.A. § 13-8-2.1.
7. W.R. Grace and Company v. Mouyal, 262 Ga. 464, 422 S.E.2d 529 (Ga. 1992); *also see* Wylie v. Royal Cup, Inc., 258 Ga. 357, 370 S.E.2d (1988); Orkin Exterminating Company v. Pelfrey, 237 Ga. 284, 227 S.E.2d 251 (1976).
8. O.C.G.A. § 10-1-760 *et seq.*; Equifax Services, Inc. v. Examination Management Services, Inc., 216 Ga. App. 35, 453 S.E.2d 488 (1994).

3.15

Confidentiality of Peer Review Organizations and Medical Review Committees

In 1980, the Georgia General Assembly enacted the peer review and medical review committee statutes that are intended to encourage in-house review of health care services. The statutes provide protection to members of peer review groups and protects the confidentiality of the records generated in the peer review process.[1] *Peer review* is defined as "the procedure by which professional health care providers evaluate the quality and efficiency of services ordered or performed by other professional health care providers."[2] The services subject to review include practice analysis, "inpatient hospital and extended care facility utilization review, medical audit, ambulatory care review, claims review and the compliance of a hospital, nursing home, convalescent home or other health care facility . . . with the standards set by an association of health care providers and with applicable laws, rules and regulations."[3] A *professional health care provider* is defined as any licensed individual or approved organization that practices in the health care field in Georgia and specifically includes psychologists, physicians, and nurses.[4]

The term *review organization* is used throughout the statutes and refers to the Joint Commission on Accreditation of Healthcare Organizations (JCAHO) or any national accreditation body or "any panel, committee, or organization which is primarily composed of professional health care providers . . . and which engages in or utilizes peer reviews and gathers and reviews information relating to the care and treatment of patients for the

---

1. The Peer Review Groups Act is codified at O.C.G.A. § 31-7-130 *et seq.*
2. O.C.G.A. § 31-7-131(1).
3. *Id.*
4. O.C.G.A. § 31-7-131(2).

purposes of evaluating and improving the quality of health care rendered, or reducing morbidity or mortality."[5]

No professional health care provider may be held liable, criminally or civilly, for performance of peer review activities unless motivated by malice toward any person affected by any such activity.[6] Similarly, no witness who provides information to a professional health care provider or to a review organization may be held liable unless the witness knowingly provides false information.[7]

All proceedings and records of a review organization shall be held in confidence and shall not be subject to discovery or introduction into evidence in civil actions. Initially, the only exception to this confidentiality provision was in a proceeding alleging violations of the peer review act. In 1991, an additional exception was enacted to allow disclosure of documents provided for licensure purposes.[8] It is important to note that if peer review documents are available from original sources, they are not immune from discovery merely because they were also considered by the review organization.

No person who attends a review organization meeting shall be permitted or required to testify regarding any evidence or other matters produced or presented during the proceeding or as to any findings, recommendations, evaluations, or other actions taken by the organization.[9] However, a person who presents information to the review organization is not barred from testifying in a civil or criminal proceeding. That person is merely prohibited from testifying about the conduct of the review organization proceedings.

The confidentiality provision for information considered by peer review groups was strictly construed in the leading case on the issue, *Emory Clinic v. Houston*.[10] The *Houston* case was a medical malpractice action brought after surgery was allegedly performed on the patient's wrong eye. The court held that the General Assembly had placed "an absolute embargo on the discovery of all proceedings, records, findings, and recommendations of a peer review group."[11] Even though newspaper reports

---

5. O.C.G.A. § 31-7-131(3). Also included in the definition of review organization is an organization that provides professional liability insurance for health care providers and engages in peer review to evaluate claims and make underwriting decisions.
6. O.C.G.A. § 31-7-132(a).
7. O.C.G.A. § 31-7-132(b).
8. O.C.G.A. § 31-7-133(b).
9. O.C.G.A. § 31-7-133(a).
10. 258 Ga. 434, 369 S.E.2d 913 (1988).
11. Emory Clinic et al. v. Houston, 369 S.E.2d at 913 (1988).

of the peer review information had been published, the prohibition on discovery for use in litigation was enforced.

MHPs should also be aware that in addition to peer review groups, there are medical review committees.[12] A *medical review committee* is defined as a committee of a state or local professional society or of a medical staff of a licensed hospital, nursing home, medical foundation, or peer review committee, provided the medical staff operates pursuant to written bylaws that have been approved by the governing board of the hospital. The medical review committee must also be formed for the purposes of evaluating and improving the quality of health care rendered or of determining whether health services rendered were professionally indicated or were performed in compliance with the applicable standard of care.[13] A medical review committee's function is narrower than a peer review committee's function, as a medical review committee is designed to review only the quality of health care services, whereas a peer review committee looks at efficiency, facility utilization, and claims review in addition to quality of health care. A psychologist who is part of a medical staff operating pursuant to approved written bylaws is eligible to sit on a medical review committee. As with a peer review committee, members of a medical review committee are also immune from liability for acts undertaken or performed within the scope of the committee if the members act without malice or fraud. The immunity is narrower, however, than the immunity for peer review committee members as medical review committee members are immune only from suits by providers of health services, not from suits by patients or the patients' successors.[14]

The medical review committee proceedings and records are not discoverable, nor may they be used in any civil action against a provider of health services that arises out of the matters that the committee reviews. Medical review committee members may not be permitted or required to testify in civil actions as to matters produced or presented during the proceeding or as to any findings, recommendations, or evaluations. A committee member or a witness before the committee may testify as to matters within his knowledge, but not as to his testimony before the committee or opinions formed by him as a result of committee hearings.[15]

---

12. O.C.G.A. § 31-7-140 *et seq.*
13. O.C.G.A. § 31-7-140.
14. O.C.G.A. § 31-7-141.
15. O.C.G.A. § 31-7-143.

3.16

Family Educational and Privacy Rights Act

The Federal Educational and Privacy Rights Act requires educational institutions to make educational records available to students who are 18 years of age or older or to the student's parents if the student is under 18 years of age.[1] These requirements are applicable to any educational institution, public or private, that receives funds from any program administered by the Secretary of Education, with certain narrow exceptions set forth in the Code of Federal Regulations.[2] The Act requires that the educational institution provide the student or the student's parents with the educational records within 45 days of the request.[3] The parents or the student have the right to inspect and review the records, as well as to challenge the contents of those records.[4]

The Act's definition of educational records specifically excludes the records of a student when those records are "made or maintained by a physician, psychiatrist, psychologist, or other recognized professional or paraprofessional acting in his professional or paraprofessional capacity, or assisting in that capacity, and which are made, maintained, or used only in connection with the provision of treatment to the student, and are not available to anyone other than persons providing such treatment." However, "such records can be personally reviewed by a physician or other appropriate professional of the student's choice."[5]

The Act also generally prohibits disclosure of educational records, other than directory information, without the written

---

1. 20 U.S.C. 1232g.
2. 34 C.F.R. Part 99.
3. 20 U.S.C. 1232 g(1)(a).
4. 20 U.S.C. 1232g(1)(a) and (1)(C)(2).
5. 20 U.S.C. 1232g(4)(B)(iv).

consent of the student's parents.[6] Disclosure without consent may be made to other school officials, to other school systems in which the student seeks to enroll, for use in financial aid applications, and to accrediting organizations.[7] If a student's educational records are sought in a judicial proceeding, they may be obtained by way of subpoena or in compliance with a judicial order requiring their release.[8] The school system must make a reasonable effort to notify the parents or student prior to producing the records.[9]

6. 20 U.S.C. 1232g(b).
7. 20 U.S.C. 1232g(b)(1). Other exceptions are set forth in the statute.
8. 20 U.S.C. 1232g(b)(2).
9. 34 C.F.R. § 99.31(g).

Adults, Minors, and Families

Competency to Marry

To constitute a valid marriage in the state of Georgia, there must be parties able to contract an actual contract and there must be consummation according to law.[1] As in many states, Georgia requires a minimum mental status before one is able to marry. To be able to enter into a marriage contract, a person must

1. be of sound mind;
2. be at least 16 years of age, unless the female party is pregnant or both parties are the parents of a living child born out of wedlock, in which case the parties may marry regardless of age;
3. have no living spouses of a previous undissolved marriage; and
4. not be related to the prospective spouse by blood or marriage.[2]

Although there is a presumption that parties to a marriage have the capacity to contract, this presumption may be overcome by sufficient proof.[3] Therefore, it is conceivable that an MHP may be called upon to assist in the determination as to whether a party was of sufficiently sound mind to enter into the marriage contract if the marriage is disputed.

---

1. O.C.G.A. § 19-3-1.
2. O.C.G.A. § 19-3-2; *see also* Taylor v. Abbott, 201 Ga. 254, 39 S.E.2d 471 (1946).
3. Fanning v. State, 46 Ga. App. 716, 169 S.E. 60 (1933).

4.2

Guardianship for Adults

Individuals who are unable to conduct their day-to-day affairs because of an emotional or cognitive disability may be appointed a guardian who will control their lives much as parents oversee the lives of their children. There are two classes of individuals for whom guardianship may be obtained: minors and incapacitated adults. This chapter is limited to a discussion of guardianships for incapacitated adult persons. Chapter 4.3 discusses the appointment of guardians of the property of incapcitated adults, whereas guardianships for minors and their property are discussed in chapters 4.11 and 4.12. The MHP may become involved in the guardianship process by being asked to evaluate an individual who may be in need of a guardianship, to testify as to whether the individual meets the test for a guardianship, or to provide therapeutic services to the person after a guardianship has been imposed.

(A) Petition for Guardianship

An incapacitated individual or anyone interested in the individual's welfare may file a petition under oath for a finding of legal incapacity and the appointment of a guardian.[1] The petition must be supported by an affidavit of a physician or of a psychologist stating that he or she has examined the proposed ward within 10 days prior to the filing of the petition and that, based on the examination, the proposed ward was determined to be incapacitated by reason of mental illness, mental retardation, mental

---

1. O.C.G.A. § 29-5-6(a)(1).

disability, advanced age, physical illness or disability, chronic use of drugs or alcohol, or other cause, to the extent that the individual lacked sufficient understanding or capacity to make significant responsible decisions or the ability to communicate such decisions concerning his or her person.[2]

Upon receiving the petition, the judge must make a preliminary determination as to whether there is sufficient evidence to believe that the proposed ward is incapacitated.[3] If there is enough evidence to sustain the petition, the court must appoint an evaluating physician or psychologist, other than the physician or psychologist who completed the affidavit attached to the petition.[4] This appointed physician or psychologist must evaluate the condition of the proposed ward and then file, with the court, a written report no later than 7 days after the examination.[5] The report must

1. state the duration and circumstances of the evaluation, including a summary of questions or tests used;
2. list all individuals or other sources of information consulted in evaluating the condition of the proposed ward;
3. describe the proposed ward's mental and physical state and condition, including all observed facts considered by the physician or psychologist;
4. describe the overall social condition of the proposed ward, including support, care, education, and well-being; and
5. describe the needs of the proposed ward and the foreseeable duration.[6]

The probate court must then review the evaluation report and the petition to determine whether there is probable cause to support a finding that the proposed ward is incapacitated. If no probable cause is found, the petition will be dismissed. If the court does find that probable cause exists, a hearing on the petition must be scheduled.[7] Either the proposed ward or the individual who filed the petition may file a written response to the evaluation report at any time up to the conclusion of the hearing. The response may include, but is not limited to, an independent evaluation and affidavits of individuals with personal knowledge of the proposed ward.[8]

---

2. O.C.G.A. § 29-5-6(a)(3).
3. O.C.G.A. § 29-5-6(b).
4. O.C.G.A. § 29-5-6(c)(1).
5. O.C.G.A. § 29-5-6(c)(5).
6. O.C.G.A. § 29-5-6(c)(6).
7. O.C.G.A. § 29-5-6(d).
8. *Id.*

(B) Guardianship Hearing

The guardianship hearing is held in a regular courtroom, if available, and the court applies the rules of evidence applicable in civil cases.[9] The person alleged to be incapacitated has the right to be represented by counsel and to subpoena and cross-examine all witnesses, including the evaluating physician or psychologist.[10] At the request of the proposed ward or the ward's attorney and for good cause shown, the public may be excluded and the appearance of the ward may be waived.[11]

The court may appoint a guardian over the person of an adult if it finds the individual to be incapacitated by reason of mental illness, mental retardation, mental disability, advanced age, physical illness or disability, chronic use of drugs or alcohol, or other cause to the extent that such adult lacks sufficient understanding or capacity to make significant responsible decisions concerning his or her person or to the extent that he or she is incapable of communicating them.[12]

Furthermore, a judge of the probate court may also appoint a guardian over the property of an adult who is incapacitated. This is discussed more fully in chapter 4.3.

The judge must issue an order setting forth his or her findings supporting the grant or denial of the petition. If the guardianship is granted, the order must specify

1. the type of guardianship established, whether of the person, of property, or both;
2. the name(s) of the guardian or guardians and the reason for the selection;
3. the nature and extent of the ward's incapacity;
4. any rights retained by the ward;
5. the duration of the guardianship, whether limited or permanent;
6. the type and frequency of physical, mental, and social evaluations of the ward's condition; and
7. such other provisions of the guardianship as the court deems proper.[13]

---

9. O.C.G.A. § 29-5-6(e)(1), (3).
10. O.C.G.A. § 29-5-6(e)(3).
11. O.C.G.A. § 29-5-6(e)(1).
12. O.C.G.A. § 29-5-1(a)(1).
13. O.C.G.A. § 29-5-6(f)(1).

(C) Appointment of Emergency Guardian

In the event that an individual believes that an adult is gravely incapacitated, the individual may file a petition for an emergency guardian. In addition to the requirements set out previously, the petition must set forth

1. such facts as establish an immediate, clear, and substantial risk of death or serious physical injury, illness, or disease unless an emergency guardian is appointed; or

2. such facts as establish an immediate, substantial risk of irreparable waste or dissipation of the estate of the proposed ward unless an emergency guardian is appointed.[14]

In its review of the petition, if the court finds that there is probable cause to believe that the proposed ward is gravely incapacitated and that an emergency guardianship is necessary, the court

1. shall order an examination of the proposed ward to be made within 72 hours by a licensed physician or psychologist and a written report to be furnished to the court within such time;

2. shall order an emergency hearing to be conducted not sooner than 3 days nor later than 5 days after the filing of the petition;

3. shall immediately appoint an attorney to represent the proposed ward at the emergency hearing;

4. if the threatened risk is so immediate and irreparable that any delay is unreasonable and the existence of such a threatened risk is certified by the affidavit of a licensed physician or psychologist, shall appoint an emergency guardian to serve until the emergency hearing; and

5. in its discretion, may order that, pending the emergency hearing, no withdrawals may be made from any account on the authority of the proposed ward's signature without prior approval from the court.[15]

After receiving the examination report, the probate court shall conduct the emergency hearing to determine whether sufficient conditions exist so as to necessitate the appointment of an emergency guardian pending a full hearing.[16] The petitioner must prove the necessity for the emergency guardian by clear and

---

14. O.C.G.A. § 29-5-8(b).
15. O.C.G.A. § 29-5-8(d).
16. O.C.G.A. § 29-5-8(e).

convincing evidence.[17] An emergency guardian has only those powers and duties specifically enumerated in the order of the probate court. Such powers cannot exceed those absolutely necessary to respond to the immediate threatened risk to the ward enumerated in the petition.[18] All emergency guardianships terminate either immediately after the full hearing, 45 days after the filing of the petition, or on a date specified in the court's order appointing the emergency guardian, whichever occurs first.[19]

(D) Appointment and Authority of the Guardian

Although any competent person may be appointed as guardian, the law specifies that the choice of guardian be made according to the following preferences:

1. an individual nominated by the incapacitated adult prior to the filing of the petition for a finding of incapacity, if at the time of nomination the incapacitated adult was 18 or more years of age and had, in the opinion of the court, sufficient mental capacity to make an intelligent choice;

2. the spouse of the incapacitated person;

3. an adult child of the incapacitated person;

4. a parent of the incapacitated person or, if none is living, then a person nominated by will or other writing signed by a deceased parent and attested by at least two witnesses, whichever instrument is later;

5. a guardian of a minor child, upon the child's reaching majority, in the event he or she is then adjudicated as incapacitated; a guardian of the person in the event of an application for guardian of the property; or a guardian of the property in the event of an application for guardian of the person;

6. a relative or other individual who has provided care for the incapacitated person and with whom the incapacitated person has resided for a significant period prior to the time of application; and

7. other individuals, such as relatives; individuals nominated by a spouse, adult child, parent, or guardian; or individuals providing income or other care to the incapacitated person.[20]

---

17. *Id.*
18. O.C.G.A. § 29-5-8(f).
19. *Id.*
20. O.C.G.A. § 29-5-2(c).

If no other individual is available to be the guardian of the ward, the judge may appoint the director of the Department of Family and Children Services of the county of residence of the individual person.[21]

Guardians of the person of incapacitated adults shall have those rights and powers reasonably necessary to provide adequately for the support, care, education, and well-being of the ward and to perform all other duties imposed on such guardians by statute.[22] The law specifies that the guardian of the person

1. shall respect and maintain the dignity and the individual rights of the ward at all times;
2. is entitled to custody of the ward and may establish the ward's residence in or out of state;
3. shall provide for the support, welfare, training, and education of the ward;
4. may consent to medical or other professional treatment;
5. must be reasonably accessible to the ward and must maintain regular contact or communication with the ward;
6. shall take reasonable care of clothing, furniture, vehicles, and other personal effects of the ward that are with the ward;
7. may participate in such legal proceedings, in the name of the ward, as are appropriate for the support, care, education, or well-being of the ward;
8. may petition the court for the appointment of a guardian *ad litem* for the ward wherever, in any legal proceeding, the interest of the ward could be adverse to that of the guardian; and
9. must report on the condition of the ward as specified by court order.[23]

It should be noted that the probate court may limit any powers granted to the guardian of the person under Georgia law and that the probate court may impose any additional duties upon such guardian that under Georgia law could have been, but were not, imposed by an earlier order of the court.[24]

---

21. O.C.G.A. § 29-5-2(d).
22. O.C.G.A. § 29-5-3(a).
23. O.C.G.A. § 29-5-3(b).
24. O.C.G.A. § 29-5-9(a).

(E) Effect of Appointment of Guardian

The appointment of a guardian of an incapacitated person removes from the ward the power to

1. contract marriage;
2. make other contracts;
3. consent to medical treatment;
4. establish a residence or place of abode; and
5. bring or defend any lawsuit, except through a guardian.[25]

(F) Modification or Termination of the Guardianship

The authority and responsibility of a guardian terminates if (a) the ward or guardian dies; (b) a court determines that the guardian is incapacitated or unfit, or there is a sufficient conflict or misconduct by the guardian to warrant removal of the guardian; (c) the guardian resigns; or (d) a petition for modification is filed showing that the need for the guardianship has ended, and the guardian is thereafter removed.[26]

When a petition for modification is filed alleging that there is a change in condition of the ward, the petition must be accompanied by an affidavit of two individuals who have knowledge of the ward or of a licensed physician or psychologist setting forth facts and determinations supporting the petition.[27] The probate court may dismiss a petition to modify guardianship prior to hearing if, after reviewing the evaluation report, the court finds that there is not probable cause to believe that there are grounds for modification or termination of the guardianship.[28] If the petition is not dismissed, the same procedures as set out earlier for the initial guardianship hearing will be used.[29]

---

25. O.C.G.A. § 29-5-7(d).
26. O.C.G.A. § 29-5-9(a).
27. O.C.G.A. § 29-5-9(b).
28. *Id.*
29. *Id.*

4.3

Guardian of the Property of an Incapacitated Adult

(A) General

In addition to the appointment of a guardian of the person (see chapters 4.2 and 4.11), Georgia law allows the court to appoint a guardian to manage the estate (e.g., property, financial resources, and business enterprises) of a person who is a minor or an adult no longer able to take care of his or her property or manage his or her financial affairs. This chapter focuses on adults. Conservatorship for minors is discussed in chapter 4.12. An MHP may become involved in this process by being asked to evaluate the person and to testify as to the person's capacity to manage his or her estate, and/or by providing therapeutic services to the individual after a guardian of the property of an incapacitated adult has been appointed.

A judge of the probate court may appoint guardians over the property of adults who are incapacitated by reason of mental illness, mental retardation, mental disability, advanced age, physical illness or disability, chronic use of drugs or alcohol, detention by a foreign power, disappearance, or other cause, to the extent that such adults are incapable of managing their estates.[1] The court must also find that the appointment is necessary either because the property will be wasted or dissipated unless proper management is provided or because the property is needed to

---

1. O.C.G.A. § 29-5-6(a)(3)(B).

support and care for the well-being of the individual or those entitled to be supported by that individual.[2]

Any person not otherwise disqualified may be appointed guardian of the property of an incapacitated adult and the preference of the proposed ward is to be considered by the court in selecting the guardian. The order of preference set forth by Georgia law with regard to guardians appointed for the person of an incapacitated adult also applies to guardians of the property.[3]

(B) Procedure for Appointment of Guardian of the Property of an Incapacitated Adult

Any interested individual or individuals, including the alleged incapacitated person and the Department of Human Resources, may file a petition under oath for the appointment of a guardian. The petition is filed with the probate court in the county in which the alleged incapacitated person resides or is found. The petition for the appointment of a guardian shall set forth

1. the name, age, address, and county of residence of the proposed ward;

2. the name, address, and county of residence of the petitioner;

3. the relationship of the petitioner to the proposed ward;

4. a statement of the reasons the proposed guardianship is sought;

5. the type of and any foreseeable limits on duration of guardianship sought;

6. the names and addresses of the spouse and all adult children of the proposed ward who are living and whose addresses are known;

7. the names and addresses of the representatives of the alleged incompetent individual;

8. all known income and assets of the proposed ward;

9. the name of the county in which such property is located; and

10. the name and address of any individual or individuals nominated by the petitioner to serve as guardian.[4]

---

2. O.C.G.A. § 29-5-1(a)(2).
3. O.C.G.A. § 29-5-2(b); *see* chapter 4.2.
4. O.C.G.A. §§ 29-5-6(a)(1) and (2).

Furthermore, the petition must be supported by an affidavit of a physician licensed to practice medicine in Georgia or of a licensed psychologist stating that he or she has examined the proposed ward within 10 days prior to the filing of the petition and that, on the basis of that examination, the proposed ward was determined to be incapacitated.[5] In addition to stating the specific incapacity of the proposed ward and the facts that support the determination, the affidavit must state any foreseeable limits on the duration of such incapacity.[6] If the judge of the probate court determines that there is such evidence, the judge will (a) immediately notify the proposed ward of the proceedings by personal service; (b) inform the proposed ward of the place and time at which the proposed ward shall submit to the evaluation provided for by Georgia law and the right to independent counsel; and (c) give notice of the petition by first class mail to the spouse and to all adult children of the proposed ward whose addresses are known.[7]

(C) Hearing for Guardian of the Property of an Incapacitated Adult

If, after the review, the court finds that there is probable cause to support a finding that the proposed ward is incapacitated, the probate court will schedule a hearing on the petition. The date of the hearing must not be less than 10 days after the date on which the notice is mailed to the proposed ward. Either the proposed ward or the petitioner may file a written response to the evaluation report at any time up to the conclusion of the hearing. The response may include, but is not limited to, independent evaluations, affidavits of individuals with personal knowledge of the proposed ward, and a statement of applicable law.[8]

If, after the review, the court finds that there is no probable cause to support a finding that the proposed ward is incapacitated within the meaning of Georgia law, the probate court shall dismiss the petition.[9] If the judge does find probable cause, a hearing must be scheduled. The procedures for the hearing are set

---

5. O.C.G.A. § 29-5-6(a)(3).
6. O.C.G.A. § 29-5-6(a)(4).
7. O.C.G.A. § 29-5-6(b)(2).
8. O.C.G.A. § 29-5-6(d)(1).
9. O.C.G.A. § 29-5-6(d)(2).

out in chapter 4.2. The hearing will be held in a regular court-room, if available, or at such place as the judge may set.

If it is determined that a guardian is necessary, in its order the court must set forth the findings of facts and conclusions of law that support the grant of the petition. If a guardianship is granted, the order must specify the type of guardianship established; the name(s) of the guardian or guardians and the reason for the selection; the nature and extent of the ward's incapacity; any rights or powers retained by the ward; the duration of the guardianship (whether limited or permanent); the reasonable sums or property to be provided to the guardian; the type and frequency of physical, mental, and social evaluations of the ward's condition; any reporting requirements in addition to those required by law; any bonding requirements in addition to those required by law; and any such other and further provisions of the guardianship as the court may deem proper.[10]

After service of the court's order, the ward's counsel must make reasonable efforts to explain the order and the ward's rights to him. If the ward desires to appeal the court's order, the attorney will file the notice in the ward's behalf; and, if counsel was appointed by the probate court, the appointment will continue on appeal to the superior court.[11]

In any case involving the creation of a guardianship over the property of an adult in which the proposed ward owns real property, the judge or clerk of the probate court must file, within 30 days after issuing the order granting the petition or terminating the guardianship, a certificate with the clerk of the superior court of each county of the state in which the ward owns real property to be recorded with the deed records for the county and indexed under the name of the ward.[12]

(D) Powers and Duties of the Guardian of the Property of an Incapacitated Adult

The guardian of the property of the adult ward must give a bond when required by the judge of the probate court. The bond must be in an amount equal to the value of the estate if the bond is secured by a licensed commercial surety, and double the value of the estate if not. The guardian has similar powers, duties, com-

---

10. O.C.G.A. § 29-5-6(f)(1).
11. O.C.G.A. § 29-5-6(f)(3).
12. O.C.G.A. § 29-5-6(f)(4).

pensations, and liabilities as are set forth by Georgia law with respect to guardians of an incapacitated adult or minor.[13] More specifically, a guardian of the property of an incapacitated individual provides for the necessary support, care, or well-being of those individuals who are entitled to be supported by the ward, to the extent consistent with the needs of the ward and the resources of the ward's estate.[14] The guardian may petition the probate court for an order allowing the ward's real or personal property, or any part thereof, to be sold, leased, encumbered, or exchanged by the guardian, upon such terms as the court may order, for the following purposes:

1. payment of the ward's debts;

2. provision of the ward's care;

3. maintenance, support, and education of those who are legally dependent upon the ward; or

4. investment of the proceeds in other property.[15]

Furthermore, the court may authorize the guardian of the property of an incapacitated individual to make transfers of personal or real property, outright or in trust, on behalf of the ward, on finding that a competent person in the ward's circumstances would make the transfer and that there is no evidence that if the ward were competent, he would not make said transfer.[16] The court may also authorize the guardian of the property to apply principal or income of the ward's estate that is not required for the support of the ward during the ward's lifetime or for the support of those individuals who are legally dependent upon the ward toward the establishment of an estate plan for the purpose of minimizing income, estate, inheritance, or other taxes payable out of the ward's estate. The following factors must be taken into consideration:[17]

1. the value of the entire estate of the ward;

2. the probable expenses for the support, care, and maintenance of the ward and the support of those individuals who are legally dependent upon the ward for the remainder of the ward's lifetime in the standard of living to which the ward and such legally dependent individuals have become accustomed;

---

13. O.C.G.A. § 29-5-4.
14. O.C.G.A. § 29-5-5.
15. O.C.G.A. §§ 29-2-3, 29-5-4, and 29-5-5.1(a).
16. O.C.G.A. § 29-5-5.1.
17. *Id.*

3. the identity of the proposed transferees;

4. the purpose and estate planning benefit to be derived by the transfer, as well as the possible harm to any interested party; and

5. any previous history of or predisposition toward making similar transfers by the ward.

(E) Effect of Appointment of Guardian

Persons determined incapacitated by Georgia law or alleged to be so incapacitated shall not be deprived of any property rights without due process of law. Unless the court order specifies that one or more of the following powers are to be retained by the ward, the appointment of a guardian of the property of an incapacitated adult removes

1. the power to bring or defend any lawsuit, except through the guardian or guardian *ad litem*;

2. the power to make contracts;

3. the power to buy, sell, or otherwise dispose of or encumber real or trust property; and

4. the power to enter into other business or commercial transactions.[18]

Each ward has the right to have his property used to provide adequately for his support, care, education, and well-being.[19]

(F) Appointment of Emergency Guardians of the Property of Adults

In the event that a proposed ward is gravely incapacitated and an emergency guardian is necessary, a guardian may be appointed for the person or property, or both, of the ward in accordance with Georgia law. There must be (a) an immediate, clear, and substantial risk of death or serious physical injury, illness, or disease unless an emergency guardian is appointed; or (b) an

18. O.C.G.A. § 29-5-7(e).
19. O.C.G.A. § 29-5-7(g)(3).

immediate, substantial risk of irreparable waste or dissipation of the estate of the proposed ward unless an emergency guardian is appointed.[20]

In the event the court determines that there is probable cause to appoint an emergency guardian, the court will

1. order an examination of the proposed ward;

2. order an emergency hearing;

3. immediately appoint counsel to represent the proposed ward;

4. under extreme circumstances, appoint an emergency guardian to serve until the emergency hearing;

5. in its discretion, order that, pending the emergency hearing, no withdrawals may be made from any account on the authority of the proposed ward's signature without prior approval from the court, if there is a substantial risk of dissipation of any bank or savings and loan account in which the proposed ward has an interest and if the risk is so immediate and the potential harm so irreparable that any further delay would be unreasonable.[21]

Any emergency guardian appointed under Georgia law has only those powers and duties specifically enumerated in the order of the probate court, and such powers and duties may not exceed those absolutely necessary to respond to the immediate, threatened risk to the ward or his or her property enumerated in the petition.[22] All emergency guardianships will terminate immediately after the full hearing set forth by statute, 45 days after the filing of the petition, or on a date specified in the court's order appointing the emergency guardian, whichever occurs first.

(G) Modification or Termination of Guardianship of the Property of an Incapacitated Adult

Upon the petition of any interested individual, including the incapacitated individual, or upon the probate court's own motion after review of the guardianship reports, a guardianship of the property of an adult ward may be modified or terminated by the court in the event of

---

20. O.C.G.A. § 29-5-8(b).
21. O.C.G.A. § 29-5-8(d).
22. O.C.G.A. § 29-5-8(f).

1. a conflict of interest, unfitness that substantially impairs the guardian's ability to perform his duties, or misconduct by the guardian;
2. the resignation or death of the guardian;
3. the death of the ward;
4. a proper showing that the need for the guardianship has ended; or
5. a significant change in the extent of the incapacity of the ward or the circumstances of the ward or the guardian.[23]

A guardianship with a specific duration ends automatically upon its expiration.[24] Upon termination of the guardianship, title to all property should revert to the ward.

---

23. O.C.G.A. § 29-5-9(a).
24. O.C.G.A. §§ 29-5-9(c) and 29-5-9(d).

4.4

Annulment of Marriages

Whereas a divorce dissolves what was once a valid marriage, annulment is a process whereby a marriage is declared void and legally held to never have existed. Annulment has significant legal ramifications. A decree of annulment has the effect of total divorce between the parties that voids the marriage and returns the parties to their original status before the attempted marriage.[1] MHPs may become involved in annulment proceedings since one ground for annulment is the inability of a person to enter into a marriage contract due to mutual incompetence.

(A) Grounds for Annulment

Marriages declared void by law are marriages of individuals unable to contract, unwilling to contract, or fraudulently induced to contract.[2] Thus, with one exception, a purported marriage that is lacking in one or more of the essential elements of marriage[3] is totally invalid from its inception and may be annulled by a superior court.[4] The one exception is a marriage invalid because of fraud, duress, or non-age within which a child is born or is about to be born as a result of the union of the parties. In this event, the only available remedy is divorce.[5]

---

1. O.C.G.A. § 19-4-5.
2. O.C.G.A. § 19-3-5.
3. *See* chapter 4.1.
4. O.C.G.A. § 19-4-1.
5. Wallace v. Wallace, 221 Ga. 510, 513, 145 S.E.2d 546 (1965); Beebe v. Beebe, 227 Ga. 248, 250, 179 S.E.2d 758 (1971).

If the grounds for annulment are the same as the grounds for divorce, the parties to an invalid marriage have the option of filing a petition for annulment or a petition for divorce.[6]

(B) Procedure for Annulment

Annulment of marriage may be granted only by the superior courts of Georgia.[7] The proceeding is commenced by a petition that is filed by the party seeking the annulment or "by next friend" in the case of minors or individuals of unsound mind.[8] All matters of residence, jurisdiction, service, procedure, pleading, and practice are the same as provided by law for obtaining a divorce with the exception that a decree for annulment may be ordered by a judge at any time after 30 days after personal service regardless of the failure of the respondent to file an answer or a contest to the petition.[9]

---

6. O.C.G.A. § 19-4-2.
7. O.C.G.A. § 19-4-1.
8. O.C.G.A. § 19-4-3.
9. A court may partition or determine the rights of the parties to jointly held property, may restore the status quo as to all property brought to the purported marriage, and may "otherwise do equity as between the parties." See McKinney v. McKinney, 242 Ga. 607, 608, 250 S.E.2d 470 (1978).

No-Fault Divorce

Prior to 1973, divorce law in Georgia (and in many other states) required the petitioning party to allege fault by the other party in order to obtain a divorce. The Georgia General Assembly had established a specific list of 12 grounds, any one of which was sufficient for a total divorce.[1] In 1973, the General Assembly added a 13th ground for divorce: "that the marriage is irretrievably broken," which is commonly referred to as the "no-fault" ground for divorce.[2] Divorce litigation now generally centers around property division, child support, spousal maintenance, or child custody. MHPs may contribute to this process in numerous ways, including appearing as an expert witness for either party, making examinations on behalf of the court, or assisting the parties through counseling.

(A) Divorce Procedure

The dissolution of marriage is initiated by the filing of a complaint in one of the superior courts of the state, which courts have exclusive jurisdiction over divorce actions. Generally, the complaint must show the following specific elements:

1. that the court has jurisdiction over the subject matter;[3] specifically, that the parties are married and that the plaintiff or

---

1. Ga. Laws 1956, p. 405.
2. O.C.G.A. § 19-5-3(13).
3. Mickas v. Mickas, 229 Ga. 10, 189 S.E.2d 81 (1972).

defendant has been a resident of the state of Georgia for 6 months prior to the date of filing the complaint;[4]

2. that the court has jurisdiction of the parties;[5]

3. that the action is brought in the proper venue, either the county of residence of the defendant, if he or she is a resident of Georgia, or the county of residence of the plaintiff, if the defendant is a nonresident of the state;[6]

4. the date of the marriage;

5. that the parties are living in a *bona fide* state of separation and the date of separation;[7]

6. one or more of the 13 grounds for divorce;[8]

7. the basic elements of a claim for temporary or permanent alimony and child support, if they are being sought; and

8. the names and ages of any minor children of the party.[9]

In addition to "irretrievably broken," grounds for total divorce include adultery, willful and continued desertion for a period of 1 year, habitual intoxication, mental or physical cruel treatment, incurable mental illness, and habitual drug addiction.[10] An irretrievably broken marriage is one within which "either or both parties are unable or refuse to cohabit, and there are no prospects for a reconciliation."[11] The parties do not have to complain specifically of each other's conduct. They merely state that their marital differences are insoluble and request a change of status. The only question is whether there are prospects for a reconciliation.[12]

Upon the finding that the marriage should be dissolved, the court can reserve jurisdiction to hear evidence and to make provisions for division of property. Matters as to child support and child custody are exclusively left to the trial judge, whereas either of the parties may request a jury trial on the issues of alimony and division of property. These matters are all incorporated into a decree of divorce, which becomes final when entered.

---

4. O.C.G.A. § 19-5-5; Walton v. Walton, 223 Ga. 85, 87, 153 S.E.2d 554 (1967).
5. O.C.G.A. § 19-5-5.
6. *Id.*
7. Sutton v. Sutton, 224 Ga. 140, 160 S.E.2d 385 (1968); O.C.G.A. § 19-5-5.
8. *Id.; see also* O.C.G.A. § 19-5-3.
9. O.C.G.A. § 19-5-5.
10. O.C.G.A. § 19-5-3.
11. Harwell v. Harwell, 233 Ga. 89, 90, 209 S.E.2d 625 (1974).
12. *Id.*

4.6

Child Custody After Marital Dissolution

Child custody determinations can result from four types of changes in the legal status of a marriage: annulment, legal separation, divorce, and modification of a divorce decree. MHPs may become involved in this determination in one of two ways. First, a party or the court may request a custody evaluation that involves the parents and children, which may culminate in court appearances as an expert witness. Second, an MHP who has provided services to the family unit, whether diagnostic or therapeutic, may be subpoenaed by either party to present evidence as a witness.

(A) Criteria to Establish Court Jurisdiction in Child Custody Cases

The authority of the court to assume jurisdiction over the child is generally a factual determination based upon the domicile of the child and the parents. For instance, if a child is living in Georgia at the commencement of the proceeding, the court automatically assumes jurisdiction. If, however, the child and the parents are not domiciled in Georgia, a court of this state has jurisdiction to make a child custody determination or modification only in the following situations:

1. Georgia is the home state of the child;

2. Georgia has been the child's home state within 6 months before the commencement of the proceeding, the child is absent from this state because of his or her removal or retention by a person claiming his or her custody or for other reasons, and the parent or person acting as parent continues to live in this state;

3. It is in the "best interest of the child" that a court of this state assume jurisdiction because the child and his or her parents, or the child and at least one party, have "significant connections" with the state, and there is available in the state substantial evidence concerning the child's present or future care, protection, training, and personal relationships;

4. The child is physically present in this state, and the child has been abandoned; or it is necessary, in an emergency, to protect the child because he or she has been subjected to or threatened with mistreatment or abuse or is otherwise neglected or dependent; and

5. It appears that no other state would have jurisdiction under prerequisites substantially in accordance with the foregoing requirements, or another state has declined to exercise jurisdiction on the ground that Georgia is the more appropriate forum to determine the custody of the child, and it is in the best interest of the child that the Georgia court assume jurisdiction.[1]

When jurisdiction is disputed, an MHP may be asked to testify as to the nature and quality of the child's relationships with persons in this state, as well as the advisability of a Georgia court assuming jurisdiction compared to a court in the state in which the child resides.

(B) Standard for Custody Determinations: Best Interest of the Child[2]

In all cases in which the custody of any minor child is involved, there is no *prima facie* right to custody in the mother or father, but the court hearing the custody issue may use its sound discretion and take into consideration all of the circumstances of the case in

---

1. O.C.G.A. §§ 19-9-42 through 19-9-64.
2. O.C.G.A. § 19-9-3(a); Gambrell v. Gambrell, 244 Ga. 178, 259 S.E.2d 439 (1979).

making its award of custody.[3] Thus, in a contest between parents, the controlling issue, often very complicated but simply stated, is: whatever is for the best interest of the child must be done.[4]

In deciding what constitutes the best interest of the child, the court may consider all relevant factors, including the fitness of the parties as evidenced by the character, conduct, and reputation of either of the parties, as well as any other evidence tending to throw light on their fitness to be the custodian.[5] The wish of the child may be considered along with other relevant evidence to enable the court to determine what custody arrangement is best for the child.[6] A child who is at least 14 years of age has the right to select the parent with whom he or she desires to live, and such selection is controlling unless the parent so selected is determined not to be a fit and proper person to have custody.[7] Other factors that may be evaluated in determining what is in the best interest of a child include, but are not limited to, the interaction and relationship of the child with the parents, siblings, and any other person who may significantly affect the child's interests; the child's adjustment to home, school, and community; and the mental and physical health of all individuals involved. On any number of these issues, an MHP could be called upon to testify as an expert to assist the parties or the trial court by evaluating the parties or the child involved, or both.

A parent not granted custody of the child or children is entitled to reasonable visitation rights unless the court finds that visitation would not be in the best interest of the child or that the noncustodial parent is morally unfit.[8] There are no preset formulas or guidelines for determining visitation, and the court will usually consider the same factors as used in the custody determination to assign reasonable visitation rights.

3. O.C.G.A. § 19-9-3(a); Turner v. Turner, 150 Ga. 191, 103 S.E. 413 (1920).
4. Ottinger v. Pelt, 217 Ga. 758, 125 S.E.2d 52 (1962).
5. Adams v. Heffernan, 217 Ga. 404, 122 S.E.2d 735 (1961); Lindsey v. Lindsey, 238 Ga. 685, 235 S.E.2d 6 (1977); Eller v. Matthews, 216 Ga. 315, 116 S.E.2d 235 (1960); Gambrell v. Gambrell, 244 Ga. 178, 259 S.E.2d 439 (1979).
6. Chunn v. Graham, 117 Ga. 551, 43 S.E. 987 (1903); Wills v. Glunts, 222 Ga. 122, 149 S.E.2d 106 (1966).
7. O.C.G.A. § 19-9-1.
8. Schowe v. Amster, 236 Ga. 720, 225 S.E.2d 289 (1976); Griffin v. Griffin, 226 Ga. 781, 177 S.E.2d 696 (1970); see, generally, O.C.G.A. §§ 19-9-1 and 19-9-3.

(C) Mental Status and Custody Evaluations: Mandatory and Voluntary

When the parents cannot agree on custody, requiring the court to make the determination, there are several means by which the parties, including the children, may be required to undergo a psychological evaluation. First, the law allows the court to order a mental examination whenever the mental or physical condition of a party is at issue.[9] This code section provides, "When the mental or physical condition (including the blood group) of a party, or of a person in the custody or under the legal control of a party, is in controversy, the court in which the action is pending may order the party to submit to a physical or mental examination by a physician or to produce for examination the person in his custody or legal control."[10] Only a physician is allowed to conduct a mental evaluation under this rule. Second, the court handling a divorce or alimony case involving the custody of a child or children may transfer the question of the determination of custody to the juvenile court for investigation or report back to the superior court.[11] An MHP may be appointed by the court to perform a custody evaluation and make a report as to what custody arrangement is in the child's best interest. Finally, in a proceeding involving the determination of custody when there has been an allegation of abuse or neglect of the child, the court may direct, on its own motion or upon the motion of one of the parties, an investigation of the home life and environment of the parents. An evaluation by an MHP, including a social worker, may be a part of the investigation of the home life.[12] The court may also order a psychological evaluation of either or both parents, as well as the child.[13]

---

9. O.C.G.A. § 9-11-35(a).
10. *Id.*
11. O.C.G.A. § 15-11-6.
12. O.C.G.A. § 19-9-4.
13. Rowe v. Rowe, 393 S.E.2d 750, 195 Ga. App. 493 (1990).

4.7

Reporting of Adult Abuse

The law requires certain professionals to report known or suspected abuse, neglect, or exploitation of disabled adults. Abuse and neglect generally refer to behavior resulting in physical harm, whereas exploitation concerns economic matters. This is a mandatory law that carries criminal sanctions for noncompliance. Furthermore, failure to follow this law may result in civil liability arising from suits brought by the adults whom this law is designed to protect.

(A) Terms and Definitions

Before discussing the reporting requirements, it is helpful to understand the terms used in this law.

1. *Disabled adult* means a person 18 years of age or older who is not a resident of a long-term care facility, but who is mentally or physically incapacitated.[1] *Mental incapacity* generally means an impairment by reason of mental illness, mental deficiency, mental disorder, physical illness or disability, advanced age, chronic use of drugs, chronic intoxication, or other cause to the extent that the individual lacks sufficient understanding or capacity to make or communicate responsible decisions concerning his or her person.

---

1. O.C.G.A. § 30-5-3(6).

2. *Abuse* means the willful infliction of physical pain, physical injury, mental anguish, unreasonable confinement, or the willful deprivation of essential services to a disabled adult.[2]
3. *Neglect* means the absence or omission of essential services to the degree that it harms or threatens the physical or emotional health of a disabled adult.[3]
4. *Exploitation* means the illegal or improper use of a disabled adult or that adult's resources for another's profit or advantage.[4]
5. *Caretaker* means a person who has the responsibility for the care of a disabled adult as a result of family relationship, contract, voluntary assumption of that responsibility, or by operation of law.[5]

(B) Who Must Report

The law requiring reporting of abuse of a disabled adult applies to any physician, osteopath, intern, resident, or other hospital or medical personnel, dentist, psychologist, podiatrist, nursing personnel, social work personnel, day care personnel, or law enforcement personnel.[6] Additionally, any other person having information regarding a disabled adult may report such information to an adult protection agency providing protective services or to an appropriate law enforcement authority or district attorney.[7]

(C) When a Report Must Be Made

A report must be made by a mandatory reporter when he or she has reasonable cause to believe that a disabled adult has had a physical injury or injuries inflicted upon him or her, other than by accidental means, by a caretaker or has been neglected or exploited by a caretaker. The duty to report concerns only past incidents. However, it attaches regardless of the source of the harm.

---

2. O.C.G.A. § 30-5-3(1).
3. O.C.G.A. § 30-5-3(10).
4. O.C.G.A. § 30-5-3(9).
5. O.C.G.A. § 30-5-3(2).
6. O.C.G.A. § 30-5-4(a)(1).
7. O.C.G.A. § 30-5-4(a)(2).

(D) How a Report Must Be Made

A report must be made to the Director of the County Department of Family and Children Services in the county in which the disabled adult resides or is present, by either oral or written communication.[8] The report must include the name and address of the disabled adult and should include the name and address of the disabled adult's caretaker; the age of the disabled adult; the nature and extent of the disabled adult's injury or condition resulting from abuse, neglect, or exploitation; and any other pertinent information.[9]

(E) Immunity From Liability

Anyone who makes a report pursuant to this law, who testifies in any judicial proceeding arising from the report, who provides protective services, or who participates in a required investigation under the provisions of the law is immune from any civil or criminal liability on account of such report, testimony, or participation, unless the person acted in bad faith or with a malicious purpose.[10]

(F) Confidentiality and Privilege

Most services provided by an MHP are confidential, either through law or the ethics of the profession (see chapter 3.3). Confidentiality is waived, however, to the extent that the MHP is required to report suspected adult abuse. In addition to requiring an MHP to report suspected adult abuse, the law requires the staff and physicians of local health departments, mental health clinics, and other public agencies to cooperate fully with the director of the county Department of Family and Children Services.[11] The director may contract with an agency or private physician for the purpose of providing immediate, accessible medical evaluations at the location that the director deems to be most appropriate. Again, if an MHP is called on by the director to assist in an evaluation of a disabled adult, the services are not confidential to the extent that the MHP is required to provide information to the director, the court, or others involved in the process with a need

---

8. O.C.G.A. § 30-5-4(b).
9. *Id.*
10. O.C.G.A. § 30-5-4(c).
11. O.C.G.A. § 30-5-6(a).

to know. An MHP is not, however, free to disclose information to third parties not directly involved in the case. All records pertaining to the abuse, neglect, or exploitation of disabled adults in the custody of the Department of Human Resources are confidential, and access thereto by persons other than the department personnel, the director, or the district attorney, may be only by valid subpoena or order of court of competent jurisdiction.[12]

(G) Failure to Report

A person required by the law to report a case of disabled adult abuse who fails knowingly and willfully to make such a report is guilty of a misdemeanor and may be punished by a fine not to exceed $1,000.00 or by confinement in jail for a total term not to exceed 12 months, or both.[13]

---

12. O.C.G.A. § 30-5-7.
13. O.C.G.A. §§ 30-5-8(b) and 17-10-3(a).

Reporting of Child Abuse

Georgia law requires certain professionals to report known or suspected incidents of child abuse.[1] The purpose of this law is to provide for the protection of children whose health and welfare are adversely affected and threatened by the conduct of those responsible for their care and protection. It is declared to be the intent of the legislature that the mandatory reporting of such cases will cause the protective services of the state to be brought to bear on the situation in an effort to prevent further abuse, to protect and enhance the welfare of these children, and to preserve family life whenever possible.[2] Although the initial duty to report is discharged once the report is properly filed, the MHP may also have to appear in court proceedings as a witness on these issues.

(A) Who Must Report

The law applies to any physician, licensed osteopathic physician, intern, resident, and all other hospital or medical personnel, dentist, psychologist, podiatrist, nursing personnel, professional counselors, social work personnel, school teachers and school administrators, school guidance counselors, child care personnel, day care personnel, child counseling personnel, child service organization and personnel, or law enforcement personnel.[3]

---

1. O.C.G.A. § 19-7-5.
2. O.C.G.A. § 19-7-5(a).
3. O.C.G.A. § 19-7-5(c).

(B) When a Report Must Be Made

The duty to report arises when a mandatory reporter has reasonable cause to believe that a child under the age of 18 years has had physical injury or injuries inflicted upon him or her by a parent or caretaker by other than accidental means, has been neglected or exploited by a parent or caretaker, or has been sexually assaulted or sexually exploited. A child is sexually exploited when the child's parent or caretaker allows, permits, encourages, or requires such child to engage in prostitution or to engage in sexually explicit conduct for the purpose of producing any visual or print medium depicting such conduct.[4] The abuse report must be made "as soon as possible" after the discovery of the alleged abuse.[5] The law pertains only to past events, not to acts of child abuse that may occur in the future.

The reporting requirement does not distinguish between harm caused by parents and harm caused by others. More important, the fact that a parent is seeking treatment for the child does not absolve the professional of the duty to report. Thus, when a parent brings a child to an MHP for psychological problems that qualify as "emotional damage," there is a duty to report unless the situation was "accidental."

The duty to report is fulfilled by making an oral report as soon as possible by telephone or other means, which is to be followed by a report in writing, if requested, to a child welfare agency providing protective services, as designated by the Department of Human Resources, or, in the absence of such agency, to an appropriate police authority or district attorney.[6] If a report of child abuse, sexual assault, or sexual exploitation is made to the child welfare agency or independently discovered by the agency, and the agency has reasonable cause to believe such report is true, then the agency shall immediately notify the appropriate police authority or district attorney.

The report must contain the following:

1. the names and addresses of the child and his or her parents or caretakers, if known;
2. the child's age;
3. the nature and extent of the child's injuries, including any evidence of previous injuries; and

---

4. O.C.G.A. § 19-7-5(b)(4).
5. O.C.G.A. § 19-7-5(e).
6. *Id.*

4. any other information that the reporting individual believes may be helpful in establishing the cause of the injuries and the identity of the perpetrator.[7]

(C) Immunity From Liability

Any individual, partnership, firm, corporation, association, hospital, or other entity participating in the making of a report to a child welfare agency pursuant to this law or participating in any judicial proceeding shall be immune from any civil or criminal liability that might otherwise be incurred or imposed. There is no immunity, however, when the reporting individual acts in bad faith[8] or has been charged with or is suspected of harming the child or children in question.[9]

In *Michaels v. Gordon*,[10] the Georgia Court of Appeals held that the statutory grant of immunity includes not only making a report of child abuse, but participating in judicial proceedings as well. Dr. Gordon, a licensed psychologist, was asked by the county Department of Family and Children Services to perform an evaluation of a child's condition in connection with an investigation of suspected child molestation. Dr. Gordon submitted a report and later testified regarding her conclusions that the child had been sexually abused. After the juvenile court concluded that the evidence did not support a finding of child abuse, the parents sued Dr. Gordon for professional malpractice. The Court of Appeals concluded that the statutory grant of immunity applied not only to a person who makes a report of abuse, but also to a person who participates in subsequent proceedings connected with a child abuse report. The court further concluded that evidence of unprofessional conduct or negligence was not sufficient to show that Dr. Gordon had acted in bad faith.[11]

(D) Confidentiality and Privilege

Information gained by an MHP in therapy is confidential, either through law or the ethics of the profession (see chapter 3.3). However, under the child abuse reporting law, there is a specific provision that provides that suspected child abuse shall be re-

---

7. *Id.*
8. O.C.G.A. § 19-7-5(f).
9. Austin v. State, 179 Ga. App. 235, 345 S.E.2d 688 (1986).
10. 39 S.E.2d 722 (Ga. App. 1993).
11. *Id.* at 725.

ported notwithstanding the fact that the reasonable cause to believe such abuse has occurred or is occurring is based in whole or in part on any privileged or confidential communication.[12] Thus, the privilege is waived to the extent that the MHP is required to report the child abuse or to testify regarding the child abuse. The waiver of the privilege is limited, and an MHP is not permitted to divulge confidential or privileged information to third parties not involved in the child abuse reporting process.

(E) Sanctions for Failure to Report

Any individual or official required to report a suspected case of child abuse who knowingly and willfully fails to do so is guilty of a misdemeanor punishable by a fine of up to $1,000.00 or imprisonment of up to 12 months, or both.[13]

---

12. O.C.G.A. § 19-7-5(g).
13. *Id.*

4.9

Abused and Neglected Children

Procedures for handling cases involving abused, neglected, or deprived children typically involve three stages:[1]

1. carrying out a preliminary investigation, taking the child into temporary custody, or both;
2. holding an adjudicatory hearing on a petition; and
3. holding a hearing on an appropriate disposition.

It is generally a hierarchical process may stop at any point at which it is determined that the allegations are unfounded or that the parents are currently capable of raising their children in a responsible manner. Each stage may involve a mental health evaluation of the child or parents, or both. In addition, the MHP may be called to testify as an expert witness at a hearing at any of these stages. Finally, the MHP may be called as an expert witness to testify at a hearing regarding termination of parental rights. (See chapter 4.10.)

---

1. The Juvenile Code uses the term *deprived child*, defined as a child who is without proper parental care or control, subsistence, education as required by law, or other care or control necessary for his physical, mental, or emotional health or morals; has been placed for care or adoption in violation of law; has been abandoned by his parents or other legal custodian; or is without a parent, guardian, or custodian. *See* O.C.G.A. § 15-11-2(8).

(A) Investigation and Temporary Custody Intervention by Department of Human Resources

The Department of Human Resources is authorized and empowered to investigate complaints of deprivation, abuse, or abandonment of children by parents, guardians, custodians, or individuals serving in the place of parents.[2] On the basis of the findings of an investigation, social services may be offered to the parents, guardians, custodians, or other persons to attempt to resolve any problems that are being experienced in raising the child.[3] The appropriate personnel, usually a representative of the Department of Family and Children Services for the county in which the child is located, may also bring the situation to the attention of a law enforcement agency, an appropriate court, or other community agency for appropriate action.[4] During such investigation or attempt to provide assistance, employees of the Department of Human Resources may request assistance from an MHP for evaluation or advice. Additionally, juvenile court probation officers are empowered to make investigations and reports regarding complaints and charges of delinquency, unruly conduct, or deprivation of a child.[5]

A probation officer is directed to take into custody or to supervise and assist a child on probation or corrective supervision if the officer has reasonable cause to believe that the child's health or safety or that of another is in imminent danger or that the child may abscond or be removed from the court's jurisdiction, or by an appropriate court order. A probation officer may not conduct an accusatory proceeding against a child under the probation officer's care or supervision. Likewise, an officer is not liable for failure to take into custody or detention a child who later commits some act for which he or she could be detained if, in the probation officer's judgment, detention or custody was not warranted. Probation officers are authorized to make appropriate referrals to other private or public agencies of the community if the assistance of those agencies appears to be needed or desirable.[6] The probation officer may also give advice to parties with a view toward an informal adjustment of a problem involving an allegedly deprived child if it appears that this course of action is

---

2. O.C.G.A. § 49-5-8(a)(2)(B).
3. Id.
4. Id.
5. O.C.G.A. § 15-11-8.
6. Id.

in the best interest of the public and of the child. Advisory actions and informal adjustments may be taken prior to the filing of any formal petition regarding the child, but such informal adjustments cannot extend beyond 3 months without a court order allowing the extension.[7]

The probation officer may also take into custody and detain a child who is under the officer's supervision or care as a delinquent, unruly, or deprived child if the probation officer has "reasonable cause" to believe that the child's health or safety is in imminent danger, that the child may abscond or be removed from the jurisdiction of the court, or when an appropriate court has so ordered.[8] A child may also be taken into custody by a law enforcement officer or other duly authorized officer of the juvenile court pursuant to the laws of arrest if there are reasonable grounds to believe that the child has committed a delinquent act, is suffering from illness or injury, or is in immediate danger from his or her surroundings and removal is necessary.[9]

As a matter of public policy, no accused child shall be restrained prior to adjudication without probable cause to believe that the accused is, in fact, guilty and there is clear and convincing evidence that the child's freedom should be restrained. Interim contact or detention is used to protect the jurisdiction and process of the court, to protect against the likelihood of infliction of severe bodily harm to others, or, upon the child's request, to protect the juvenile from imminent bodily harm. Interim control or detention cannot be imposed to punish, treat, or rehabilitate the juvenile; to allow the parents to avoid their legal responsibilities; to satisfy demands by the victim, police, or community; or to permit convenient access or investigation. If unconditional release is not feasible, a conditional or supervised release that provides the least interference with the juvenile's liberty is favored over more intrusive alternatives. In all situations, the exercise of the court's authority should protect the privacy, dignity, and individuality of the accused juvenile and his or her family, as well as the mental and physical health of the child; ensure a tolerance of diverse values and preferences, together with equal treatment regardless of race, class, ethnicity, and gender; and avoid regimentation, depersonalization, and stigmatization.[10] Finally, the juvenile shall be informed of his or her right to consult with an attorney.[11]

An officer taking a child into custody must deliver the child to a medical facility if the child is believed to suffer from a serious

---

7. O.C.G.A. § 15-11-14.
8. O.C.G.A. § 15-11-8(2)-(5).
9. O.C.G.A. §§ 15-11-17(a)(4) and 15-11-18.
10. O.C.G.A. § 15-11-18.1.
11. *Id.*

physical condition or illness that requires immediate treatment and must promptly notify a juvenile court or intake officer. The intake officer must then determine whether the child should be released or detained.[12] The officer taking the child into custody must also give prompt notice that the child has been taken into custody, together with a statement of the reasons, for taking the child into custody, to a parent, guardian, or other custodian and to the juvenile court.[13] Bail is given to a juvenile as a matter of right, the same as is given to an adult.[14]

A child alleged to be delinquent, unruly, or deprived may be placed and detained only in a licensed foster home or a home approved by the juvenile court, which may be a public or private home, the home of the noncustodial parent or of a relative, a facility operated by a licensed child welfare agency, or a detention center that is under the supervision of the court or agency approved by the court.[15] The actual physical placement of a child who is alleged to be deprived requires the approval of the judge of the juvenile court or his designee.[16]

Once the child is brought before the court or delivered to a detention or shelter care facility, the intake or other authorized juvenile court officer must immediately make an investigation and release the child unless it appears that his detention or shelter is required.[17] If the child is not released, an informal detention hearing must be held not later than 72 hours after the child is placed in shelter care to determine whether the child's detention is required.[18] If the child alleged to be deprived is not released after the formal detention hearing, a formal petition for release must be presented to the juvenile court within 5 days of the hearing.[19]

(B) Commencement of Formal Proceedings

The juvenile court of each county has the exclusive jurisdiction over juvenile matters and is the sole court for initiating action concerning any child who is delinquent, unruly, incorrigible, or

---

12. O.C.G.A. § 15-11-19(a)(2).
13. O.C.G.A. § 15-11-19(c).
14. O.C.G.A. § 15-11-19(d).
15. O.C.G.A. § 15-11-20(a).
16. O.C.G.A. § 15-11-20(f).
17. O.C.G.A. § 15-11-21(a).
18. O.C.G.A. § 15-11-21(c)(1)(2)(3).
19. O.C.G.A. § 15-11-21(e).

deprived,[20] or conducting any proceedings for the termination of the parent–child relationship.[21] A formal proceeding in the juvenile court regarding a case of alleged child delinquency, unruliness, or deprivation is initiated by the filing of a petition.[22] The petition is filed in the county in which the child resides or in which the child is present when the deprivation action is commenced.[23] If delinquent or unruly conduct is alleged, the proceeding may be commenced in the county in which alleged delinquent or unruly acts occurred.[24] A petition alleging misconduct or deprivation of a child may be made by any person, including a law enforcement officer, who has knowledge of the facts alleged or is informed and believes that they are true.[25] However, the petition cannot be filed unless the juvenile court or a person authorized by the court has determined that the filing of the petition is in the best interest of the public and the child.[26]

The petition itself must set forth a statement that it is in the best interest of the child and the public that the proceeding be brought; the name, age, and address of the child on whose behalf the petition is brought; the names and addresses of the parents, guardian, or custodian of the child and of the child's spouse, if any; and, if the child is in custody, the place of his detention and the time he was taken into custody.[27]

(C) The Conduct of Hearings

Once the juvenile court takes jurisdiction of the matter, hearings are conducted at which the child and other interested parties have a right to representation by counsel.[28] The first hearing (called an adjudicatory hearing) is conducted without a jury. The judge is clothed with wide discretion because of the particular nature of the matters before the court and may adjourn the hearing, dismiss the petition, discharge the child from detention, or order restrictions placed on the child. After hearing the evidence, the court can proceed immediately to a disposition if it determines beyond a reasonable doubt that the child is deprived, needs treatment or rehabilitation, or is a delinquent or unruly child. This finding triggers a dispositional hearing within 30 days of the adjudicatory

---

20. O.C.G.A. § 15-11-5(a)(1).
21. O.C.G.A. § 15-11-5(a)(2)(C).
22. O.C.G.A. § 15-11-11(4).
23. O.C.G.A. § 15-11-15.
24. Id.
25. O.C.G.A. § 15-11-24.
26. O.C.G.A. § 15-11-23.
27. O.C.G.A. § 15-11-25.
28. O.C.G.A. § 15-11-30(b).

hearing. In juvenile court proceedings, the court is governed and directed in all instances by what it perceives to be the "best interests of the child" and conducive to the child's welfare.[29] The court has the duty to advise parties of their entitlement to be represented by legal counsel at all stages of any proceedings alleging delinquency, unruliness, incorrigibility, or deprivation, and, if the party is an indigent person or under "undue hardship" and cannot afford counsel, the court will provide legal representation if requested to do so.[30]

(D) Adjudicatory Hearings

The initial hearing is a nonjury proceeding recorded by stenographic notes (unless waived), which is conducted with only the parties, witnesses, court personnel, and family or persons assisting the child present. The court has discretion to exclude the child from the hearing at any time, except while inquiring into allegations of delinquency or unruly conduct.

In the adjudicatory phase of the process, either the juvenile court solicitor or someone from the district attorney's office will conduct the hearing. In the event that no one from the district attorney's office is available, a court-appointed legal counsel may be substituted. The district attorney, as the state's representative, is provided full access to all files, documents, reports, and hearing transcripts, and may, on the basis of the pretrial investigation, file a motion to dismiss the petition based on an insufficiency of evidence.[31]

(E) Additional Rights of the Child and Parties

Georgia law ensures that any party to a juvenile court hearing has the basic due process right to introduce evidence and to be heard in his or her own behalf and to confront and cross-examine witnesses.[32] The law provides that a child charged with delinquency cannot be a witness against or otherwise incriminate himself or herself. Illegally obtained out-of-court statements are specifically excluded, as is evidence seized illegally. An out-of-

---

29. O.C.G.A. § 15-11-1(2).
30. O.C.G.A. § 15-11-3(a).
31. O.C.G.A. § 15-11-28.
32. O.C.G.A. § 15-11-31.

court confession alone is deemed to be insufficient to establish a determination of delinquency.[33]

(F) Social Study and Report

When the petition alleges delinquency, unruliness, or deprivation, and such assertions are admitted by a party, or if notice of a hearing under Georgia law has been given,[34] the court may direct a social study and report in writing to be made by the probation officer concerning the child, his environment, and his family. Also, the probation officer may order an examination of the child by a physician or psychologist. In an appropriate case, medical or surgical treatment may be ordered on the basis of the opinion of a licensed physician that prompt medical attention is needed. The treatment may be ordered whether or not the parents or guardian have given consent.[35]

(G) The Dispositional Hearing

After the adjudicatory phase is concluded, the court will direct that a second, dispositional hearing be conducted for delinquent or unruly children, for deprived children, or for children committing delinquent acts constituting an AIDS-transmitting crime.[36] The appropriate remedy will be fashioned by the court. The child may be held in custody between the two hearings for a period of not more than 30 days (unless written statements regarding a need for delay are filed, at which time inquiries into the need for treatment, rehabilitation, or supervision are made). Information and reports used by the court must be made available to the parties. The individuals making the report are subject to cross-examination. Those portions of the report not relied on by the court in reaching its decision may be withheld if release would be prejudicial to the child or other parties. The court, in its discretion, may keep sources of information confidential.[37]

---

33. *Id.*
34. O.C.G.A. § 15-11-39.
35. O.C.G.A. § 15-11-32.
36. O.C.G.A. §§ 15-11-33, 15-11-34, 15-11-35, and 15-11-35.1.
37. O.C.G.A. §§ 15-11-33(c) and (d).

(H) A Deprived Child

The disposition for a deprived child focuses on which parents, guardian, or custodian, including a putative father, is best suited to care for the child and what type of supervision is indicated for the child. The probation officer or agency designated by the court recommends to the court those individuals who are qualified to care for the child. While awaiting the formulation of a placement plan, deprived children are not confined with delinquent children.[38]

Delinquent children may receive the same disposition as deprived children. Alternatively, they may be placed on probation under conditions and limitations, under the supervision of a public agency authorized by law or any community rehabilitation center willing to accept responsibility for the child. The court may also place the child in an institution, camp, or facility operated under the direction of the court or commit the child to the Department of Children and Youth Services. Continued education, restitution, community service, and driver's license suspension are considered alternative or additional remedies available to the court.[39]

(I) Victim Impact Statement

A victim impact statement is a statement that generally describes the victim, the physical injury or economic loss sustained by the victim, and the effect of the child's act on the victim's personal welfare or family relationships. The victim is also asked to identify any psychological services sought by him or the family as a result of the offense and to supply any additional information the court requires. This statement may be used by the district attorney or the judge at any stage of the proceedings.

If the victim is unable to provide the information, the victim's attorney or a family member may complete the form on the victim's behalf. The statement will be attached to the case file and used by the district attorney or judge during any stage of the proceeding involving predisposition, disposition, or determination of whether to grant restitution or not. In no event, however, does the failure to comply with the provision of this law invalidate the proceeding or create a separate cause of action for any party or establish grounds for appeal.[40]

---

38. O.C.G.A. § 15-11-34.
39. O.C.G.A. § 15-11-35.
40. O.C.G.A. § 15-11-28(f)(1) and (2).

4.10

Termination of Parental Rights

After child abuse or deprivation has been reported and the Georgia Department of Human Resources has made an investigation, the question will sometimes arise as to whether parental rights should be terminated. This is an extreme measure that occurs rarely, particularly if it is the first allegation of abuse or deprivation. If the determination is made to petition for termination of parental rights, the parent is afforded the same range of procedural due process rights as when a deprivation petition is filed (see chapters 4.9 and 4.16). Because such a decision inevitably involves consideration of the child's emotional well-being and of the parent–child relationship, MHPs are frequently called on to undertake individual and family evaluations to assist the court in its decision.

(A) Filing the Termination Petition: Petition Requirements

The petition must be verified, but may be based on information and belief. It must set forth the facts that bring the child within the jurisdiction of the court, with a statement that it is in the best interest of the child and the public that the proceeding be brought. The petition must also include the name, age, and residence address of the child on whose behalf the petition is brought and the names and residence addresses, if known, of the parents, guardian, or custodian of the child.[1] The petition must also state

---

1. O.C.G.A. §§ 15-11-82(a) and O.C.G.A. 15-11-25.

clearly that an order for termination of parental rights is requested.[2] Finally, the petition must also assert one of the following grounds that support termination of parental rights:

1. The parent has abandoned the child;

2. The child is a deprived child, and the conditions and causes of the deprivation are likely to continue; by reason thereof, the child is suffering or probably will suffer serious physical, mental, moral, or emotional harm;

3. The parent has given written consent acknowledged before the court; or

4. A decree has been entered by a court of competent jurisdiction ordering the parent, guardian, or other custodian to support the child, and the parent, guardian, or other custodian has wantonly and willfully failed to comply with the order for a period of 12 months or longer.[3]

(B) Effect of Order Terminating Parental Rights

An order terminating the parental rights of a parent terminates all his or her rights and obligations with respect to the child and all rights and obligations of the child to the parent arising from the parental relationship, including rights of inheritance. The parent is not thereafter entitled to notice of proceedings for the adoption of the child and does not have the right to object to the adoption or to participate in the proceedings.[4]

If there is no parent having parental rights after the termination order is entered, the court must commit the child to the custody of the Department of Human Resources or a licensed child-placing agency for the purpose of placing the child for adoption or, in the absence of an adoption, in a foster home. The new custodian of the child has the authority to consent to the adoption of the child, his or her marriage, enlistment in the armed forces of the United States, and surgical and other medical treatment for the child.[5]

---

2. O.C.G.A. § 15-11-82.
3. O.C.G.A. § 15-11-81.
4. O.C.G.A. § 15-11-80.
5. O.C.G.A. § 15-11-90.

4.11

Guardianship for Minors

A guardian may be appointed for a minor when the custodial parent is unable to care for the child as a result of death, legal termination of parental rights, or other circumstances. MHPs become involved in the guardian selection process and follow-up treatment, if any, for the children. The power of a guardian over the person of his or her ward is the same as that of the parent over the child. It is the duty of the guardian to protect and maintain and, according to the circumstances of the ward, to educate the child.[1]

(A) Application for Guardianship

There are two methods for appointing a guardian of a minor. The first is by testamentary appointment in which the parents indicate in their will whom they wish to be guardians of their children.[2] If one parent is dead, the surviving parent, by will, may appoint a guardian for the person of his or her minor child or children.[3] A testamentary guardian stands on the same footing as other guardians.[4] Children who do not have a guardian and who are over the age of 14 years before a guardian is appointed have the privilege of selecting a guardian. If the selection is judicious, the judge of the probate court will appoint the guardian so selected. Once this privilege has been exercised, the ward may not do so again,

---

1. O.C.G.A. § 29-2-1.
2. O.C.G.A. § 29-4-3(a).
3. O.C.G.A. § 29-4-3(b).
4. O.C.G.A. § 29-4-3(d).

except upon cause shown for the removal of the guardian first selected.[5] A testamentary appointment becomes effective when the guardian files an acceptance in the court in which the will is probated.

The second method of appointment is by application for appointment as guardian. Every application for appointment of a guardian of a minor under the age of 14 years who is not the child of the applicant must be made to the judge of the probate court and served upon three nearest adult relatives of the child who reside in Georgia or a notice of the application must be published once a week for 4 weeks. The guardianship may be granted to the applicant or to some other person in the court's discretion.[6] If there is no application for letters of guardianship and the necessity for a guardian exists, the judge of the probate court, after giving notice for 30 days, "may vest the guardianship in the county guardian, the clerk of the superior court of the county, or any person or persons residing in the county, whom he, in his discretion, deems fit and proper."[7]

The nearest relative will be preferred for guardianship of the minor. Among collateral relatives applying for the guardianship of a minor child, the nearest kin by blood, if otherwise unobjectionable, is preferred. However, the judge of the probate court may exercise his or her discretion and grant the letters of guardianship to one who is not a blood relative.[8]

(B) The Guardianship Process

Before entering upon the duties of his or her appointment, every guardian appointed by the probate court must take an oath or affirmation before the judge to perform well the duties required of the guardianship and to account faithfully to the ward for the estate. A guardian must give bond when required with good and sufficient security, approved by the probate judge. If the guardian is for the person only, the court, in its discretion, may dispense with the requirement that the guardian give bond; and, in the event that bond is required, it may not exceed $1,000.00.[9]

When the appointment of a guardian is made at a regular term, the taking of the oath or affirmation and the giving of the

---

5. O.C.G.A. § 29-4-4.
6. O.C.G.A. § 29-4-10.
7. O.C.G.A. § 29-4-11.
8. O.C.G.A. § 29-4-8.
9. O.C.G.A. § 29-4-12.

bond may be done at any time thereafter. The bond, when taken, shall be recorded by the judge in a book to be kept for that purpose, and the original is kept on file in the judge's office.[10]

Unless otherwise provided by Georgia law, if both parents are alive, either parent is the natural guardian of a minor child. If a parent is dead or if the parents are legally separated or divorced, the parent having legal custody of the child is the natural guardian.[11]

The law does not clearly specify what "circumstances" are sufficient to authorize the appointment of a guardian. Presumably, this would involve a situation in which the parents are unable to carry out their parental responsibilities and their powers and duties are given to a guardian.

The court next determines who should be appointed guardian. In considering a given candidate, courts usually consider what would be in the best interest of the minor. Although there are specific statutes for custody determinations following marital dissolution (which use a "best interest" standard), there is no specific statutory provision setting forth the factors to be considered. Furthermore, although there are numerous cases applying the best interest standards in custody disputes, it is not clear that the standard will be the same when at least one parent is deceased. Finally, it is clear that when one parent is deceased, there is a presumption in favor of the other parent. When there are specific circumstances indicating that the best interest of the child would be served by placing guardianship in another, the presumption is overcome.[12]

Although there is no statutory law regarding duties and liabilities of guardians of minors, guardians should have the same powers and responsibilities as parents, except that guardians should not be legally obligated to provide their own funds for the children and should not be liable to third persons for acts of the children. The law also does not specify the exact duties of guardians of minors. However, consistent with Georgia law with regard to guardians of adults, guardians of minors are expected to

1. take reasonable care of the child's personal effects;
2. receive money for the support of the child;
3. facilitate the child's education, and social and other activities;
4. authorize medical or other professional care, treatment, or advice;

---

10. O.C.G.A. § 29-4-13.
11. O.C.G.A. § 29-4-2.
12. *See* Whitlock v. Barrett, 158 Ga. App. 100, 279 S.E.2d 244 (1981); Girtman v. Girtman, 191 Ga. 173, 11 S.E.2d 782 (1940).

5. consent to marriage or adoption of the child; and

6. report on the condition of the child if required by court order.

Pursuant to Georgia law, every guardian is allowed all reasonable disbursements and expenses suitable to the circumstances of the ward committed to his care, as well as the necessary expenses of maintaining, supporting, and educating those who may be legally dependent on the ward. The expenses of maintenance and education must not exceed the annual profits of the estate, absent the prior approval of the judge of the probate court. The judge, in his discretion, may allow the corpus of the estate, in whole or in part, to be used for the maintenance and education of the ward and for the necessary expenses of maintaining, supporting, and educating those who may be legally dependent on the ward.[13]

(C) Termination of the Guardianship

Although the statutory law with regard to the termination of the guardianship of minors is vague, the following principles would be consistent with Georgia law with regard to guardianship of adults. A guardian's authority and responsibility should terminate upon the death, resignation, or removal of the guardian; upon the child's death, adoption, or marriage; or upon the child's attainment of majority. Any person interested in the welfare of the child should be able to petition for removal of the guardian on the ground that removal would be in the best interest of the child. The court should then hold a hearing to determine whether it is in the child's best interest to terminate the guardianship. If the court determines that it is, the court should then appoint a new guardian.

It should be noted that pursuant to Georgia law,[14] if the judge of the probate court knows or is informed that any guardian wastes or in any manner mismanages the property of his or her ward, does not take care of the maintenance and education of his or her ward according to his circumstances, fails or refuses to make returns as required by law, or for any cause is unfit for his trust, the judge shall require the guardian to answer the charges against him or her and in the judge's discretion may

1. revoke the guardian's letters;

---

13. O.C.G.A. § 29-2-2.
14. O.C.G.A. § 29-2-45.

2. require the guardian to appear and submit to a settlement of his or her accounts; and/or

3. pass such other order as in his judgment is expedient under the circumstances of the case.

Letters of dismission may also be granted by the judge of the probate court to any guardian. The guardian makes an application in writing for letters of dismission, setting forth his full discharge of the duties of his trust. The judge examines the guardian's accounts and vouchers to verify the truth of the application. The application must be published one time in the public newspaper in which legal notices of the office of the judge of the probate court are usually published. Thereafter, the judge examines any objections filed. Proof is offered to show that the ward is of age or that there is no longer a necessity for continuing the guardianship.

In all cases in which the estate does not exceed $2,500.00, a guardian may be granted letters of dismission without compliance with the described application procedures if

1. the guardian was appointed for a minor ward who would not otherwise require a guardian but for that minority;

2. the ward has reached the age of majority;

3. the guardian has filed verified application for letters of dismission setting forth the guardian's full discharge of the duties of that trust; and

4. the guardian has made a satisfactory final accounting to the judge of the probate court.[15]

---

15. O.C.G.A. § 29-2-84(b).

4.12

Guardians of the Property of Minors

While guardians of the person are appointed to undertake parental responsibilities for minors when the parents are absent or incapacitated (see chapter 4.11), guardians of the property are charged with the responsibility of managing or protecting the estate (e.g., money, property, and business enterprises) of a minor. There is no requirement that the minor also have a guardian of the person appointed. Although this is primarily a financial determination, MHPs may be involved in the guardian selection process and follow-up treatment for the child.

(A) Application for Guardians of the Property of Minors

The judge of the probate court of the county in which a minor is domiciled has the power to appoint a guardian of the property of the child.[1] Although Georgia law is vague as to the exact contents of the petition for guardian of the property of a minor, the petition should describe:

1. the interest of the petitioner:
2. the name, age, residence, and address of the person to be protected;
3. the name and address of the guardian, if any, of the person to be protected;

---

1. O.C.G.A. § 29-4-4.

4. the name and address of the nearest relative of the person to be protected known to the petitioner;

5. a general statement of the property of the person to be protected with an estimate of the value, including any compensation, insurance, pension, or allowance that is due to the person;

6. reasons why appointment of a guardian of the property of the minor is necessary; and

7. reasons for the appointment of a particular person as guardian of the property of the minor.

Although Georgia law is silent as to the particular circumstances that justify the appointment of a guardian for the property of a minor, other jurisdictions have specified that the court may appoint a guardian of the property of a minor if it determines that

1. the minor owns money or property that requires management or protection that cannot otherwise be provided;

2. the minor may have business affairs that may be jeopardized or prevented by minority; or

3. funds are needed for support and education, and protection is desirable to provide said funds.

(B) Authority and Responsibilities of the Guardian of the Property

The court may appoint an individual or a corporation as guardian of the estate. The order of preference, which the court may bypass with a good reason, is the nearest of kin by blood.[2] The judge of the probate court, however, may exercise his discretion according to the circumstances of each case and, if necessary, may grant guardianship to one who is not a blood relative.

(C) Sale, Lease, or Exchange of a Minor Ward's Property

Whenever any guardian deems it necessary or in the best interests of his or her ward to sell, lease, exchange, or encumber the estate of the ward, or any part thereof, the guardian shall file with the judge of the probate court of the county of the guardian's appointment or of the county in which the property is situated in the case

---

2. O.C.G.A. § 29-4-8.

of a foreign guardian, a petition for authority to dispose of the property. The court, on such terms as it deems appropriate, may order the property to be sold, leased, exchanged, or encumbered for the following purposes:

1. payment of the ward's debts;
2. provisions for the ward's care;
3. maintenance, support, and education of those who are legally dependent on the ward; or
4. investment of the proceeds in other property.[3]

---

3. O.C.G.A. § 29-2-3.

Foster Care

Foster care provides residential housing and support under the supervision of the Department of Human Resources for children and adults who are not able to live at home. The person may be placed in a foster home for as little as one night or as long as several years. MHPs may be involved in the licensing of a home and in assessment and therapeutic services to those placed in them.

(A) Certificate at the Foster Home

Before any child is brought or sent into the state for the purpose of placing him in a foster home, the person so bringing or sending such child shall first notify the Department of Human Resources of his intention and must obtain from the Department of Human Resources a certificate stating that such home is, in the opinion of the Department of Human Resources, a suitable home for the child. Such notification must state

1. the name, age, and personal description of the child;
2. the name and address of the person with whom the child is to be placed; and
3. such other information as may be required by the Department of Human Resources.[1]

The person bringing or sending such child into the state must report at least once each year and at such other times as the

---

1. O.C.G.A. § 49-5-16.

Department of Human Resources shall direct as to the location and well-being of the child so long as such child remains within the state and until he has reached the age of 18 years or has been legally adopted.[2]

(B) Licensing and Inspection of Private and Public Child Welfare Agencies

Single or married persons may apply to the Department of Human Resources for licensure to provide foster care services using the department's form for licensure of a foster home. The Department of Human Resources will consider applicant's age; the applicant's criminal record, if any; the applicant's income; and the applicant's physical and mental health. A licensed medical practitioner should describe the applicant's general physical and mental health, including any emotional problems that would prevent him or her from properly caring for foster children.

Georgia also licenses child welfare agencies, which, for purposes of Georgia law, are defined as any child-caring institution, child-placing agency, maternity home, group day care home, and day care center.[3]

The Department of Human Resources assists applicants or licensees as child welfare agencies in meeting departmental standards. If a licensee is denied renewal of a license, if a license is revoked, or if any applicant for a license cannot meet the department's standards, the department assists in the placement of the children in the agency's custody or in some other licensed child welfare agency, returns them to their own homes, or makes other plans or provisions as may be necessary and advisable to meet the particular needs of the children involved.[4] Application for a license must be made to the Department of Human Resources on forms furnished by the department. Upon receipt of an application for a license and upon presentation by the applicant of evidence that the child welfare agency meets the standards prescribed by the Department of Human Resources, the department will issue the child welfare agency a license for a 1-year period.[5]

---

2. *Id.*
3. O.C.G.A. § 49-5-12(a).
4. O.C.G.A. § 49-5-12(c).
5. O.C.G.A. § 49-5-12(d).

In the event that the Department of Human Resources finds that any child welfare agency applicant does not meet the department's standards, but is attempting to meet such standards, the department may, in its discretion, issue a temporary license to the agency. A temporary license shall not be issued for more than a 1-year period. Upon presentation of satisfactory evidence that the agency is making progress toward meeting prescribed standards, the department may, in its discretion, reissue the temporary license for one additional period not to exceed 1 year. As an alternative to a temporary license, the department, in its discretion, may issue a restricted license that states the restrictions on its face.[6]

The department may refuse a license upon a showing of the following:[7]

1. noncompliance with the rules and regulations for day care centers, family day care homes, or group day care homes as adopted by the Board of Human Resources, which are designated in writing to the facilities as being related to health and safety;

2. flagrant and continued operation of an unlicensed facility in contravention of the law; or

3. prior license denial or revocation within 1 year of application.

All licensed child welfare agencies must prominently display the license issued to the agency by the Department of Human Resources at some point near the entrance of the premises in a manner that is open to view by the public. The department's action revoking or refusing to renew or issue a license required by law must be preceded by notice and an opportunity for a hearing and constitutes a contested case within the meaning of the Georgia Administrative Procedure Act, except that only 30 days' notice in writing is required prior to license revocation. Hearings relating to license denial or revocation may be closed to the public if the hearing officer determines that an open hearing would be detrimental to the physical or mental health of any child who will testify at the hearing.[8]

Child-caring institutions and child-placing agencies, when licensed in accordance with Georgia law, may receive needy or dependent children from their parents for special, temporary, or continued care. Parents, guardians, custodians, or persons serving *in loco parentis* to such children may sign releases or agreements giving such institutions or agencies custody and control

---

6. O.C.G.A. § 49-5-12(e).
7. O.C.G.A. § 49-5-12(f).
8. O.C.G.A. § 49-5-12(h).

over the children during the period of care.[9] Child-placing agencies, in placing children in foster family homes, must safeguard the welfare of the children by thoroughly investigating each home and the character and reputation of the persons residing therein and must adequately supervise each home during the period of care. All children placed in foster family homes must, as far as is practicable, be placed with persons of the same religious faith as the children or the children's parents.[10]

It is the duty of the department to inspect at regular intervals all licensed child welfare agencies within the state, including all family boarding homes, foster family homes, and family day care homes. The department has the right of entrance, privilege of inspection, and right of access to all children under the care and control of the licensee.[11] If any flagrant abuses, derelictions, or deficiencies are made known to the department or its duly authorized agents during their inspection of any child welfare agency or if, at any time, violations are reported to the department, the department is required to immediately investigate and take such action as may be required.[12] In the event that abuses, derelictions, or deficiencies are found in the operation and management of any child welfare agency, they must be brought immediately to the attention of the management of such agency. If not corrected within a reasonable time, the department will revoke the license of such agency in the manner prescribed by law.[13]

Each child welfare agency makes a periodic report of its work to the Department of Human Resources in such form and at such time as the department prescribes. The department prepares and supplies child welfare agencies with all forms needed for the purpose of providing the department with such information as may, from time to time, be required by the department.[14]

Child welfare agencies and other facilities and institutions in which children and youths are detained that are operated by any department or agency of state, county, or municipal government are not subject to licensure under Georgia law, but the Department of Human Resources may, through its authorized agents, make periodic inspections of such agencies, facilities, and institutions. Reports of such inspections must be made privately to the proper authorities in charge of such agencies, facilities, or institutions. The department is required to cooperate with such authorities in the development of standards that will adequately protect

---

9. O.C.G.A. § 49-5-12(i).
10. O.C.G.A. § 49-5-12(j).
11. O.C.G.A. § 49-5-12(k).
12. O.C.G.A. § 49-5-12(l).
13. O.C.G.A. § 49-5-12(m).
14. O.C.G.A. § 49-5-12(n).

the health and well-being of all children and youths detained by such agencies, facilities, or institutions.

The department may recommend changes in programs and policies and if, within a reasonable time, the standards established by the department and the recommendations of the department are not met, it is the duty of the commissioner to make public the inspection and departmental recommendations. If any serious abuses, derelictions, or deficiencies are found and are not corrected within a reasonable time, the commissioner must report them in writing to the governor.[15]

Any child welfare agency that operates without a license issued by the department is guilty of a misdemeanor and, upon conviction thereof, shall be punished by a fine. Each day of operation without a license constitutes a separate offense.[16] In addition, no person, official, agency, hospital, maternity home, or institution, public or private, in Georgia may receive or accept a child under 17 years of age for placement or adoption or place such a child, either temporarily or permanently, in a home other than the home of the child's relatives without having been licensed by the Department of Human Resources.[17]

In addition to being in good mental health, foster parents should also have good parenting skills. These include an ability to provide nurturance, warmth, intellectual stimulation, and protection of the children from harm; an understanding of and the ability to handle the emotional, physical, developmental, educational, and intellectual needs of children; and a wholesome attitude toward and an understanding of habit training, discipline, health, nutrition, sex education, and the various experiences that a child may have and with which a child may need assistance and guidance.

A foster home may also qualify to receive children with special needs such as physical handicaps, an emotional disability, or a delinquent background. Parents in these special foster homes should have had previous training or experience or a demonstrated willingness to care for children with special needs. They should also have the ability to work effectively with specialists involved in the evaluation and treatment of the child's condition.

A home may also qualify as a receiving foster home for short-term emergency placement. These parents should have a household that is exceptionally flexible and capable of accepting children of varied cultural and racial backgrounds, in all states of emotional stress, at all hours of the day and night. All foster home

---

15. O.C.G.A. § 49-5-12(o).
16. O.C.G.A. § 49-5-12(p).
17. O.C.G.A. § 49-5-12(q).

parents should be willing to participate in specialized training when offered by the Department of Human Resources.

(C) Powers and Duties of Department of Human Resources With Regard to Foster Care

The Department of Human Resources is authorized and empowered to establish, maintain, extend, and improve throughout the state, within the limits of funds appropriated therefor, programs that will provide child welfare services through boarding care or through the payment of maintenance costs in foster family homes or in group care facilities for children and youths who cannot be adequately cared for in their own homes.[18]

In addition, the Department of Human Resources regulates child-placing and child-caring agencies by

1. setting standards, providing consultation, and making recommendations concerning establishment and incorporation of child welfare agencies; and

2. licensing and inspecting regularly such agencies to ensure their adherence to established standards as prescribed by the Department of Human Resources. In the event that the foster parents should decide to submit a petition for the adoption of a foster child, the Department of Human Resources may inquire into the character and reputation of the applicants.[19]

The Department of Human Resources may also provide for miscellaneous services, such as medical, hospital, psychiatric, surgical, or dental services or provide for the payment of the costs of such services as may be considered appropriate and necessary by competent medical authority, to those children subject to the supervision and control of the Department of Human Resources without securing prior consent of parents or legal guardians.[20]

---

18. O.C.G.A. § 49-5-8(a)(1)(E).
19. O.C.G.A. § 49-5-8(a)(7)(D).
20. O.C.G.A. § 49-5-8(a)(9).

(D) Placement of Children in Foster Homes

Prior to placing a child in a foster home, the Department of Human Resources or a licensed child welfare agency must arrange for a complete medical examination and any other diagnostic evaluation as is necessary. If the investigation and medical examination disclose no physical, mental, or emotional reasons for special care, and if the child is not found to be delinquent, the child may be placed in a regular foster home. If special care is required, or if the child has been found to be delinquent, the child may be placed only in certain foster homes. The Department of Human Resources or a licensed agency will then establish a placement plan that should contain the purpose for which the child has been placed in foster care, the length of the time in which the purpose of foster care will be accomplished, the description of the services which are to be provided in order for the purposes of foster care to be accomplished, and the person within the Department of Human Resources or the agency who is directly responsible for ensuring that the plan is implemented.

4.14

Adoption

The law sets out specific procedures that must be followed in the adoption process in order to protect the rights of the child and the natural parents. Compliance with such procedures is a necessary precondition to a valid adoption. Georgia law also provides that individuals who wish to adopt a child must meet certain minimum requirements (described in the chapter that follows). MHPs may contribute to this process by providing mental health evaluations of prospective adoptive parents and children, and treatment of the adopted children, if necessary.

(A) Adoption Requirements: Adoptive Parents

Any adult resident of Georgia, whether married, unmarried, or legally separated, may try to qualify to adopt a child. A husband and wife may jointly adopt. More specifically, any adult person may petition to adopt a child if the person

1. is at least 25 years old or is married and living with a spouse;
2. is at least 10 years older than the child;
3. has been a bona fide resident of Georgia for at least 6 months immediately preceding the filing of the petition; and
4. is financially, physically, and mentally able to have permanent custody of the child.[1]

---

1. O.C.G.A. § 19-8-3.

(B) Investigation by Agency

Unless otherwise provided by law, prior to the date set by the court for a hearing on the petition for adoption, it is the duty of a child-placing agency or other independent agent appointed by the court to verify the allegations in the petition for adoption, to make a complete and thorough investigation of the entire matter, and to report its findings and recommendations.[2]

Under Georgia law, the report and findings of the investigating agency must include

1. verification of allegations contained in the petition;
2. circumstances under which the child came to be placed for adoption;
3. whether the proposed adoptive parent(s) is financially, physically, and mentally able to have the permanent custody of the child;
4. the physical and mental condition of the child, insofar as this can be determined by a competent medical authority;
5. whether or not the adoption is for the best interest of the child;
6. suitability of the home to the child;
7. whether the identity and location of the putative father are known or are ascertainable and whether the requirements pertaining to such as set forth by Georgia law were complied with, if applicable; and
8. any other information that might be disclosed by the investigation that would be of value or interest to the court in deciding the case.[3]

In the event that it appears to the court that the interests of the child may conflict with those of the petitioner(s), the court may, in its discretion, appoint a guardian *ad litem* to represent the child.[4]

The goal in the adoption process is to duplicate the relationship that most persons have with their natural parents.[5] With regard to the adoptive parents, the court should review a complete social history of the applicants, including information about their financial condition, moral fitness, religious background, physical and mental condition, and any court actions involving child abuse.

---

2. O.C.G.A. § 19-8-16.
3. O.C.G.A. § 19-8-17(a).
4. O.C.G.A. § 19-8-17(c).
5. *See* Drummond v. Fulton County Department of Family and Children Services, 563 F.2d 1200 (5th Cir. 1977), *cert. denied*, 437 U.S. 910, 98 S. Ct. 3103 (1978).

(C) Adoptive Child

Only children who are under the age of 18 years (the age of majority) at the time a petition for adoption is filed may be adopted. In the case of a child 14 years of age or older, the written consent of the child to the adoption must be given and acknowledged in the presence of the court.[6] With regard to the adoptive child, the court should review the following factors:

1. whether the natural parents, if living, are willing to have the child be adopted and the reasons for such willingness;

2. whether the natural parents have abandoned the child or are unfit to have custody of the child;

3. whether the parent–child relationship has been previously terminated by court action and the circumstances of the termination;

4. the heritage of the child and of the natural parents, and the mental and physical condition of the child and of the natural parents;

5. the existing and proposed arrangements as to the custody of the child; and

6. the adoptability of the child and the suitability of the child's placement with the applicants.

(D) Petition for Adoption

The petition, duly verified, together with one conformed copy thereof, must be filed with the clerk of the superior court having jurisdiction. Generally, the petition must set forth the following information:

1. the name, age, and place of residence of the petitioner(s);

2. the name by which the child is to be known should the adoption ultimately be completed;

3. the date of birth and the sex of the child;

4. the date and circumstances of the placement of the child with the petitioner(s);

---

6. O.C.G.A. § 19-8-4(b).

5. whether the child is possessed of any property and, if so, a full and complete description thereof;

6. whether the child has one or both parents living; and

7. whether the child has a guardian of his or her person.[7]

When required by law, applicable affidavits from the Department of Human Resources or from a licensed child-placing agency, required consents, and required certifications must be provided or attached when the petition is filed. If the petition is filed in a county other than that of the petitioner's residence, the reason therefor must be set forth in the petition.[8] Except as otherwise provided by law, the petitioner(s) in any proceeding for the adoption of a minor must file with the petition, in a manner acceptable to the court, a report fully accounting for all disbursements of anything of value made or agreed to be made, directly or indirectly, by, on behalf of, or for the benefit of the petitioner(s) in connection with the adoption. The report must show any expenses incurred in connection with

1. the birth of the minor;

2. the placement of the minor with the petitioner(s);

3. medical or hospital care received by the mother or by the minor during the mother's prenatal care and confinement; and

4. services relating to the adoption or to the placement of the minor for adoption that were received by or on behalf of the petitioner(s), either natural parent of the minor, or any other person.[9]

Every attorney for the petitioner(s) in any proceeding for the adoption of a minor, in which proceeding the petitioner(s) is required to file an accounting pursuant to law, must file, in a manner acceptable to the court, before the decree of adoption is entered, an affidavit of all sums paid or promised to him or her, from whatever source, for all services of any nature rendered or to be rendered in connection with the adoption; provided, however, that if the attorney received less than $500.00, the affidavit need only state that fact.[10] Whenever a petitioner is a grandparent or blood relative of the child to be adopted and another grandparent has visitation rights with the child granted pursuant to Georgia law, the petitioner must forward a copy of the petition for adop-

---

7. O.C.G.A. § 19-8-13.
8. O.C.G.A. § 19-8-13(a).
9. O.C.G.A. § 19-8-13(c).
10. O.C.G.A. § 19-8-13(d).

tion to the grandparent with visitation rights or to such person's attorney.[11]

Upon the filing of the petition for adoption, the court will fix a date on which the petition shall be considered, which date is not less than 60 days from the date of filing. Copies of the petition, the order fixing the date on which the petition is to be considered, and all exhibits, surrenders, or certificates required by law are then forwarded to the Department of Human Resources, together with a request that a report and investigation be made as required by law.[12]

In the event that the court wishes more information, it may direct that a social study be made by the Department of Human Resources, an agency, or other qualified personnel. The social study should include information regarding the child's social history, the child's present condition and placement, and adjustment in the home of the petitioners (if any), as well as the suitability of the adoptive parents' home.

The natural parents must consent in writing to releasing their child for adoption except when the parental rights have been judicially terminated.[13] Furthermore, if after a hearing about which all persons who may be affected by the adoption have been given notice, the court may waive the requirement of consent if it determines that the interests of the child are promoted by a waiver. The court may not, however, waive consent when the parent objects absent a showing of cause. In essence, this means that a court may not grant a petition for adoption when the natural parents object unless there are grounds for termination of parental rights (see chapter 4.10).

For the consent to be valid, it must be in writing, signed by the individual giving consent and witnessed. The form for the consent is set forth in the Georgia code.[14] The consent should fully describe the consenting party, the child, the adoptive parents, and the Department of Human Resources or the agency that places the child for adoption.

---

11. O.C.G.A. § 19-8-13(f).
12. O.C.G.A. § 19-8-14.
13. O.C.G.A. § 19-8-4.
14. O.C.G.A. § 19-8-26.

(E) Hearing and Decree of Adoption

On the scheduled date, the court will conduct to a full hearing on the petition in chambers. The court will examine the parties under oath and give consideration to the investigation report and the recommendations contained therein. The court will also examine the petition for adoption, the affidavit, and the financial disclosures. The court is free to make such examination of the petitioner(s) and his attorney as it deems appropriate.[15]

The court must find that each living parent or guardian of the child has surrendered or had terminated all rights to the child in the manner provided by law prior to the filing of the petition for adoption; that the petitioner(s) has satisfied his burden of proof required by law that he is capable of assuming responsibility for the care, supervision, training, and education of the child; that the child is suitable for adoption in a private family home; and that the adoption is in the best interest of the child. The court may then enter a decree of adoption, terminating all the rights of the parent(s) or guardian(s) to the child, granting the permanent custody of the child to the petitioner(s), naming the child as prayed for in the petition, and declaring the child to be the adopted child of the petitioner(s).[16]

If the court determines that the petitioner(s) has not complied with the requirements for adoption, it may dismiss the petition for adoption without prejudice, or it may continue the case. In the event that the court is not satisfied that the adoption is in the best interest of the child, it will deny the petition. If the petition is denied, the court may commit the child to the custody of the Department of Human Resources or to a licensed child-placing agency. The court may permit the child to remain in the custody of the petitioner(s) if the petitioner(s) is fit to have custody, or the court may place the child with the Department of Human Resources for the purpose of determining whether or not a new petition should be initiated.[17]

---

15. O.C.G.A. § 19-8-18(a).
16. O.C.G.A. § 19-8-18(b).
17. O.C.G.A. §§ 19-8-18(c) and (d).

(F) Surrender of Parental Rights

A surrender of parental rights to the Department of Human Resources or to a licensed child-placing agency must be executed in the presence of a representative of the department or the agency, under oath, and following the birth of the child. A copy will be delivered to the parent(s) or guardian(s) signing the surrender at the time of its execution.[18]

A parent or guardian signing a surrender has the right to withdraw the surrender by written notice within 10 days after signing, and the surrender document shall not be valid unless it so states. After 10 days, a surrender may not be withdrawn. The notice of withdrawal of surrender must be delivered in person or by registered or certified mail to the person or agency to whom the child was surrendered, at the address designated in the surrender document.[19] Furthermore, the procedure for surrender of parental rights requires strict compliance.[20]

(G) Notice to Putative Father

In the event that the identity and location of the putative father of a legitimate child or a child born out of wedlock are known and he has not executed a surrender as provided for by law, then he must be notified of the mother's surrender or of the proceeding to terminate her parental rights by registered or certified mail, return receipt requested, at his last known address.[21]

If the identity and location, or either, of the putative father of a legitimate child or a child born out of wedlock is not known and he has not executed a surrender as provided by law, then a petition to terminate the biological father's rights to the child must be filed.[22] When the rights of a parent or guardian of the child have been surrendered or terminated in accordance with the law, the Department of Human Resources, a licensed child-placing agency, or the person petitioning for adoption may file such a petition with the court. The court must, within 30 days of such filing, conduct a hearing in chambers to determine the facts in the matter. The court will enter an order terminating the rights of the putative father if the court finds from the evidence that reasonable effort has been made to identify and locate him with-

---

18. O.C.G.A. § 19-8-4(c).
19. O.C.G.A. § 19-8-9(b).
20. *See* Johnson v. Smith, 251 Ga. 1, 302 S.E.2d 542 (1983).
21. O.C.G.A. § 19-8-12(a).
22. O.C.G.A. § 19-8-12(b).

out success and if it finds that he has not lived with the child, nor contributed to the child's support, nor made any attempt to legitimate the child, and that he did not provide support for the mother (including medical care) either during her pregnancy or during her hospitalization for the birth of the child. If the court finds from the evidence that reasonable effort has not been made to identify and locate the putative father, it will direct the Department of Human Resources or a licensed child-placing agency to expend additional efforts to identify and locate the putative father and to report the results of the additional efforts to the court. The court will continue the hearing until the additional effort has been expended and the results reported. If the court finds from the evidence that the putative father either lived with the child, or contributed to the child's support, or attempted to legitimate the child, or provided support for the mother (including medical care) during her pregnancy or during her hospitalization for the birth of the child, then the court must determine from the evidence whether such conduct by the putative father was sufficient to establish a familial bond between the putative father and the child. If the court finds that the conduct was sufficient to establish a familial bond, then the court will enter an appropriate order designed to afford the putative father notice of the surrender, consent, or proceeding to terminate parental rights.[23]

When notice to the putative father is to be given pursuant to law, it must advise the putative father that he loses all rights to the child and will neither receive notice nor be entitled to object to the adoption of the child unless, within 30 days of receipt of such notice, he files

1. a petition to legitimate the child pursuant to law; and
2. a notice of the filing of the petition to legitimate with the court in which the adoption is pending.[24]

In the event that the putative father does not file a legitimation petition and give notice as required by law within 30 days of his receipt of the notice or, if after filing the petition he fails to prosecute it to final judgment, he loses all rights to the child. He may not thereafter object to the adoption and is not entitled to receive notice of the adoption. If the child is legitimated by the putative father, the adoption will not be permitted.[25]

---

23. O.C.G.A. § 19-8-12(b).
24. O.C.G.A. § 19-8-12(c).
25. O.C.G.A. §§ 19-8-12(d) and (e).

(H) When Termination of Parental Rights Is Not Required

Surrender or termination of parental rights, as provided by law, is not a prerequisite to the filing of a petition for adoption pursuant to law when

1. the child has been abandoned by a parent;
2. the parent of a child cannot be found after a diligent search has been made; or
3. the parent is insane or otherwise incapacitated from surrendering such rights, when the court is of the opinion that the adoption is in the best interest of the child.[26]

Surrender or termination of parental rights, as provided by law, is not a prerequisite to the filing of a petition for adoption in the case of a parent who, for a period of 1 year or longer immediately prior to the filing of the petition for adoption, has failed

1. to communicate or make a bona fide attempt to communicate with the child; or
2. to provide for the care and support of the child as required by law or judicial decree, when the court is of the opinion that the adoption is in the best interest of the child.[27]

Whenever it is alleged by the petitioner(s) that the surrender or termination of parental rights is not a prerequisite to the filing of a petition for adoption, the parent(s) must be personally served with a conformed copy of the adoption petition, together with a copy of the court's order thereon.[28]

(I) Programs and Protection for Adopted Children

Adoption subsidy is a program that provides monetary assistance and special services for children who otherwise might not be adopted by making it possible to secure adoptive homes with people who meet all but the financial standards for adoptive parents.[29] Children adopted under this program would otherwise remain in foster care at state expense. Financial assistance may be

---

26. O.C.G.A. § 19-8-10(a).
27. O.C.G.A. § 19-8-10(b).
28. O.C.G.A. § 19-8-10(c).
29. O.C.G.A. § 49-5-8(a)(7)(F).

granted only for hard-to-place children with physical, mental, or emotional handicaps or with other problems for whom it is difficult to find a permanent home. Financial assistance may not exceed 75% of the amount paid for boarding such child and for special services such as medical care not available through insurance or public facilities. Supplements are available only to families who could not provide for the child adequately without continued financial assistance. The department may review the supplements paid at any time, but shall review them at least annually to determine the need for continued assistance.[30] The child must be in the custody of the Department of Human Resources or an agency and be legally free for adoption; that is, parental rights must have been terminated.

(J) General Considerations

The condition of a child who is suspected of having an emotional disturbance or of being vulnerable to one should be evaluated by a psychologist or psychiatrist. Also, proof that children have become attached to their foster parents may be shown by psychological or psychiatric examination indicating that a child is unable to readily accept another family. The Department of Human Resources or social worker may also determine that a meaningful relationship with the foster parents has been established and that the most appropriate plan is adoption by them. These factors should be considered by the court in the adoption process.

---

30. *Id.*

4.15

Delinquency and Persons in Need of Supervision

The juvenile court is a special court of limited jurisdiction with the responsibility of hearing matters relating to minors. These matters include resolving complaints about children who are alleged to be delinquent, unruly, deprived, mentally ill, or mentally retarded; granting consent for the marriage, employment, or enlistment of a minor when required by law; waiving requirements for parental notification prior to abortion; hearing petitions for the termination of parental rights, except in connection with adoption; and determining issues of custody and support either initially or when transferred from the superior court.[1] Most judicial circuits in the state have juvenile court judges, either full or part time, who are appointed by the superior court judges. However, in some circuits, particularly rural ones, a superior court judge may also act as the juvenile court judge.[2] The overriding purpose of the juvenile court is to protect the best interests of the child whenever possible.[3]

The juvenile court has exclusive original jurisdiction over matters concerning juveniles under the age of 17[4] if alleged to be delinquent, unruly, mentally ill or retarded, or having committed

---

1. O.C.G.A. § 15-11-5.
2. O.C.G.A. § 15-11-3.
3. O.C.G.A. § 15-11-1. *See, e.g.,* In re. M.A.F., 254 Ga. 748, 334 S.E.2d 668 (1985).
4. P.R. v. State, 133 Ga. App. 346, 210 S.E.2d 839 (1974).

a juvenile traffic offense and under the age of 18 years if alleged to be deprived.[5]

The juvenile court has concurrent jurisdiction with the superior court over a child who is alleged to have committed a criminal offense punishable by loss of life, life imprisonment, or life imprisonment without parole.[6] However, the superior court has exclusive jurisdiction over any child 13 to 17 years of age who is alleged to have committed the offenses of murder, voluntary manslaughter, rape, aggravated sodomy, aggravated child molestation, aggravated sexual battery, or armed robbery with a firearm.[7] Such cases may be transferred to the juvenile court for "extraordinary cause"[8] (see chapter 4.19). As to those offenses for which the juvenile court has concurrent jurisdiction, jurisdiction attaches to the court that first begins to process the case.[9] In certain cases where the juvenile court first assumes jurisdiction, the matter may be transferred to the superior court after a hearing (see chapter 4.18).

Children who appear before the juvenile court may see an MHP for evaluation, most often during the dispositional phase. An MHP may also become involved during the informal adjustment process in an effort to avoid the filing of a formal petition. MHPs are frequently active in the treatment phase after formal disposition of the child.

(A) Terms and Definitions

Before considering how the law operates, it is important to understand the terms it employs and their legal meanings:

1. A *delinquent child* is one who has committed an act that would be a criminal offense if committed by an adult and whom the court determines to be in need of treatment or rehabilitation.[10]

---

5. The juvenile court also has jurisdiction over a juvenile between the ages of 17 and 21 years who committed an act of delinquency before reaching the age of 17 years and who has been placed under the supervision of the court or on probation; *see* O.C.G.A. § 15-11-2(2)(B). However, the juvenile court does not have jurisdiction to initiate any new action against an individual for acts committed after his 17th birthday; *see* O.C.G.A. § 15-11-5(d).
6. O.C.G.A. § 15-11-2(2).
7. O.C.G.A. § 15-11-5(b)(1). The death penalty may not be imposed on one who was under 17 years at the time of the commission of the offense; *see* O.C.G.A. § 17-19-3.
8. O.C.G.A. § 15-11-5(b)(2)(A).
9. O.C.G.A. §§ 15-11-5(b)(2)(B) and (C); Relyea v. State, 236 Ga. 299, 223 S.E.2d 638 (1976).
10. Jurisdiction attaches upon the filing of a petition alleging delinquency; *see* Hartley v. Clack, 239 Ga. 113, 236 S.E.2d 63 (1977).

2. A *deprived child* is one who

   a. is without proper parental care or control, subsistence, education as required by law, or other care or control necessary for his physical, mental, or emotional health or morals;

   b. has been placed for care or adoption in violation of law;

   c. has been abandoned by his parents or other legal custodian; or

   d. is without a parent, guardian, or custodian. (No child who in good faith is being treated solely by spiritual means through prayer in accordance with the tenets and practices of a recognized church or religious denomination is, for that reason alone, considered to be a deprived child.)[11]

3. An *unruly child* is one who[12]

   a. although subject to compulsory school attendance is habitually and without justification truant from school;[13]

   b. is habitually disobedient of the reasonable and lawful commands of his parent, guardian, or other custodian and is ungovernable;

   c. has committed an offense applicable only to a child;

   d. without just cause and without the consent of his parent or legal custodian, deserts his home or place of abode;

   e. wanders or loiters about the streets of a city, or in or about a highway or a public place, between the hours of 12:00 midnight and 5:00 a.m.;

   f. disobeys the terms of supervision contained in a court order that has previously been directed to the child; or

---

11. O.C.G.A. § 15-11-2(6) and (7).
12. A child may also commit a delinquent act if he has previously been determined to be delinquent and violates a court-ordered term of probation, or if a child fails to appear in court as required by a citation for possession of alcoholic beverages; *see* O.C.G.A. § 15-11-2(6)(B) and (C). O.C.G.A. § 15-11-2(8). Some states refer to such children as *dependent children. See, e.g.,* Ariz. Rev. Stat. Ann. § 8-201 (Supp. 1987).
13. O.C.G.A. § 15-11-2(12). *Status offender* is the generic term used to refer to a child who has committed an "unruly" act. *See* O.C.G.A. § 15-11-2(11). Other states use a variety of specific legal terms to describe these children: "Incorrigible" (Arizona) Ariz. Rev. Stat. Ann. § 8-201 (Supp. 1987); "Minors habitually disobedient or truant" (California) Cal. Welf. & Inst. Code § 601 (West 1984); "Children in need of services (CHINS)" (Massachusetts) Mass. Gen. Laws Ann. ch. 119, § 39E; "Persons in need of supervision (PINS)" (New York) N.Y. Soc. Serv. Law § 371 (McKinney 1983); "Juvenile-family crisis" (replacing the 1974 concept of "Juvenile in need of supervision (JINS)" (New Jersey) N.J. Stat. Ann. § 2A:4A-22(g) (West 1987); "Child in need of care" (Kansas) Kan. Stat. Ann. § 38-1502 (1986).

g. patronizes any bar in which alcoholic beverages are being sold, unaccompanied by such child's parents, guardian, or custodian, or possesses alcoholic beverages.

In addition to having committed any of the foregoing acts, the child must also be in need of supervision, treatment, or rehabilitation to be found unruly. A child who has committed a delinquent act and who is in need of supervision, but not treatment or rehabilitation, can also be found unruly.

(B) Complaint

Proceedings commonly are initiated in juvenile court when a person having knowledge of an alleged act of delinquency, deprivation, or unruliness, or who is informed and believes that such an act has occurred, including a police officer, signs a written complaint against the child.[14] All complaints must be reviewed by a juvenile court intake officer who screens the complaint and makes a recommendation to the court to dismiss the complaint, make a referral to an agency for appropriate services, informally adjust the case, or file a petition.[15] If a petition is filed, the child is then processed formally through the court.

(C) Informal Adjustment

If a child has committed a nonserious delinquent act or an unruly act, the intake officer may recommend that the case be informally adjusted, in which event no petition will be filed. In addition, the juvenile court judge may direct the withdrawal of a filed petition when it appears that informal adjustment best suits the needs of the child and the public. When informal adjustment is appropriate, a juvenile court probation officer may counsel with the child and the parents at an informal hearing or conference or may place the child on a program of counsel and advise for an initial period of not more than 3 months, with one 3-month extension permitted. *Counsel and advise* is an informal type of probation and may include specific requirements, such as attending traffic

---

14. Although the parent is responsible for ensuring that the child attends school (O.C.G.A. § 20-3-6901), the courts have found a child to be unruly based upon the parents' failure to send the proper excuse note to school. In the interest of A.D.F., 176 Ga. App. 5, 335 S.E.2d 144 (1985).

15. Uniform Juvenile Court Rules, Rule 4.1 (West 1988) [hereinafter Rules]. A proceeding may also be initiated by filing a petition, by a transfer from another court, or by the filing of a traffic citation. *Id*. Rule 4.2.

school or working at community service. A child may also be referred for counseling, and the successful completion of the counseling may be made a condition of the informal adjustment.[16]

(D) Filing of Petition

If an intake officer determines that a child alleged to be delinquent, deprived, or unruly should be formally processed through the juvenile court, a petition must be filed with the clerk of the juvenile court, and a court officer must endorse upon the petition that its filing is in the best interest of the public and the child.[17] A petition may be filed by any person, including a law enforcement officer, who has knowledge of the facts or who has been informed of the facts.[18] The petition is a formal document filed under oath; it must include a jurisdictional statement; a description of the act or acts alleged; the name, age, and residence of the child; the names and addresses of the child's parents or guardian; whether the child is in custody and, if so, the place of detention and the time he was taken into custody.[19] If a child is placed in detention, a petition must be filed within 72 hours.[20] If the child is not detained, the petition must be filed within 30 days.[21]

(E) Detention Hearing

If certain specific standards are met, a child alleged to be delinquent or unruly may be taken into custody and placed in a secure juvenile detention facility.[22] Rigorous restrictions are imposed by statute on where a child may be detained, for how long he may be detained, and the nature of the acts for which he may be detained. Official approval of the child's detention and notice of the detention to the child's parents are also required.[23]

If a child is placed in detention, he must be given a formal detention hearing within 72 hours of placement in detention.[24]

---

16. O.C.G.A. § 15-11-14 and Rules, *supra* note 15, Rule 4.3.
17. O.C.G.A. § 15-11-25 and Rules, *supra* note 15, Rules 6.1, 6.3.
18. O.C.G.A. § 15-11-24.
19. Rules, *supra* note 13, Rule 6.5.
20. O.C.G.A. § 15-11-21(e).
21. O.C.G.A. § 15-11-21(b).
22. *See* O.C.G.A. § 15-11-18.
23. A deprived child may not be placed in a secure facility. *See* O.C.G.A. §§ 15-11-20(f) and § 15-11-19-20.
24. O.C.G.A. § 15-11-21(c)(1) to (3). The time limits vary somewhat based on the nature of the act alleged, whether delinquent, unruly, or deprived. *Id.*

The purposes of the detention hearing are to determine whether the child should be released or detained pending further court proceedings and whether reasonable grounds exist to believe that the allegations in the complaint or petition are true.[25] Children may not be detained unless

1. their detention is required to protect the person or property of others or to protect the child;
2. they abscond or are removed from the jurisdiction of the court;
3. they have no parent, guardian, or custodian able to provide supervision and care for them and return them to the court; or
4. the court has ordered detention or shelter care pursuant to some other provision of the Juvenile Code.

Before the commencement of the detention hearing, the court will inform the parties of their right to counsel and of their right to have counsel appointed for them if they are indigent. The child shall also be informed of his right to remain silent.[26] The court will also rule on an application for bond if such an application has been filed. If necessary, a separate bond hearing may be scheduled.[27]

(F) Arraignment Hearing

The arraignment hearing is an optional formal hearing that may be conducted in conjunction with the detention hearing or in a separate hearing.[28] The purpose of the arraignment hearing is to formally advise the child of his rights to counsel, to remain silent and to have a hearing before the judge; to advise him of the allegations as they are stated in the petition; and to offer the child an opportunity to enter a plea to the charges against him.[29] Counsel for the child or the child's parents may waive the formal arraignment hearing and proceed to an adjudicatory hearing or may enter an admission to the charges and proceed to a dispositional hearing.[30]

---

25. Rules, *supra* note 15, Rule 8.1, O.C.G.A. § 15-11-18.1.
26. Rules, *supra* note 15, Rule 8.3.
27. Rules, *supra* note 15, Rule 9.1.
28. Rules, *supra* note 15, Rule 10.1.
29. *Id.*
30. Rules, *supra* note 13, Rule 10.3.

(G) Adjudicatory Hearing

The adjudicatory hearing is a fact-finding hearing, the purpose of which is to determine whether the allegations contained in the petition are true.[31] The prosecution must prove beyond a reasonable doubt that the acts were committed before the child can be adjudicated delinquent or unruly.[32] A child can be adjudicated as deprived if there is clear and convincing evidence of deprivation.[33]

In an adjudicatory hearing in juvenile court, a child has many of the rights that are afforded to an adult criminal defendant,[34] except the rights to have a trial by jury[35] and to have the public present.[36] A child's parent is considered to be a party to proceedings involving the child.[37]

(H) Dispositional Hearing

After hearing the evidence in the adjudicatory hearing, the court must make written findings as to whether the child is deprived or whether the child committed a delinquent or unruly act.[38] The court may then proceed immediately or at a postponed hearing to

---

31. O.C.G.A. §§ 15-11-28 and 15-11-30.
32. *See, generally,* Rules, *supra* note 13, Rule 11.1 *et seq.;* Rules, *supra* note 13, Rule 11.2(a).
33. This standard for the determination of guilt is the same as the standard applied in an adult criminal trial. *See* In re Winship, 397 U.S. 358 (1970).
34. Rules, *supra* note 13, Rule 11.3.
35. For example, a child has the right to counsel, the right to examine and cross-examine witnesses, the right against self-incrimination, and the right to exclude illegally seized evidence. *See* O.C.G.A. §§ 15-11-30 and 15-11-31 and Rules, *supra* note 13, Rule 11.3 These rights flow from the landmark Supreme Court decision of In re Gault, 387 U.S. 1, 87 S. Ct. 1428 (1967). There the Court held that a juvenile facing the possible loss of his liberty has the right to written notice of the charges against him and the specific law that has been violated, a right to counsel at every stage of the proceedings, the privilege against self-incrimination, and the opportunity to examine and cross-examine witnesses. *Id.* at 29-59. Later, in In re Winship, 397 U.S. 358, 90 S. Ct. 1068 (1970), the Court held that the standard of proof must be beyond a reasonable doubt. *See* O.C.G.A. § 15-11-28. The Supreme Court ruled in McKeiver v. Pennsylvania, 403 U.S. 528, 91 S. Ct. 1976 (1971) that there is no constitutional right to a trial by jury in juvenile cases.
36. Rules, *supra* note 15, Rules 11.3 and 11.6.
37. The Supreme Court has clarified this issue in Smith v. Daily Mail Pub. Co., 443 U.S. 97, 99 S. Ct. 2667 (1979). *See also* Florida Publishing Co. v. Morgan, 253 Ga. 467, 322 S.E.2d 233 (1984); Sanchez v. Walker Co. Dep't of Family and Children Services, 237 Ga. 406, 229 S.E.2d 66 (1976).
38. O.C.G.A. § 15-11-33(a).

make a disposition of the case.[39] The purpose of the dispositional hearing is to hear evidence on whether the child is in need of treatment, rehabilitation, or supervision and, if in such need, what is the appropriate disposition.[40] During the pendency of a postponed dispositional hearing, the court may order the child to be examined by a physician or a psychologist. The court may also direct that a social study and report be made concerning the child, his family, his environment, and other matters relating to disposition. An MHP may be designated to make such a report.[41]

The court may consider a report by an MHP in making a disposition of the case even though such reports might not be admissible evidence in an adjudicatory hearing.[42] The parties or their counsel have the right to examine and controvert the written report and to cross-examine the individual making the report.[43] However, the court may withhold from the parties portions of reports not relied on by the court in reaching its decision, if revealing those portions would be prejudicial to the child. The court may also refuse to disclose confidential sources of information.[44]

(I) Disposition by Way of Counseling

A juvenile court may order counseling for the parents and the child when a child appears for the first time and is found by the court to have committed a delinquent act, to be deprived or unruly, or to have committed specified juvenile traffic offenses. The county is required to pay for the counseling services.[45]

(J) Disposition of a Deprived Child

If the court finds the child to be a deprived child, an order of disposition may be entered for the purpose of protecting the physical, mental, and moral welfare of the child. Such an order may include the following:

---

39. A dispositional hearing is not necessary if a petition for termination of parental rights alleges only that the child is deprived. In interest of J.C., 242 Ga. 737, 251 S.E.2d 299 (1978); O.C.G.A. § 15-11-33(b).
40. O.C.G.A. § 15-11-33(c).
41. The finding that the child is in need of treatment or rehabilitation must be based on clear and convincing evidence. A.C.G. v. State, 131 Ga. App. 156, 205 S.E.2d 435 (1974); O.C.G.A. § 15-11-32.
42. O.C.G.A. § 15-11-33(d).
43. *Id.*
44. *Id.*
45. O.C.G.A. §§ 15-11-36.1 and 15-11-56, as amended by House Bill 1977 (1992).

1. permitting the child to remain with his parents, guardian, or other custodian subject to certain prescribed conditions;

2. transferring temporary legal custody to another individual or to a private or public agency; or

3. transferring custody to the court of another state.[46]

Unless a child found to be deprived is also found to be delinquent, he may not be committed to or confined in an institution or other facility designed for delinquent children.[47]

(K) Disposition of a Delinquent Child

If the court finds that the child has committed a delinquent act and determines further that the child is in need of treatment or rehabilitation, the court may make any of the following orders of disposition:

1. an order authorized by code section 15-11-34 for the disposition of a deprived child;

2. an order placing the child on probation under conditions prescribed by the court, which may include supervision by a public agency;

3. an order placing the child in an institution, camp, or other facility for delinquent children operated under the direction of the court or a local public authority;

4. an order committing the child to the Department of Children and Youth Services;

5. an order requiring the child to make restitution; or

6. an order suspending the child's license to drive or prohibiting the issuance of a license until the child turns 18 years.[48]

A child 13 to 17 years of age convicted of murder, voluntary manslaughter, rape, aggravated sodomy, aggravated child molestation, aggravated sexual battery, or armed robbery with a firearm is sentenced to the custody of the Department of Corrections. However, the child must be housed in special "youth confinement" until he reaches the age of 17 years.[49] A 13- to 15-year-old child who is convicted of those offenses and who is mentally ill or

---

46. O.C.G.A. § 15-11-34(a). As to termination of parental rights, see chapter 4.10.
47. O.C.G.A. § 15-11-34(b). House Bill 1549 (1992) created the Department of Children and Youth Services to carry out the functions formerly performed by the Division of Youth Services of the Department of Human Resources. *See* O.C.G.A. Chapter 49-4A.
48. O.C.G.A. § 15-11-35.
49. O.C.G.A. § 15-11-5.1.

mentally retarded shall be committed to the Department of Human Resources rather than the Department of Corrections.[50]

(L) Disposition of an Unruly Child

If the child is found to be unruly, the court may make any disposition authorized for a delinquent child, except that if commitment to the Department of Children and Youth Services is ordered, the court must first find that the child is not amenable to treatment or rehabilitation by probation or by placement in a facility operated under supervision of the court or a local public authority.[51]

---

50. O.C.G.A. § 15-11-40(e).
51. O.C.G.A. § 15-11-36.

4.16

Competency of Juveniles to Stand Trial

When a plea is filed in an adult criminal trial asserting that the defendant is mentally incompetent to stand trial, the court will convene a special jury to determine the mental status of the defendant at the time of the trial.[1] The plea of incompetency raises the issue of whether the defendant is capable of understanding the nature and object of the proceedings, whether he comprehends his own situation in relation to the proceedings, and whether he is capable of rendering assistance to his attorney.[2] Although it is clear that a juvenile defendant who is tried in superior court as an adult has the right to file a plea of incompetency to stand trial,[3] the Georgia Juvenile Court Code contains no provision for the filing of a plea of incompetency to stand trial nor a procedure for handling such a plea. There are no reported cases in Georgia that raise the issue of competency to stand trial in the juvenile court setting.

The Juvenile Court Code does contain a provision that if, at any time, the evidence indicates that a child may be suffering from mental illness or mental retardation, the court may commit the child to an appropriate institution, agency, or individual for evaluation. Presumably, the court could use this authority to have the child's condition evaluated in those instances in which the child appeared to be incompetent to stand trial. If it appeared

---

1. O.C.G.A. § 17-7-130; *see also* Echols v. State, 149 Ga. App. 620, 255 S.E.2d 92 (1979); Allanson v. State, 158 Ga. App. 77, 279 S.E.2d 316 (1981). For a more detailed discussion of competency to stand trial for adults, *see infra* chapter 7.5.
2. *See, e.g.,* Allanson v. State, 158 Ga. App. 77, 279 S.E.2d 316 (1981).
3. Crawford v. State, 240 Ga. 321, 240 S.E.2d 824 (1977) (16-year-old tried in superior court was first found competent to stand trial by a special jury).

from the report that the child was committable as mentally ill or mentally retarded, the court could then institute commitment proceedings.[4]

The Juvenile Court Code also contains a provision requiring the court to determine whether the juvenile is committable as mentally ill or mentally retarded prior to deciding whether to transfer the juvenile to superior court to be tried as an adult.[5] Although the legal standard for commitment is not the same as the standard for competency to stand trial, the question of whether a child is committable as mentally ill or retarded may depend, in part, on whether the child is competent to stand trial. For example, the Georgia Supreme Court held in *In re K.S.J.*[6] that the finding that the 13-year-old defendant was competent to stand trial was a factor that could properly be considered in determining that he was not committable to a mental institution and, therefore, subject to transfer to the superior court for trial as an adult.[7] By implication, if the child was not competent to stand trial, he could not be transferred for trial as an adult, but would be committed instead.[8]

The U.S. Supreme Court has held that when juveniles face the potential loss of liberty, they are entitled to the same basic procedural protections that adults are entitled to in criminal proceedings.[9] It would raise a serious constitutional question to try a juvenile for a delinquent or unruly act when the juvenile could not understand the nature of the proceedings nor assist counsel in his defense. Unlike an adult, however, a juvenile would not be entitled to a special jury trial on the issue of competency.[10]

A child who is sufficiently ill to be incompetent to stand trial would seem to be a strong candidate for informal adjustment. If the delinquent act is of a serious nature, prompt intervention to head off transfer to the superior court and to secure appropriate treatment would be in order.

---

4. O.C.G.A. § 15-11-40; *see infra* chapter 4.19.
5. O.C.G.A. § 15-11-39; *see infra* chapter 4.18.
6. 258 Ga. 52, 365 S.E.2d 820 (1988).
7. *Id.* at 53, 365 S.E.2d at 821.
8. Other states have used the standard adult competency test in juvenile proceedings. *See, e.g.,* State *ex rel.* Dandoy v. Superior Court, 127 Ariz. 184, 619 P.2d 12 (1980); State v. Wilkins, 736 S.W.2d 409 (Mo. 1987). *See also* chapter 7.5.
9. In re Gault, 387 U.S. 1, 87 S. Ct. 1428 (1967); In re Winship, 397 U.S. 358, 90 S. Ct. 1068 (1970).
10. McKeiver v. Pennsylvania, 403 U.S. 528 (1971).

4.17

Nonresponsibility Defenses in Juvenile Court

(A) Insanity

There is no express statutory authority in the Juvenile Court Code for a child charged with a delinquent act to assert the insanity defense. The Criminal Procedure Code, as applicable to adults, expressly provides for the defense[1] and sets out the procedures[2] for invoking it. Although it is apparent that juveniles who are tried as adults may invoke the insanity defense,[3] there are no Georgia cases deciding this issue in a juvenile court proceeding.[4]

Considering the U.S. Supreme Court's holding *In re Gault*[5] that juveniles facing loss of liberty for delinquent acts must be afforded the same basic procedural protections as adults, it would seem logical that the juvenile court would apply essentially the

---

1. O.C.G.A. §§ 16-3-2 and 16-3-3.
2. O.C.G.A. §§ 17-7-130.1 and 17-7-131. These provisions will be discussed *infra* chapter 7.9.
3. *See* Couch v. State, 253 Ga. 764, 325 S.E.2d 366 (1985) (trial court properly excluded evidence of 16-year-old defendant's mental capacity as irrelevant because he never pleaded not guilty by reason of insanity nor guilty but mentally ill).
4. In re K.S.J., 258 Ga. 52, 365 S.E.2d 820 (1988), the Georgia Supreme Court, in an appeal from a transfer order, stated that the 13-year-old defendant was not committable to an institution for the mentally retarded or mentally ill, in part, because he "could distinguish right from wrong, and that he was not suffering from any mental disorder or mental defect."*Id.* at 53, 365 S.E.2d at 821. These factors are the traditional bases for determining whether an adult criminal defendant is not guilty by reason of insanity. *See* O.C.G.A. § 16-3-2.
5. 387 U.S. 1, 87 S.Ct. 1428 (1967); *see also* Freeman v. Wilcox, 119 Ga. App. 325, 167 S.E.2d 163 (1969).

same substantive law for the insanity defense as is applied in superior court. The main differences are likely to be procedural ones, such as the juvenile court's following the provision for disposition of a mentally ill or mentally retarded child[6] rather than the procedures outlined in the criminal code for the commitment of adults found not guilty by reason of insanity.[7]

Whether the insanity defense should be asserted in any particular case requires a joint determination by the child; the child's parents, if appropriate; the lawyer; and the MHP as to the risks and benefits of the defense and the effect of a successful defense on the child. Given the authority of the juvenile court to commit a mentally ill child, coupled with the nature of the evidence that must be presented in order to achieve a successful insanity defense, it is likely that a finding of not guilty by reason of insanity would result in civil commitment. One possible benefit to the child of a successful insanity defense is that commitment is for an initial period of 6 months, whereas an order of disposition of a delinquent or unruly child generally continues in force for at least 2 years.[8]

(B) Criminal Capacity

Another nonresponsibility defense, uniquely available to juveniles, provides that a person shall not be found guilty of a crime unless he has reached the age of 13 years at the time of the act.[9] Georgia has, thus, provided statutory authority for the common law defense of "infancy."[10] Under Georgia law, under no circumstances may a child under the age of 13 years be tried as an adult. Children between the ages of 13 and 17 years may, under specified circumstances, be tried as adults, either by transfer to the superior court[11] or by the provisions for exclusive criminal jurisdiction.[12] Infancy is considered to be a nonresponsibility defense because a child under the age of 13 years is considered to be unable to form the requisite criminal intent.[13] Georgia has no

---

6. O.C.G.A. § 15-11-40. *See infra* chapter 4.1.
7. O.C.G.A. §§ 17-7-130.1 and 17-7-131.
8. O.C.G.A. § 15-11-41(a).
9. O.C.G.A. § 16-3-1.
10. *See* W. Lafave & A. Scott, *Handbook on Criminal Law*, Section 46 (1972).
11. O.C.G.A. § 15-11-39; *see infra* chapter 4.18.
12. O.C.G.A. § 15-11-5; *see supra* chapter 4.15.
13. Lafave & Scott, *supra* note 10, Section 46; *but see* K.M.S. v. State, 129 Ga. App. 683, 200 S.E.2d 916 (1973) (section does not provide that an individual under 13 years of age is incapable of performing an act that is designated as a crime under laws of Georgia; it simply raises a defense for such person because of the social desirability of protecting those no more than 12 years of age from the consequences of criminal guilt).

provision setting forth a minimum age of capacity to commit a delinquent or unruly act.[14] Under the common law, however, children under the age of 7 years would be immune from prosecution even in juvenile court.[15] Some commentators have argued that the traditional concept of incapacity has no application in juvenile court, given the court's purported purpose of acting in the best interests of the child.[16]

14. *But see* Corley v. Russell, 92 Ga. App. 417, 88 S.E.2d 470 (1955). ("It is elementary law well established that a child three and one-half years old is incapable of violating any law. . . .")
15. Lafave & Scott, *supra* note 10, Section 46.
16. *Id.*

4.18

Transfer of Juveniles to Stand Trial as Adults

In 1994, the Georgia General Assembly enacted the School Safety and Juvenile Justice Reform Act. The Act changed prior law by mandating that children charged with certain violent felonies be tried and sentenced as adults in superior court. The Juvenile Court Code now provides two methods by which children under the age of 17 years can be tried in superior court as adults:

1. by the superior court under its exclusive jurisdiction for specified serious felonies, or
2. by the juvenile court transferring a juvenile to superior court for prosecution.

(A) Concurrent Jurisdiction of the Juvenile and Superior Courts

The Juvenile Court Code provides that the juvenile court has concurrent jurisdiction with the superior court over a child who is alleged to have committed a delinquent act that would be considered a crime if tried in the superior court and for which the child may be punished by loss of life, confinement for life in a penal institution, or imprisonment for life without parole.[1] However, the superior court has exclusive jurisdiction over any matter involving a child 13 to 17 years of age who is alleged to have

---

1. O.C.G.A. § 15-11-5(b). However, the death penalty cannot be imposed on a child who was under 17 years of age at the time of the commission of the offense. *See* O.C.G.A. § 17-9-3; Bankston v. State, 258 Ga. 188, 367 S.E.2d 36 (1988).

committed any of the following offenses: murder, voluntary manslaughter, rape, aggravated sodomy, aggravated child molestation, aggravated sexual battery, or armed robbery with a firearm.[2] Prior to indictment, the district attorney may, after investigation and for extraordinary cause, decline to prosecute in superior court a child charged with the aforementioned offenses. There is no provision for review of this decision, as it appears to be within the district attorney's discretion. The case is then transferred to the juvenile court where it is subject to disposition as a designated felony.[3]

After indictment, the superior court judge may, after investigation and for extraordinary cause, transfer a case involving the aforementioned offenses that are not punishable by death, life imprisonment, or life imprisonment without parole. Cases punishable by death or life imprisonment are not transferable by the judge. The decision to transfer may be appealed by the district attorney. Any case that is transferred is also subject to the designated felony provisions in the juvenile court.[4]

In addition, if a child is tried in the superior court, but convicted of a lesser included offense not punishable by death, life imprisonment, or life imprisonment without parole, the case may be transferred to the juvenile court for disposition. Upon transfer the superior court's jurisdiction is terminated.[5]

(B) Transfer to Superior Court

In addition to the exclusive jurisdiction of the superior court in violent felony cases, the Juvenile Court Code provides for the transfer to the superior court of a juvenile charged with a delinquent act for prosecution as an adult, if certain conditions are met. First, the juvenile court may not merely waive jurisdiction, but it must conduct a full evidentiary hearing to determine if there are reasonable grounds for the transfer.[6] The transfer hearing is a critical determination affecting the juvenile's subsequent treatment in the courts, and the child must, therefore, be afforded the basic panoply of due process rights.[7]

---

2. O.C.G.A. § 15-11-5(b)(2)(A).
3. O.C.G.A. § 15-11-5(b)(2)(C).
4. O.C.G.A. § 15-11-5(b)(2)(B).
5. O.C.G.A. § 15-11-5(b)(2)(D).
6. O.C.G.A. § 15-11-39(a)(1); see R.S. v. State, 156 Ga. App. 460, 274 S.E.2d 810 (1980); In the interest of T.J.M., 142 Ga. App. 415, 236 S.E.2d 152 (1977).
7. C.L.A v. State, 137 Ga. App. 511, 224 S.E.2d 491 (1976).

The state bears the burden of proof[8] in a transfer hearing to establish the existence of the statutory criteria for transfer.[9] The court must find that there are reasonable grounds to believe that the stated criteria are met before a transfer may be made. These criteria are

1. that the child has committed the delinquent act alleged;[10]

2. that the child is not committable to an institution for the mentally retarded or mentally ill (The application of this factor has been the subject of a number of appellate decisions. However, it is difficult to defeat the court's statutory discretion to find that the child is not committable to an institution for the mentally retarded or mentally ill. A case in point is *In the interest of L.L.*,[11] in which the court of appeals rejected the claim that the child, a 15-year-old charged with murder, was committable even though the evidence was undisputed that he was moderately retarded with an IQ of 44 and with a mental age of 8 years, and that he was a diagnosed schizophrenic. In addition, the court rejected the testimony of experts who had examined L.L. that he should be placed in a facility for the mentally retarded.);[12]

3. that the interests of the child and the community require that the child be placed under legal restraint and transferred to the superior court for trial;[13] whether the child is amenable to treatment in the juvenile system is a factor to be considered in determining the best interests of the community and the child. Even if a child is amenable to treatment, he may still be transferred to superior court if the community's interest outweighs the child's interest in remaining in the juvenile system;[14] and

4. that the child was at least 15 years of age at the time of the delinquent act or, if the alleged act was one for which the

---

8. *Id. See, generally,* Kent v. United States, 383 U.S. 541 (1966).

9. O.C.G.A. § 15-11-39(a)(3); D.L.M. v. State, 160 Ga. App. 424, 287 S.E.2d 355 (1981).

10. O.C.G.A. § 15-11-39(a)(3)(A); In re. K.S.J., 258 Ga. 52, 365 S.E.2d 820 (1988) (court found that there were reasonable grounds to believe the defendant committed felony murder).

11. 165 Ga. App. 49, 299 S.E.2d 53 (1983).

12. 165 Ga. App. at 50; O.C.G.A. § 15-11-39(a)(3)(B); *see also* In re K.S.J., 258 Ga. at 53, 365 S.E.2d at 821 (the court was presented with competent evidence that the child suffered from a conduct disorder and an attention deficit disorder, was of average intelligence and not psychotic, was competent to stand trial, could distinguish right from wrong, and was not suffering from a mental disorder or mental defect and held he was not committable).

13. O.C.G.A. § 15-11-39(a)(3)(C).

14. State v. M.M., 259 Ga. 637, 386 S.E.2d 35 (1989).

punishment is loss of life or confinement for life in prison, that he was 13 or 14 years of age.[15]

Transfer terminates the jurisdiction of the juvenile court with regard to the delinquent acts alleged in the petition.[16] The decision transferring the juvenile to the superior court to be tried as an adult is appealable as a final order.[17] Once a child is convicted in superior court, it would be a violation of the double jeopardy clause of the Fifth Amendment to try him again in juvenile court for the same offense.[18]

Once a transfer is made, a juvenile who is tried in superior court is subject to all the criminal sanctions that may be imposed by that court, with the exception of the death sentence if the offense was committed before the age of 17 years.[19] Juveniles under the age of 17 years who are convicted of a felony and who are sentenced to life imprisonment or to a term of imprisonment must be placed in a juvenile institution operated by the Department of Children and Youth Services, until they are 18 years of age, at which time they will be transferred to the Department of Corrections to serve the remainder of their sentence. A juvenile convicted of aggravated assault may be sentenced to the Department of Corrections, but must be housed in a designated youth confinement unit until age 17 years. A child convicted of the violent felonies discussed earlier must be sentenced to the Department of Corrections and will be housed in a youth confinement unit until age 17 years.[20]

(C) The Designated Felony Act: Restrictive Custody and Mandatory Transfer

The Juvenile Code also contains a section that provides for a special order of disposition for a child who has committed spe-

---

15. O.C.G.A. § 15-11-39(a)(4); *see* In re K.S.J., *supra* note 10 (13-year-old charged with felony murder).
16. O.C.G.A. § 15-11-39(b).
17. Fulton County Dep't of Family and Children Services v. Perkins, 244 Ga. 237, 259 S.E.2d 427 (1978); J.T.M. v. State, 142 Ga. App. 635, 236 S.E.2d 764 (1977).
18. Lincoln v. State, 138 Ga. App. 234, 225 S.E.2d 708 (1976); *see also* Breed v. Jones, 421 U.S. 519, 95 S. Ct. 1779 (1975).
19. Carrindine v. Rickets, 236 Ga. 283, 223 S.E.2d 627 (1976); the U.S. Supreme Court has upheld the constitutionality of imposing the death penalty on a person who was as young as 16 years of age at the time of the commission of the crime.
20. Stanford v. Kentucky, 492 U.S. 361, 109 S. Ct. 2969 (1989).

cific acts, as well as a procedure for transferring certain cases to superior court for trial.[21] Under the Designated Felony Act, if a juvenile is tried in juvenile court and is adjudicated guilty of specific offenses ("a designated felony act"),[22] he may be committed to the Department of Children and Youth Services for a period of 5 years, rather than the normal 2 years, if the court determines that restrictive custody is warranted.[23] In determining whether restrictive custody is required, the court shall consider

1. the needs and interest of the juvenile;
2. the juvenile's record and background;
3. the circumstances of the offense, including the extent of any injury inflicted on the victim;
4. the need for community protection; and
5. the age and physical condition of the victim.

In addition, if the delinquent felony act involved the infliction of serious physical injury on a person 62 years of age or older, or if the juvenile has committed two or more previous burglaries, the court shall order restrictive custody.

When a juvenile is placed in restrictive custody, he must be initially confined in a juvenile institution for a period of 12 to 60 months[24] with mandatory intensive supervision for at least 12 months after release from the institution.[25] In a case involving a serious felony, placement of the child in restrictive custody is a possible alternative to transfer to the superior court for trial as an adult.

Another provision of the Designated Felony Act mandates transfer in certain cases of burglary. A mandatory transfer to superior court is initiated when a petition is filed alleging that a child aged 15 years or older has committed an act of burglary and has been found, at previous court proceedings, to have committed burglary on three or more previous occasions.[26] The juve-

---

21. O.C.G.A. § 17-10-14. In 1992, the Department of Children and Youth Services was created to perform the detention functions formerly carried out by the Department of Human Resources Division of Youth Services.
22. O.C.G.A. § 15-11-37. Designated felony acts include any of the violent felonies over which the superior court has exclusive jurisdiction and offenses of kidnapping, arson, aggravated assault, arson in the second degree, aggravated battery, robbery or armed robbery, and other serious felonies. See O.C.G.A. § 15-11-37(a)(2). In addition, if the juvenile has three prior delinquency detentions based on felony offenses, he can be treated under the designated felony provisions.
23. O.C.G.A. § 15-11-37(e)(1)(A). See O.C.G.A. § 15-11-41(b) (order of disposition committing a delinquent or unruly child to the Department of Children and Youth Services continues in force for 2 years).
24. O.C.G.A. § 15-11-37(e)(1)(B).
25. O.C.G.A. § 15-11-37(e)(1)(C).
26. O.C.G.A. § 15-11-39.1(a).

nile court must hold a transfer hearing and determine whether there are reasonable grounds to believe that the child committed the act alleged. If so, it must order the transfer.[27] There is no requirement that the court find that the child is not committable as mentally retarded or mentally ill or that it is in the best interest of the child and the community to make the transfer. Once the transfer has been made, the district attorney must investigate the case and report to the judge whether the matter should be transferred back to juvenile court.[28] On the basis of the report, or on its own motion, the superior court may order the case transferred back to the juvenile court.[29]

---

27. O.C.G.A. § 15-11-39.1(b) and (c).
28. O.C.G.A. § 15-11-39.1(d).
29. *Id.*

4.19

Voluntary Admission and Civil Commitment of Minors

Georgia law sets out different procedures for the voluntary and involuntary treatment of mentally ill and mentally retarded adults. In the case of individuals under the age of 18 years, these distinctions are not generally important because the law allows a parent to commit a child "voluntarily" to a mental health facility without the requirement of a court hearing or a court order. Involuntary civil commitment proceedings are necessary only when the parent is unable or unwilling to commit the child or when a hearing is required in connection with a juvenile court proceeding. In general, a parental "voluntary" admission is done extrajudicially. There is no requirement that a court become involved even if the minor objects to being committed. However, under both the Mental Health Code and the Mental Retardation Code, any individual detained by a facility, or a relative or friend on the person's behalf, may at any time file a petition for a writ of *habeas corpus* to question the cause and legality of the detention and to request release.[1] Because minors are persons, a *habeas corpus* proceeding is an available method to obtain court review of their commitment.

(A) Voluntary Admission: Mentally Retarded Minors

The parent or guardian of a minor child may apply to the Department of Human Resources to have the child examined by an

---

1. O.C.G.A. §§ 37-3-148 and 37-4-108.

evaluation team.[2] If a majority of the team concludes that the child is mentally retarded and in need of appropriate care, training, education, or specialized services, the team may recommend an individualized program plan for the child, and the department may provide inpatient services in accord with the plan.[3] The parent or guardian of a minor child admitted to a facility on a voluntary basis may request the child's discharge in writing at any time after his admission.[4] The child must be discharged within 72 hours of delivery of the written request unless the hospital superintendent finds that the discharge would be unsafe to the child or others, in which case proceedings to receive involuntary services must be initiated.[5]

A retarded minor may also be admitted to a facility for temporary or "respite care" for a period of up to 2 weeks when the person with whom the child normally resides is ill or absent from home.[6] Admission for the sole purpose of receiving dental care is also possible on a temporary basis.[7]

(B) Voluntary Admission: Mentally Ill Minors

Any child between the ages of 12 and 17 years may make a request to a mental health facility that he be admitted for observation and diagnosis, but the child's parent or guardian must give written consent for treatment.[8] Additionally, the parent or guard-

---

2. O.C.G.A. § 37-4-20(a).
3. *Id.*
4. O.C.G.A. § 37-4-20(b).
5. *Id.*
6. O.C.G.A. § 37-4-21.
7. O.C.G.A. § 37-4-22. *Also see* Rules of the Department of Human Resources, Admission, Treatment and Release of Minors From Mental Health Facilities, Chapter 290-4-7.
8. O.C.G.A. § 37-3-20(a).

ian of any minor under age 18 years may make a similar request.[9] If the child is found to show evidence of mental illness and to be suitable for treatment, the facility may retain the child for treatment.[10]

The hospital must discharge any voluntary patient who has recovered from his mental illness or who has significantly improved so that he is determined to no longer require inpatient hospitalization.[11] A voluntary patient who has admitted himself or any voluntary patient's representative, guardian, parent, spouse, attorney, or adult next of kin may request his discharge in writing at any time after his admission.[12] However, if the patient is a minor child for whom admission has been sought by his parents or guardian, only the child's representative, parents, guardian, attorney, or adult next of kin may request his discharge.[13] In other words, the child's parents or guardian may override the child's request for discharge, and no court proceeding is needed for the hospital to retain the child.

When the parent or guardian requests discharge, the patient must be discharged within 72 hours after delivery of the written request, unless the chief medical officer finds that the discharge would be unsafe for the patient or others, in which case proceedings for involuntary treatment must be initiated.[14] At the time of admission and every 6 months thereafter, a voluntary patient must be notified in writing of his right to discharge.[15]

---

9. *Id.* The provisions for the voluntary admission of children to Georgia mental health facilities were challenged in a class action suit filed in federal court in 1975. The plaintiffs claimed that the statutory scheme deprived children of their liberty in violation of the Due Process Clause of the Fourteenth Amendment. J.R. v. Parham, 412 F. Supp. 112 (M.D. Ga. 1976) *rev'd sub nom.* Parham v. J.R., 442 U.S. 584, 99 S. Ct. 2493 (1979). The district court agreed with the plaintiffs. However, the Supreme Court reversed and, applying the balancing test of Mathews v. Eldridge, 424 U.S. 319, 96 S. Ct. 893 (1976), held that the statutory scheme, which authorized the admission of minors upon the application of parents or guardians, together with certification by an examining physician that the child is mentally ill, provided adequate procedural safeguards. Parham v. J.R., 442 U.S. 584 (1979). The Supreme Court found unpersuasive the substantial evidence produced by the plaintiffs that state hospitals were being used as a "dumping ground" for problem and unwanted children. For additional discussion of Parham v. J.R., *see* comment, Juveniles Committed to State Mental Hospitals Upon Application of Parents or Guardians Are Not Entitled to Adversarial Hearing to Determine Their Need for Institutionalization, Parham v. J.R., 442 U.S. 584 (1979); Secretary of Public Welfare v. Institutionalized Juveniles, 442 U.S. 640 (1979)., 29 *Emory Law J.* 517 (1980).
10. O.C.G.A. § 37-3-20(a).
11. O.C.G.A. § 37-3-21(a).
12. O.C.G.A. § 37-3-22(a).
13. *Id.*
14. *Id.*
15. O.C.G.A. § 37-3-23.

(C) Involuntary Commitment: Mentally Retarded Minors

The Juvenile Court Code provides for the involuntary commitment of mentally retarded juveniles. If at any time during a juvenile court proceeding the evidence indicates that a child may be mentally retarded, the court may commit the child to an appropriate institution, agency, or individual for an evaluation and report on the child's mental condition.[16] If it appears from the report that the child is "committable under the laws of this state" as a mentally retarded child, the court may order the child detained and committed to the Division of Mental Retardation of the Department of Human Resources.[17] The phrase, "committable under the laws of this state," refers to the standards contained in the Mental Health Code.[18] Thus, the juvenile court may consider the commitment of a mentally retarded child in conjunction with a delinquency, unruliness, or deprivation proceeding, or a transfer hearing, or the proceeding may be instituted for the sole purpose of securing specialized services for the retarded child. In either case, the procedures outlined in the Mental Health Code are followed.

The parent, guardian, or person standing *in loco parentis*[19] may also file a petition stating that he believes that the child is mentally retarded and that the petitioner is unable to obtain appropriate services for the child.[20] Additionally, any person may file a similar petition asserting that the parent or guardian of the child has failed or is unable to secure such services.[21] The court will review the petition and, if the court finds reasonable cause to believe that the child might be mentally retarded and not receiving adequate and appropriate care, the court will issue an order within 72 hours of the filing of the petition directing that the child be examined by a comprehensive evaluation team.[22]

The evaluation team will file its written report with the court within 10 days after examining the child. If a majority of the team concludes that the child is mentally retarded and that he needs

---

16. O.C.G.A. § 15-11-40(a).
17. O.C.G.A. § 15-11-40(c).
18. *See* 1976 Op. Att'y Gen. 204 (1976).
19. *In loco parentis* means in the place of a parent. It normally refers to a person who puts himself in the situation of a lawful parent by assuming the obligations incident to the parental relation without having gone through the formalities necessary for legal adoption. *See Barron's Law Dictionary* 233 (2d ed. 1984).
20. O.C.G.A. § 37-4-40(a).
21. *Id.*
22. O.C.G.A. § 37-4-40(b). It should be noted that this is essentially the same process as outlined in O.C.G.A. § 15-11-40(a).

specialized services, the report will be in the form of an individualized program plan for the child.[23]

The court is to hold a full and fair hearing no later than 15 days after the report is filed.[24] If the court finds that the child is not mentally retarded or that he is not in need of additional care, training, or specialized services, the court will dismiss the petition.[25] If the proceeding is being held in conjunction with a delinquency, unruliness, deprivation, or transfer hearing, the court will then proceed to disposition under the appropriate provision of the Juvenile Court Code.[26]

If the court finds that the child is mentally retarded and in need of additional services, the Department of Human Resources shall recommend an habilitative program for the child that is an alternative to care in a facility.[27] If the court finds that such an alternative program is available and that the program presents a reasonable expectation of accomplishing the stated goals of the individualized plan, the court will order the child to comply with the plan.[28] If the court concludes from the evidence that the least restrictive available alternative that would accomplish the goals of the plan is for the child to be admitted to a facility, the court may not order such admission unless it further finds that

1. the child requires direct medical services;
2. the child needs 24-hour training in a residential care facility; and
3. the court has been notified by the department that a bed is available and that the plan, as recommended, can be provided.[29]

The court may then order admission to a facility for a period not to exceed 6 months, subject to the power of the superintendent to discharge the child.[30] If continued care as a resident is felt by the facility staff to be necessary at the end of 6 months, the person in charge of the child's habilitation must apply to the court for an order authorizing such continued care.[31]

In addition to the described procedures, any physician, psychologist, or clinical social worker licensed in the state can certify that he has found a child to be mentally retarded and in need of

---

23. O.C.G.A. § 37-4-40(c).
24. O.C.G.A. § 37-4-40(d).
25. O.C.G.A. § 37-4-40(e).
26. O.C.G.A. § 15-11-40(c).
27. O.C.G.A. § 37-4-40(e).
28. *Id.*
29. *Id.*
30. O.C.G.A. § 37-4-40(f).
31. *Id.*

temporary and immediate care.[32] The certificate expires 7 days after it is executed.[33] Any responsible family member or representative of the child named in the certificate may transport the child to the nearest mental health facility, or a peace officer may deliver the child to the facility.[34]

If a physician or psychologist examines the child at the facility and determines that the child is mentally retarded and in need of temporary and immediate care, a petition for a full and fair hearing must then be filed in the juvenile court of the county in which the facility is located.[35]

(D) Involuntary Commitment: Mentally Ill Minors

The same Juvenile Court Code provision that authorizes the involuntary commitment of a mentally retarded juvenile also authorizes the commitment of a mentally ill juvenile.[36] As is the case with the mentally retarded, the provisions of the Mental Health Code provide detailed procedures for such a commitment.

A child's possible need for involuntary commitment as a mentally ill child may come to the attention of the court in one of several different ways:

1. by evidence of mental illness being presented during any delinquency, unruliness, deprivation, or transfer hearing;[37]

2. by the execution of a certificate from a physician, psychologist, or clinical social worker stating that he has personally examined the child within the preceding 48 hours and has found that the child appears to be mentally ill and in need of emergency treatment;[38]

3. by a peace officer who takes a child into custody for the alleged commission of a criminal act and who has probable cause to believe that the child is mentally ill;[39]

4. by any person signing an application, under oath, with the county board of health alleging that the child is mentally ill and in need of involuntary treatment. If the board finds proba-

---

32. O.C.G.A. § 37-4-40.1.
33. Id.
34. O.C.G.A. § 37-4-40.1.
35. O.C.G.A. § 37-4-40.2.
36. O.C.G.A. § 15-11-40. Also see Ga. Comp. R. & Regs. r. 290-4-7-.07.
37. See O.C.G.A. § 15-11-40(a).
38. See O.C.G.A. § 37-3-41.
39. See O.C.G.A. § 37-3-42. The peace officer must deliver the person to a physician or psychologist for examination under § 37-3-41.

ble cause to believe that the allegation is true, it shall file a petition with the juvenile court seeking involuntary admission for an evaluation;[40]

5. by any person filing a petition with the juvenile court alleging that a child within the county is a mentally ill person requiring involuntary treatment. The petition must be accompanied by a certificate of a physician or psychologist stating that he has examined the child within the preceding 5 days and has found that the child may be a mentally ill person requiring involuntary treatment.[41]

Once a petition is filed, the juvenile court will hold a full and fair hearing on the petition and may order that a full mental status evaluation be conducted.[42] If, after evaluation, it is determined that proceedings for involuntary treatment should be initiated, facility staff will develop an individualized service plan for the patient.[43] Another hearing will then be held, at which time the court will determine whether the patient is a mentally ill person requiring involuntary treatment and, if so, whether the patient is to be an inpatient or outpatient.[44] Thus, in order to commit a child to a hospital for inpatient treatment in the absence of a voluntary admission by the parent or guardian, the court must find that the child is mentally ill and in need of inpatient services.[45] The court may order hospitalization for a period not to exceed 6 months, subject to the power of the chief medical officer to discharge the patient earlier.[46] If hospitalization is deemed necessary beyond 6 months, the chief medical officer must apply for a court order authorizing continued hospitalization for up to 12 months.[47] Whenever a patient is found, by the chief medical officer, to no longer need inpatient services, he may either discharge the patient outright, discharge the patient and require outpatient services,[48] or transfer the patient to voluntary status at the patient's request.[49]

---

40. O.C.G.A. § 37-3-61(1).
41. O.C.G.A. § 37-3-61(2).
42. O.C.G.A. § 37-3-62.
43. O.C.G.A. § 37-3-64(c).
44. O.C.G.A. § 37-3-81.1(a).
45. The Court of Appeals has ruled that a finding that a criminal defendant is "insane" meets the definition of "mental illness for purposes of civil commitment." Clark v. State, 151 Ga. App. 853, 261 S.E.2d 764 (1979); Moses v. State, 167 Ga. App. 556, 307 S.E.2d 35 (1983).
46. See supra text accompanying note 9. O.C.G.A. § 37-3-81.1(c).
47. Id.; see also O.C.G.A. § 37-3-83.
48. See O.C.G.A. §§ 37-3-90 to 37-3-95.
49. O.C.G.A. § 37-3-85(b).

4.20

Education for Handicapped and Intellectually Gifted Children

(A) Introduction

Under the federal Individuals With Disabilities Education Act (Education Act), all handicapped children are entitled to a free appropriate public education that includes special education and related services designed to meet their unique needs.[1] The Education Act requires local school systems to identify handicapped children; to evaluate each child's educational needs properly in relation to the handicap; to develop an individualized education plan (IEP) for the handicapped child that addresses the child's unique needs; to provide each handicapped child with free educational and related services in the least restrictive environment; and to maintain appropriate procedural safeguards during the evaluation, formulation, and implementation of the IEP. The federal Department of Education has promulgated detailed regulations implementing the Education Act and its procedural safeguards.[2]

Georgia's Quality Basic Education Act (QBEA) provides that all children who have special education needs shall be provided with free special education programs by their local school systems.[3] Children with special education needs include the physically and mentally handicapped, as well as the intellectually

---

1. Education of the Handicapped Act, Pub. L. 94-142, 20 U.S.C. § 1400 *et seq.* The Act's name was changed in 1990.
2. 34 C.F.R. Part 300.
3. O.C.G.A. §§ 20-2-131, 20-2-133, and 20-2-152.

gifted.[4] The State Board of Education has issued comprehensive regulations implementing the special education programs mandated by the QBEA and the federal Education Act.[5] These regulations mirror, in many respects, the Education Act regulations as to evaluation, assessment, IEP formulations, and procedural safeguards.

Because special education programs include children with specific learning disabilities, behavior disorders, and mental handicaps, and children who are intellectually gifted, the MHP plays an important role in the process. MHPs may be involved in evaluating children's status; in rendering opinions as to the nature and extent of a child's handicap and special education needs; in formulating IEPs; and in participating in hearings concerning a child's status, placement, and programs.

(B) Definitions

A student aged 5 through 21 years is considered to be *exceptional* under QBEA if he meets any of the following requirements:

1. is severely emotionally disturbed;
2. is mentally handicapped (mild, moderate, severe, or profound);
3. is speech–language disordered;
4. is hearing impaired;
5. is visually impaired;
6. is orthopedically handicapped;
7. has a specific learning disability;
8. has a behavior disorder;
9. is otherwise health impaired;
10. is deaf or blind; or
11. is intellectually gifted.[6]

---

4. O.C.G.A. § 20-2-152(a) and (d).
5. Rules of the Georgia Department of Education, Special Education, Regulations and Procedures, Ga. Comp. R. & Regs., Chapter 160-4-7. In State Dep't of Education v. Kitchens, 193 Ga. App. 229, 387 S.E.2d 579 (1989), the Court of Appeals held that the Department of Education was not exempt from the rule-making requirements of the Administrative Procedure Act. The Special Education Regulations and Procedures were subsequently adopted under the Administrative Procedure Act.
6. O.C.G.A. § 20-2-152(a); Special Education Regulations, 160-4-7-.01(1). For a detailed definition of *handicapped* under the EHA, *see* 34 C.F.R. § 300.5.

Additionally, a student from birth through 4 years of age, whose handicap is so severe as to necessitate early education intervention may be eligible for special education services.[7]

(C) Referral for Evaluation

A readiness assessment must be provided to all children entering first grade within 60 days immediately prior to September 1 of the year in which they enter public school.[8] Such a readiness assessment may also be conducted during the last 40 school days of the previous school year. If the student does not achieve the test score specified by the State Board of Education, the student will be referred for consideration for special education services.[9]

Except for evaluations that are routinely administered to all students, the local school system must have a signed, informed parental consent before any student is singled out for an evaluation.[10] If the student is referred for evaluation, the school system must then give written notice to the parent containing the following:

1. a statement that a referral has been made;
2. a statement that informs the parents of the place and date of the evaluation and that the appropriate school official will meet with the parents to discuss the reasons for the referral and the nature of the evaluation;
3. a statement that the parents will be informed within 30 school days of the results of the evaluation and the right to challenge the results by presenting an independent evaluation by an approved examiner;
4. a statement that the parents may be present at all placement committee meetings;
5. a statement that the parents may grant or refuse consent for the evaluation;
6. a statement that if no response is received, an appropriate school official will contact the home to determine the reason for the lack of response or the necessity of assigning a surrogate parent;

---

7. Spec. Ed. Regs. 160-4-7-.01(2).
8. O.C.G.A. § 20-2-151(b)(2).
9. *Id.*
10. *Id.*

7. a statement that no change will be made in the student's educational program until notification is given to the parents and due process procedures are fulfilled; and

8. a statement that either party may appeal to the local system for mediation or a hearing regarding lack of parental consent.[11]

(D) Evaluation and Recommendation for Placement

All students who are evaluated for possible special education services are reviewed by a placement committee.[12] If the committee determines that a student is handicapped and needs special education services, an IEP must be developed. The IEP forms the basis of the student's special education program.[13] A student's parents must sign an informed consent form before placement can occur.[14]

When a student is recommended for placement, the local school system will send a notice to the parents containing the following:

1. a statement that the placement committee minutes and other pertinent records and reports pertaining to the student will be available for inspection and copying at reasonable cost;

2. a statement of reasons for the proposed action, including specific tests or reports on which the proposed action is based;

3. a description of options and other factors that the school considered and the reasons why those options were rejected;

4. a statement that appropriate school officials will meet with the parents to discuss the recommended placement;

5. a statement that the parents may obtain for their child an independent evaluation by a certified or licensed examiner;

6. a statement that no change will be made in the student's status until the proposed placement is accepted by both parties;

7. a statement indicating that the parents may accept or reject the proposed placement;

8. a statement that either party may appeal the placement decision to the local board of education for mediation or for a due process hearing; and

---

11. Spec. Ed. Regs. 160-4-7-.03(3)(a).
12. Spec. Ed. Regs. 160-4-7-.03(3)(b).
13. *Id.*
14. *Id.*

9. a statement that, in the event no response is received, a school official will contact the home to determine the reasons for the lack of response or the necessity of assigning a surrogate parent.[15]

(E) Independent Evaluations

A parent has the right to an independent educational evaluation at public expense if the parent disagrees with an evaluation obtained by the local school system.[16] However, the school may initiate a hearing to show that its evaluation is appropriate.[17] If the final decision is that the evaluation is appropriate, the parent may obtain an independent evaluation at personal expense.[18]

If the parents obtain an independent evaluation at personal expense, the results of the evaluation must be considered by the school in any decision made with regard to the child's education.[19]

(F) Hearing Procedures

Each local school system must provide an opportunity for concerned parties to mediate their differences regarding the identification, evaluation, placement, and provision of a free appropriate public education to handicapped students.[20] If the mediation fails to resolve the differences, the parents may request a local due process hearing to resolve the differences. This hearing must be held within 20 calendar days of the receipt of the request.[21] Both the parents and the school may be represented by counsel, and both parties may present evidence and subpoena witnesses.[22] Parents have the right to receive written findings of fact, as well as the right to appeal the decision to a regional hearing officer. The regional hearing officer's decision may be appealed to the State Board of Education hearing officer.[23] The decision of the state hearing officer may be appealed directly to the courts.[24]

---

15. *Id.*
16. Spec. Ed. Regs. 160-4-7-.03(5)(a).
17. *Id.*
18. *Id.*
19. Spec. Ed. Regs. 160-4-7-.03(5)(b).
20. Spec. Ed. Regs. 160-4-7-.03(6)(a).
21. Spec. Ed. Regs. 160-4-7-.03(6)(b)(3).
22. Spec. Ed. Regs. 160-4-7-.03(6)(b)(4).
23. Spec. Ed. Regs. 160-4-7-.03(6)(b)(3).
24. *Id.*

(G) Least Restrictive Environment

One of the central features of both the Education Act and the QBEA special education regulations is that handicapped students be educated, to the maximum extent appropriate, in regular classes with nonhandicapped students.[25] Special classes or separate schooling is permitted only when the nature or severity of the handicap is such that education in regular classes cannot be satisfactorily achieved.[26] The need for removal from regular classes must be based on documented evidence, and the placement committee must consider various placement options to meet individual student needs.[27] A continuum of alternative placements must be available to every student, including regular classes, special classes, special schools, home instruction, and instruction in hospitals and institutions when necessary.[28] Psychological counseling and social work services are covered services under the Education Act.[29]

25. Spec. Ed. Regs. 160-4-7-.04.
26. *Id.*
27. *Id.*
28. *Id.*
29. 34 C.F.R. § 300.13.

4.21

Consent, Confidentiality, and Services to Minors

As discussed in detail in chapter 3.1 (this volume), the general rule is that unless a person gives consent to certain types of medical treatment and procedures, including treatment incident to the care of the mentally ill and mentally retarded, the health care provider may be subject to liability in tort for malpractice, assault, and battery. To avoid liability, the consent must be legally effective. If a person lacks the capacity to consent, as in the case of a minor or a person who is incompetent, the consent given by the individual will not be effective to prevent liability. The general rule is that a minor does not possess the legal capacity to consent to medical treatment. However, the law recognizes certain instances in which a minor may consent to certain types of treatment. In addition, it is often possible to obtain the consent of someone legally authorized to act on the minor's behalf, such as a natural parent or legal guardian.[1]

(A) The Georgia Medical Consent Law

The Georgia Medical Consent Law[2] provides generally that any parent may give consent to a licensed physician to provide medical or surgical treatment procedures to his minor child.[3] In the

---

1. *See, generally,* W. Keeton, *Prosser and Keeton on the Law of Torts,* Section 18 (5th ed. 1984).
2. O.C.G.A. § 31-9-1 *et seq.*
3. O.C.G.A. § 31-9-2(a)(2); *see also* O.C.G.A. § 31-9-4 (providing that the Medical Consent Law also applies to mental health services).

landmark case of *In re Jane Doe*, the Georgia Supreme Court addressed the issue of how to reconcile conflicts between parents over the decision to withdraw medical treatment from a terminally ill, unconscious child.[4] The court first noted that as a general rule, medical decision-making for incompetent patients, including minors, is best left to the patient's family and physician. The parents, as the individuals legally responsible for Jane Doe, could have refused treatment without seeking prior judicial approval because the child was terminally ill and without any reasonable hope for recovery or improvement. As to a "Do Not Resuscitate (DNR) Order," the court concluded that the consent of one parent is legally sufficient if the other parent is not present or merely prefers not to participate in the decision. However, if there is a second custodial parent who disagrees, that parent may revoke consent to a DNR order.[5] The court held that "[w]here two parents have legal custody of a child, each parent shares equal decision-making responsibility for that child."[6]

In addition to parents, a guardian may consent to services to his minor ward, and a person standing *in loco parentis* may consent for a minor under his care.[7] In addition, a married minor may consent to services for himself or his spouse;[8] a minor parent may consent to services for his minor child;[9] a minor female, regardless of marital status, may consent to family planning services.[10] Surgical and medical treatment may also be provided without express consent in an emergency when delay would jeopardize the life or health of the patient.

The Medical Consent Law by its terms deals only with surgical and medical treatment and procedures "suggested, recommended, prescribed, or directed by a duly licensed physician."[11] It is also applicable to the care and treatment of patients in mental health facilities.[12] Thus, a child between the ages of 12 and 17 years may request admittance to a mental health facility, but the

---

4. In re Jane Doe, No. S92A0325 (July 6, 1992).
5. O.C.G.A. § 31-39-1 *et seq.* If a child is of sufficient maturity to understand the nature and effect of a DNR order, then the child must also consent. *See* O.C.G.A. § 31-39-4(d).
6. *See* chapter 4.23 as to the rights of custodial and noncustodial parents.
7. O.C.G.A. § 31-9-2(a)(4); *see also* O.C.G.A. § 15-11-32 (1985) (authority of juvenile court to order a child to undergo medical treatment); O.C.G.A. § 15-11-40 (authority of juvenile court to commit mentally ill or retarded juvenile to mental health facility).
8. O.C.G.A. § 31-9-2(a)(3).
9. O.C.G.A. § 31-9-2(a)(2).
10. O.C.G.A. § 31-9-2(a)(5). The Act expressly provides that it does not apply to abortion procedures. O.C.G.A. § 31-9-5 (1982). *See* chapter 4.22 for consent to abortion.
11. O.C.G.A. § 31-9-2(a).
12. O.C.G.A. § 31-9-4.

child's parent or guardian must give written consent.[13] Any services deemed surgical or medical that are provided while in the facility would also require the parent or guardian's consent. This would presumably include consent to the administration of medication.

(B) Consent to Treatment by a Nonphysician MHP

The Medical Consent Law does not address the provision of psychotherapeutic care to minors by psychologists and other nonphysician MHPs. There is no law in Georgia that addresses directly the question of whether a minor can consent to receive such services. As a general proposition, the therapist–patient relationship is, in part, a contractual relationship. That is, there is an agreement between the therapist and the patient for the provision of psychotherapeutic services, usually for a fee. An unemancipated minor is generally not competent to contract. Moreover, providing psychotherapeutic services to a minor without the parents' consent, if consent is required, could also expose the therapist to potential tort liability.

(C) Exceptions to Parental Consent

There are also exceptions in separate statutes that permit a minor to consent to certain services for himself. A minor child seeking treatment for a venereal disease may provide consent to a physician for treatment and therapy relating to such a condition.[14] Any such consent cannot later be disaffirmed because it was given by a minor.[15] Parental consent or the consent of a guardian is not required.[16] However, the physician may, in his own discretion, and over the express objection of the minor, notify the spouse, parent, custodian, or guardian of the minor of the treatment given or needed.[17] Thus, the provision for a minor's consent to treatment does not create a right to keep the nature and fact of the treatment confidential as to the minor's parents.

Another statutory exception to the general law of consent exists for treatment relating to drug abuse. A minor seeking ser-

---

13. O.C.G.A. § 37-3-20.
14. O.C.G.A. § 31-17-7(a).
15. *Id.*
16. *Id.*
17. O.C.G.A. § 31-17-7(b).

vices for drug abuse may consent to the provision of medical or surgical care or services by a hospital, public clinic, or other licensed physician if the treatment involves procedures and therapy related to conditions or illnesses arising out of drug abuse.[18] No parental consent is required.[19] As with the general Medical Consent Law, this statutory exception applies only to medical care provided by or under the direction of a physician. It does not encompass services provided by nonphysician MHPs who are not acting under a physician's direction.

(D) Confidentiality

As in the case of treatment for venereal disease, the physician has the discretion to notify the child's parent or guardian of the treatment for a drug or alcohol abuse even over the child's objection.[20] Additionally, a minor between the ages of 12 and 17 years may apply for voluntary admission to a hospital or facility for treatment of drug or alcohol abuse, but the parents or guardian must give written consent to such inpatient treatment.[21]

As discussed in detail in Section 3 of this volume, communications between MHPs and their patients are privileged, that is, communications and records developed in the course of the relationship may not be disclosed except with consent, or pursuant to specified exceptions to consent. The privilege also applies to communications between the MHPs and their minor patients and prevents disclosure to third parties. The question arises, however, as to the disclosure of information to minor's parents or guardian.

As noted, although a child may receive drug abuse and venereal disease treatment without parental consent, the physician can inform the parent or guardian without the minor's consent and in spite of his objections. The records of a child receiving treatment in a mental health facility may also be released to the child's parent or guardian. Although there are no Georgia cases dealing with the issue, it would appear that when a parent's or guardian's consent is required for a child to receive treatment, then the parent would have the right to examine the child's records and to be informed of the nature and course of the treatment. This is because the child can act only through the

---

18. O.C.G.A. § 37-7-8(b). This provision does not, however, apply to a minor seeking services for alcohol abuse. There is no provision in Georgia law that permits a minor to consent to treatment for alcohol abuse absent parental consent or pursuant to some other general exception.

19. *Id.*

20. O.C.G.A. § 37-7-8(c).

21. O.C.G.A. § 37-7-20(a).

parent, and the parent has the right to be informed as to the care given the child.[22] However, the confidential nature of the MHP–patient relationship exists regardless of the fact that the patient is a minor and disclosure to third parties, other than the parent or guardian or when otherwise permitted by law, would be actionable under the same principles as those that govern the disclosure of privileged communications with adult patients.

---

22. As to the disclosure of medical records, *generally see* O.C.G.A. § 24-9-40, which provides that medical information may be released to a minor's parent or guardian. This code section does not apply to psychiatrists.

4.22

Consent for Abortion

Georgia law requires that a minor seeking an abortion either notify her parents or obtain a court order waiving notice. MHPs may become involved in judicial bypass proceedings concerning the minor's ability to make her own decision and the impact requiring notice would have on her child.

(A) History of Parental Notification

In 1987, the Georgia General Assembly passed the Parental Notification Act[1] requiring a minor seeking an abortion to notify her parent or guardian or to petition the juvenile court for a waiver of parental notification. The Act was challenged in the U.S. District Court for the Northern District of Georgia, which granted the plaintiffs' motion for a preliminary injunction enjoining the implementation of the Act.[2] The court reasoned that

---

1. 1987 Ga. Laws 1013 (codified as amended at O.C.G.A. §15-11-110 *et seq.*).
2. Planned Parenthood Ass'n of Atlanta Area v. Harris, 670 F. Supp. 971 (N.D. Ga. 1987). For an excellent discussion of abortion litigation in Georgia, *see* Appley, *Two Decades of Reproductive Freedom Litigation*, 28 Ga. St. B.J. 34 (Aug. 1991).

1. the verification procedures of the Act were unconstitutionally burdensome and failed to provide adequate alternative means of verification;[3] and

2. the Universal Juvenile Court Rules requiring the inclusion on certain documents of the minor's name and social security number failed to guarantee adequate anonymity in seeking judicial waiver by not requiring that the juvenile court record be sealed.[4]

The legislature amended the Parental Notification Act in 1988[5] in an effort to cure the defects noted by the district court. The amended Act met with the same fate as the original Act. The district court once again issued a preliminary injunction enjoining implementation of the amended Act.[6] On appeal, the Eleventh Circuit Court of Appeals vacated the injunction and upheld the statute on all grounds.[7]

(B) Parental Notification Requirements

The Parental Notification Act, as it is currently codified, provides that a physician cannot perform an abortion upon an unemancipated minor under the age of 18 years unless

1. the minor furnishes a statement from a parent, guardian, or individual standing *in loco parentis* stating that he or she has been notified that the child is seeking an abortion; or

2. the physician gives 24 hours' actual notice, in person or by telephone, to a parent, guardian, or individual standing *in loco parentis* of the pending abortion; or

---

3. Verification could be accomplished either by the minor's parent or legal guardian accompanying the minor to the abortion facility and furnishing an affidavit that he or she was the minor's parent or guardian, or by the minor finding another adult to accompany her to the abortion facility and furnish an affidavit that the minor's parent, or guardian, or individual standing *in loco parentis* had been notified. See O.C.G.A. §§ 15-11-112(a)(1)(A)-(1)(C) (Supp. 1987).

4. 670 F. Supp. at 994. The court also stayed further proceedings in the case pending the outcome in the U.S. Supreme Court of Zbaraz v. Hartigan. *Id.* Zbaraz v. Hartigan was subsequently affirmed without an opinion; 763 F.2d 1532 (7th Cir. 1985), *aff'd mem.*, 484 U.S. 1082 (1987).

5. 1988 Ga. Laws 13; 1988 Ga. Laws 661 (codified at O.C.G.A. § 15-11-110 *et seq.*).

6. Planned Parenthood Ass'n of Atlanta Area v. Harris, 691 F. Supp. 1419 (N.D. Ga. 1988).

7. Planned Parenthood Ass'n v. Miller, 934 F.2d 1462 (11th Cir. 1991).

3. the physician gives written notice of the pending abortion, sent by regular mail, addressed to a parent, guardian, or individual standing *in loco parentis* of the child. Such notice is deemed to be delivered 48 hours after mailing, and the abortion may be performed 24 hours after the delivery of the notice; and

4. the minor signs a consent form stating that she consents, freely and without coercion, to the abortion.[8]

If the minor or the physician does not wish to provide notice to the parent or guardian, or if the parent or guardian cannot be located, the minor may petition any juvenile court in the state for a waiver of the notice requirements.[9] The hearing on the petition must be held within 3 days of the date of filing, and if not held within that time frame, the petition is deemed granted.[10] The court must take steps to preserve the anonymity of the minor.[11]

The notification requirements will be waived if the court finds either that the minor is mature enough to make the abortion decision in consultation with her physician independently of the wishes of the parent or guardian, or that the notice requirements would not be in the best interests of the minor.[12] The court may wish to use the expert testimony of an MHP in determining if the child is mature enough to make the abortion decision or to provide information concerning whether it would be in the best interests of the child that her parents not be notified. The court must render its decision within 24 hours of the conclusion of the hearing, or the petition is deemed granted.[13]

The U.S. Supreme Court has held that the state may not impose a blanket provision requiring the consent of a parent as a condition for abortion of an unmarried minor.[14] However, it has held that the state has a legitimate interest in promoting parental consultation with a minor who is seeking to obtain an abortion because of the minor's presumed inability to make important decisions in an informed, mature manner and the serious concerns implicated by a decision to have an abortion.[15] The U.S. Supreme Court has specifically upheld statutes that

---

8. O.C.G.A. § 15-11-112(a).
9. O.C.G.A. § 15-11-112(b).
10. O.C.G.A. § 15-11-113.
11. O.C.G.A. § 15-11-114(b).
12. O.C.G.A. § 15-11-114(c).
13. O.C.G.A. § 15-11-114(d).
14. Planned Parenthood of Central Missouri v. Danforth, 428 U.S. 52 at 74, 96 S. Ct. 2831 (1976).
15. Bellotti v. Baird, 443 U.S. 622 at 634, 99 S. Ct. 3035 (1979).

require the consent of one parent, but that also provide for a judicial bypass procedure.[16]

---

16. Planned Parenthood of Southeastern Pennsylvania et al. v. Casey et al., 112 S. Ct. 2791 (1992); City of Akron v. Akron Center for Reproductive Health, Inc., 462 U.S. 416, 103 S. Ct. 2481 (1983) (Akron I); Ohio v. Akron Center for Reproductive Health, 497 U.S. 502 (1990) (Akron II); Bellotti v. Baird, 443 U.S. 622 (1979) (Bellotti II).

4.23

Involvement of Noncustodial Parents in the Evaluation and Treatment of Their Children

When divorcing parents have minor children, Georgia law provides for joint legal custody, joint physical custody, both joint legal and physical custody, and sole custody. MHPs may be asked to provide services to children at the request of noncustodial parents. Furthermore, noncustodial parents may request information regarding the evaluation and treatment of their children. The question arises whether MHPs, in complying with such requests, violate any law or professional duties if they fail to obtain consent from the custodial parent for cooperating with the noncustodial parent.

Joint legal custody gives both parents equal rights and responsibilities for major decisions concerning the child, including health care.[1] In the absence of some provision in the court's custody order to the contrary, parents with joint legal custody would have equal rights to make decisions concerning a child's mental health care and would have equal rights of access to the child's medical records. The granting of sole custody to one parent does not terminate the parental rights of the noncustodial parent but the Georgia Code specifies that a parent with sole custody of a child has the rights and responsibilities for major decisions concerning the child, including health care, unless otherwise provided.[2] Although there are no court decisions interpreting this code section, the Georgia courts have indicated that a noncustodial parent can legitimately make decisions regarding a minor child during visitation periods.[3] Furthermore, it is unlikely

---

1. O.C.G.A. § 19-9-6.
2. O.C.G.A. § 19-9-6(4).
3. *See, e.g.,* Applebaum v. Hanes, 159 Ga. App. 552 (1981).

that a court would find that the noncustodial parent has the right to examine the child's records absent consent of the parent with sole custody. If an MHP faces a dispute between parents, the safest course would be to ask the non-custodial parent for a court order giving him or her the right to direct the MHP.

If there is a court order in effect regarding the custody of the minor child, it may modify the statutory rights and obligations of parents and limit their right to consent to treatment and may impose obligations as to the payment of medical expenses. Therefore, any MHP who is being asked to treat a child whose parents are divorced or separated should inquire as to whether there is a court order dealing with custody, consent to treatment, medical care, and financial responsibility. If such an order exists, it should be examined to determine the extent of both parents' rights and responsibilities.

4.24

Family Violence

As used in the Georgia Code, the term *family violence* refers to the occurrence of one or more of the following acts between past or present spouses, parents and children, stepparents and stepchildren, foster parents and foster children, or other individuals living in the same household:

1. any felony; or
2. commission of the offenses of battery, assault, criminal damage to property, unlawful restraint, or criminal trespass.[1]

The term *family violence* does not include reasonable discipline administered by a parent to a child in the form of corporal punishment, restraint, or detention.[2] Georgia law provides a method for relief from family violence about which MHPs should be aware so that they may advise clients who are experiencing such difficulties.

(A) Procedures for Relief From Family Violence

An individual may seek relief from family violence by filing either on his or her behalf or on behalf of a minor a petition with the superior court of the county in which the individual responsible for the family violence resides, alleging one or more specific

---

1. O.C.G.A. § 19-13-1.
2. *Id.*

acts of family violence.[3] Upon the filing of a verified petition in which the petitioner alleges with specific facts that probable cause exists to establish that family violence has occurred in the past and may occur in the future, the court may order such temporary relief as it deems necessary to protect the petitioner or a minor of the household from violence.[4] The court may issue an order without a hearing and without giving the individual allegedly responsible for the family violence advance notice or time to respond to the allegations (an *ex parte* order). If the court issues an *ex parte* order, a copy of the order must be immediately furnished to the respondent.

Within 10 days of the filing of the petition, a hearing must be held at which the petitioner must prove the allegations of the petition by a preponderance of the evidence, as in all other civil cases. If a hearing is not held within 10 days, the petition shall be dismissed unless the parties otherwise agree.[5]

(B) Granting of Protective Orders

Upon the filing of a verified petition, the court may grant any protective order or approve any consent agreement to bring about a cessation of acts of family violence.[6] The order or agreement may

1. direct a party to refrain from such acts;
2. grant a spouse possession of the residence or household of the parties and exclude the other spouse from the residence or household;
3. require a party to provide suitable, alternate housing for a spouse and his or her children;
4. award temporary custody of minor children and establish temporary visitation rights;
5. order the eviction of a party from the residence or household and order assistance to the victim in returning to it or order assistance in retrieving personal property of the victim if the respondent's eviction has not been ordered;
6. order either party to make payments for the support of a minor child as required by law;

---

3. O.C.G.A. § 19-13-3(a).
4. O.C.G.A. § 19-13-3(b).
5. O.C.G.A. § 19-13-3(c).
6. O.C.G.A. § 19-13-4.

7. order either party to make payments for the support of a spouse as required by law;

8. provide for possession of personal property of the parties;

9. order a party to refrain from harassing or interfering with the other;

10. award costs and attorneys' fees to either party; and

11. order either or all parties to receive appropriate psychiatric or psychological services as a further measure to prevent the recurrence of family violence.[7]

A copy of the order is issued by the clerk of the court to the sheriff of the county in which the order was entered and is then retained by the sheriff as long as that order is to remain in effect.[8] The court issuing any protective order may order the sheriff, any deputy sheriff, or any other state, county, or municipal law enforcement officer or official to enforce or carry out such order.[9] Any such order granted remains in effect for not more than 6 months.[10]

A violation of an order issued pursuant to this law may be punished by an action for contempt.[11] Any individual who violates the provisions of a domestic violence order that excludes or evicts that person from a residence or household shall be guilty of a misdemeanor.[12]

---

7. *Id.*
8. *Id.*
9. O.C.G.A. § 19-13-4(d).
10. O.C.G.A. § 19-13-6(c).
11. O.C.G.A. § 19-13-6(a).
12. O.C.G.A. § 19-13-6 (b).

Other Civil Matters

5.1

Mental Status of Licensed Professionals

The state of Georgia, like other states, provides for an examining board's investigation, examination, and scrutiny of professionals who are required to be licensed. Increasingly, the laws governing licensure include provisions concerning the mental status of professionals, including mental health professionals (MHPs). These laws generally pertain to the regulation of licenses (i.e., discipline, suspension, and revocation). MHPs may be asked to evaluate and testify before a licensing board or a court concerning the professional's mental status and its effect on his or her ability to practice the profession properly.

As a general rule, Georgia's licensure laws contain a provision that a license may be suspended, revoked, or not issued if the person is unable to practice with reasonable skill and safety.[1] Clearly, some mental disorders and nervous conditions could hinder or prevent a practitioner from performing competently. Most laws provide that the applicant or professional, by virtue of his application for license, has granted to the examining board the right to require a physical or mental examination. Examining boards are given the authority and duty to inquire into the ability of professionals to perform in accordance with acceptable standards of care.

(A) Attorneys

Georgia law provides that members of the State Bar of Georgia are disciplined by the State Disciplinary Board and the Georgia

---

1. *See* O.C.G.A. § 43-1-19(a)(10).

Supreme Court. The powers and duties of the board include the duty to receive and evaluate any and all written complaints against members of the bar, to frame such a charge or complaint in compliance with the requirements of the rules, or to initiate a complaint on its own motion and to conduct investigations, and take evidence, and hold hearings.[2] Disciplinary action that may be taken includes disbarment, suspension, or reprimand.[3] Want of a sound mind or senility, when found to exist, constitutes grounds for removing the name of an attorney from the roll of attorneys who are members of the State Bar of Georgia and from the practice of law.[4]

(B) Dentists

The Practice Act for Dentists and Dental Hygienists (the Dental Practice Act) provides that the Georgia Board of Dentistry (the Dentistry Board) has the authority to refuse to grant a license to an applicant, to revoke a license, or to discipline a dentist upon a finding by a majority of the Dentistry Board that the licensee had "been adjudged mentally incompetent by a court of competent jurisdiction within or without this state."[5] Any such adjudication automatically suspends the license and prevents the reissuance or renewal of a license so suspended for so long as the adjudication of incompetence is in effect.[6]

The Dental Practice Act further provides that a dentist who has displayed an inability to practice dentistry with reasonable skill and safety to patients or who has become unable to practice dentistry with reasonable skill and safety to patients by reason of illness; use of alcohol, drugs, narcotics, chemicals, or other type of material; or as a result of a mental or physical condition; or by displaying habitual intoxication, addiction to or recurrent misuse of alcohol, drugs, narcotics, chemicals, or any similar substance, may have his or her license revoked or suspended. The Dentistry Board may, upon reasonable grounds, require a licensee or applicant to submit to a mental or physical examination by physicians designated by the Board. The results of the examination are admissible in any hearing before the Dentistry Board, notwithstanding any claim of privilege. Every person who accepts the privilege of practicing dentistry will be deemed to have given his or her

---

2. Rules and Regulations for the Organization and Government of the State Bar of Georgia, Rule 4-201.
3. *Id.*, Rule 4-102.
4. *Id.*, Rule 4-104.
5. O.C.G.A. § 43-11-47(a)(11).
6. *Id.*

consent to a mental or physical examination and to have waived all objections to the admissibility of the results in any hearing before the Dentistry Board upon the grounds that the information constitutes a privileged communication. If the licensee or applicant fails to submit to an examination when directed to do so, unless such failure is due to circumstances beyond control, the Board may enter a final order upon proper notice, hearing, and proof of such refusal. Any licensee who is prohibited from practicing under this will be afforded, after reasonable intervals, an opportunity to demonstrate to the Dentistry Board that he or she can resume or begin the practice of dentistry with reasonable skill and safety to patients.[7]

(C) Physical Therapists

The State Board of Physical Therapy (the Physical Therapy Board) is the licensing and disciplinary agent for physical therapists and physical therapy assistants. The Physical Therapy Board determines the "competence of applicants to practice as physical therapists or as physical therapist assistants by any method or procedure which the Physical Therapy Board deems necessary to test the applicant's qualifications."[8] A physical therapist who holds a license may have it revoked, suspended, or restricted on the basis of the Physical Therapy Board's determination that a physical therapist or physical therapy assistant is unable to practice his or her occupation with reasonable skill and safety by reason of illness; use of alcohol, drugs, narcotics, chemicals or other type of material; or as a result of any mental or physical condition.[9] In an effort to encourage the reporting of individuals who are unable to practice physical therapy with reasonable skill and safety, immunity from civil or criminal liability by reason of the act of reporting is accorded to anyone making a report in good faith.[10]

(D) Physicians

Applicants for medical license and physicians already licensed must possess the mental capacity necessary to practice medicine and may be required to take a physical or mental examination[11] (see chapter 1.1).

---

7. O.C.G.A. § 43-11-47(a)(12).
8. O.C.G.A. § 43-33-14.
9. O.C.G.A. § 43-33-18.
10. O.C.G.A. § 43-33-18(d).
11. O.C.G.A. § 43-34-37(a)(13).

(E) Psychiatric Nurses

A registered nurse, including registered nurses certified in advanced nursing practice such as psychiatry/mental health, may have his or her license revoked or be disciplined if the Georgia Board of Nursing finds that the licensee or applicant has displayed an inability to practice nursing with reasonable skill and safety to patients by reason of illness; use of alcohol, drugs, narcotics, chemicals, or any other type material; or as a result of any mental or physical condition (see chapter 1.2).[12]

(F) Licensed Pactical Nurses

Licensed practical nurses are required to renew their license biannually. The Georgia Practical Nurses Practice Act[13] provides for the denial of a license or sanctions should the licensee or applicant be adjudged mentally incompetent by a court of competent jurisdiction or display an inability to practice nursing with reasonable skill and safety to the public by reason of illness or the use of alcohol, drugs, narcotics, or chemicals, or as a result of any mental or physical condition.[14] The statute further provides that the Board of Examiners of Licensed Practical Nurses (LPN Board) may obtain any and all records relating to the mental or physical condition of a licensee or applicant. These records will be admissible in any hearing before the LPN Board notwithstanding any privilege to the contrary.[15]

(G) Psychologists

The State Board of Examiners of Psychologists (Psychology Board) has the authority to refuse to grant or renew a license, to suspend or revoke a license, or to discipline a licensed psychologist. The Psychology Board may take action if it determines that a psychologist has engaged in habitual intemperance in the use of alcoholic beverages, narcotics, or stimulants to such an extent as to incapacitate the psychologist in the performance of his or her duties; has been negligent or engaged in wrongful actions in the performance of duties; has been adjudged mentally incompetent by a court of competent jurisdiction; or has become unable to

---

12. O.C.G.A. § 43-26-11(2).
13. O.C.G.A. § 43-26-30.
14. O.C.G.A. § 43-26-40(a)(6).
15. *Id.*

practice a business or profession with reasonable skill and safety to the public by reason of illness, use of alcohol, drugs, narcotics, or chemicals.[16] The Board may, if it has a reasonable basis to believe that a psychologist is practicing while incapacitated by reason of substance abuse or mental or physical illness, require the licensee to submit to a mental or physical examination by an appropriate licensed practitioner. The results of such an examination will be admissible in any hearing before the Board, notwithstanding any claim of privilege.[17] Furthermore, the Board may require the psychologist to provide or give to the Board permission to obtain any and all records relating to the alleged incapacitating mental or physical condition, including the individual's psychiatric and psychological records.[18] If a psychologist fails to submit to the required examination or to provide the requested records, his or her license may be suspended by the Board.[19]

---

16. O.C.G.A. § § 43-39-13(a) and 43-1-19(a)(9), (10).
17. O.C.G.A. § 43-39-13(a)(1).
18. O.C.G.A. § 43-39-13(a)(2).
19. *Id.*

5.2

Workers' Compensation

Under the Georgia Workers' Compensation law, individuals in the service of another under any contract of hire or apprenticeship who sustain sickness, injury, or accident arising out of the scope and course of work for their employer are accorded the protection of the workers' compensation law requiring that the employer provide insurance against losses relating to work-related accidents or diseases.[1] The law provides that the employer (with certain exceptions[2]) must purchase insurance or by a certification process declare itself self-insured to provide the statutory benefits to its employees.[3] In return, the employee relinquishes the right to sue the employer under principles of fault and legal responsibility. An employee may elect to forgo benefits and retain the right to sue only if the workers' compensation coverage is formally rejected prior to the accident or sickness. Otherwise, the employee is presumed to have elected the coverage.

Psychologists, psychiatrists, and other MHPs are involved in this process, not only in terms of their own employees who may be injured, but when an employee/claimant consults a psychologist, vocational rehabilitation professional, or other MHP for diagnosis and treatment, with the cost of these services being paid by the workers' compensation carrier or the employer under a self-insured plan. Likewise, an insurance company may request a psychologist, psychiatrist, or other MHP to conduct an independent medical or psychological examination (IME or IPE) to deter-

---

1. O.C.G.A. § 34-9-120.
2. O.C.G.A. § 34-9-2.
3. O.C.G.A. § 34-9-150 *et seq.*

mine the nature and extent of the employee's injury and to testify regarding the findings before the Workers' Compensation Board.

(A) Scope of Coverage

Workers' compensation benefits are payable for accidents and disease arising out of and in the course of employment. The law draws distinctions between those compensable incidents that are accidents and those conditions that are termed occupational diseases. For an accident to be compensable, it must

1. result from an injury caused by either an external cause or an injury that is unexpected or accidental; and
2. have occurred within a reasonably definite period of time.

Although gradual injuries are compensable provided this test is satisfied, the cause and effect must be reasonably definite. The injury may be accidental if the result is repeated trauma. The notion that repeated trauma can create a compensable injury is substantiated by the idea that the injurious effect materializes on the day on which the last trauma occurs and, at that point, it becomes an accident that is subject to a claim.[4]

For an occupational disease to be compensable, it must be shown that the disease

1. has some direct causal connection with the conditions under which the work is performed;
2. is the natural incident of the work, occasioned by the nature of the employment;
3. can be fairly traced to the employment as the proximate cause;
4. does not come from a hazard to which the employee would have been equally exposed outside of the employment;
5. is incidental to the character of the business and not independent of the relation of the employer and employee; and
6. appears to have its origin in a risk connected with the employment, and flows from that source as a natural consequence, although it may not have been foreseen or expected.[5]

Compensable diseases may include those arising naturally and unavoidably from an accident.[6]

---

4. O.C.G.A. § 34-9-1(4).
5. O.C.G.A. § 34-9-280(2).
6. O.C.G.A. § 34-9-280 *et seq.*

(B) Workers' Compensation: Mental and Emotional Disorders

Workers' compensation cases involving mental stress or emotional disorders in Georgia may be classified in one of the following categories:

1. Mental or emotional illness is compensable if the mental or emotional condition results from some initial compensable physical injury.[7]

2. A psychological or nervous injury resulting from long-term stress or other job-related factor may be compensable as an occupational disease if it meets the test for an occupational disease.[8]

An emotional or physical condition emanating from stress, conversely, can produce a compensable, physical condition.[9] Purely emotionally initiated heart attacks can also constitute accidental injuries.[10] The statute also treats disability or death resulting from an occupational disease in the same manner as an injury by accident.[11]

In a situation in which two or more employers are involved, the employer and insurance carrier who last exposed the employer to any hazard is liable for payment of workers' compensation.[12]

(C) Processing a Claim

The Workers' Compensation Board is required to publish a summary of the rights, benefits, and obligations under the workers' compensation laws. The rules are required to be displayed by employers in a location accessible to employees.[13]

---

7. Employer's Insurance Company of Alabama v. Wright, 114 Ga. App. 10, 150 S.E.2d 254 (1966).
8. *See* Glynn County Board of Commissioners v. Mimbs, 161 Ga. App. 350, 291 S.E.2d 62 (1982); Howard v. Superior Contractors, 180 Ga. App. 68, 348 S.E.2d 563 (1986); Sawyer v. Pacific Indemnity Company, 141 Ga. App. 298, 233 S.E.2d 227 (1977).
9. City Council of Augusta v. Williams, 137 Ga. App. 177, 223 S.E.2d 227 (1976).
10. Travelers Insurance Company v. Neal, 124 Ga. App. 750, 186 S.E.2d 346 (1971).
11. O.C.G.A. § 34-9-281(a).
12. O.C.G.A. § 34-9-284.
13. O.C.G.A. § 34-9-81.1(a).

Notice of injury must be provided by an injured employee to the employer in written or oral form within 30 days of the occurrence of the injury or death (or in the case of a minor or mentally incompetent claimant, within 30 days of the date on which the individual has a guardian, trustee, or representative to provide such notice for him).[14] After providing such notice, a claim must be filed with the Workers' Compensation Board within 1 year from the date of injury or death. Even if the employee is injured on the job and continues working for the same employer, an aggravation of the original injury will be treated as a "new injury" and the 1-year period begins to run anew from the time of the aggravation.[15]

After the filing of the claim, an administrative law judge is assigned, and a hearing is held as soon as practicable. The judge may administer oaths and affirmations, issue subpoenas, rule upon offers of proof, regulate the course of the hearing, and set the time and place for other hearings, briefs, and otherwise exercise plenary jurisdiction over the proceeding.[16] Pleadings need not be in any specific form, and hearings are conducted as informally as possible while preserving the rights of the parties. The rules of evidence as applied in civil non-jury proceedings in the superior court are used. Hearsay evidence, no matter how it is received, is deemed to be without probative value.[17] The law does provide, however, that

> any medical report on a form prescribed by the board or in narrative form signed and dated by an examining or treating physician or other duly "qualified medical practitioner"shall be admissible in evidence insofar as it purports to represent the history, examination, diagnoses, treatment, and prognosis by the persons signing the report, as if that person were present at the hearing and testifying as a witness, subject to the right of any party to object to the admissibility of any portion of the report, and subject to the right of an adverse party to cross-examine the person signing the report and provide rebuttal testimony.[18]

Although the opinion of an expert witness is entitled to great weight in workers' compensation cases, it is not conclusive to the Board and may be either accepted or rejected.[19] In a compensation proceeding, the disability of an employee may also be proved by nonexpert testimony.[20]

---

14. O.C.G.A. § 34-9-80.
15. House v. Echota Cotton Mills, Inc., 129 Ga. App. 350, 199 S.E.2d 585 (1973).
16. O.C.G.A. § 34-9-102.
17. Merritt v. Continental Cas. Ins. Co., 65 Ga. App. 826, 16 S.E.2d 612 (1941).
18. O.C.G.A. § 34-9-102(e)(2).
19. Department of Revenue v. Graham, 102 Ga. App. 756, 117 S.E.2d 902 (1960).
20. B.P.O. Elks Lodge No. 230 v. Foster, 91 Ga. App. 696, 86 S.E.2d 725 (1955).

After the hearing, the administrative law judge enters his decision, the claimant having the burden of proof. The decision contains a concise report of the case, including findings of fact and conclusions of law, and such explanation as may be necessary. The only decision that the Workers' Compensation Board has the power to make is to grant or deny compensation.

After the decision becomes final, a party may file a certified copy of the final award for settlement agreement approved by the Board with the superior court in the county in which the injury occurred. The court will then enter a judgment in accordance with the award which will then have the same effect as if it had been determined by the court. The existence of a judgment entitles parties to enforce the award made by the Board in the same manner as other civil judgments.[21]

Review of the administrative law judge's decision may be obtained by filing an application for review within 20 days after entry of the decision. Upon the filing of an application, all members of the Workers' Compensation Board will review the evidence contained in the record, may call parties and witnesses, and proceed with a further hearing.[22]

A party may appeal the Board's final decision to the superior court of the county in which the injury occurred. If the decision of the Workers' Compensation Board is supported by any evidence, it will not be disturbed on appeal, unless it is based on fraud or an erroneous legal theory.[23]

(D) Workers' Compensation Benefits

The benefits provided under the Workers' Compensation Act generally include medical, disability, death, and, in some instances, rehabilitation benefits. Medical benefits cover immediate and long-term expenses based on medical services rendered and medical fees approved by the Workers' Compensation Board.[24] Additionally, a claimant may be awarded rehabilitation benefits.[25]

Disability payments cover the loss of income during the period when the employee is unable to work and include the terms "permanent" or "temporary," "partial" or "total" to describe the disability and the classification in which the claimant falls. A claimant may move from a temporary total condition, indicating

---

21. O.C.G.A. § 34-9-106.
22. O.C.G.A. § 34-9-103.
23. Sewell Plastics, Inc. v. Skelton, 163 Ga. App. 163, 293 S.E.2d 555 (1982).
24. O.C.G.A. § 34-9-200.
25. O.C.G.A. § 34-9-200.1.

that he cannot work at all, to a permanent partial condition should he be able to resume work on a part-time basis. The ratings of the percentage of functional impairment must be in accordance with standards recognized and applied by physicians. Although guides such as the Guide to the Evaluation of Permanent Impairment may be used, they do not permit a precise evaluation of the more discrete type of injury. Disability awards are divided into scheduled and unscheduled benefits. Scheduled benefits include loss of a body function such as loss of a limb, an eye, or hearing. Unscheduled benefits concern all other injuries and require determination of the extent and nature of the impairment. Death benefits cover burial expenses and specified payments to the employee's dependents.

Payment of Rehabilitation Benefits Under Workers' Compensation Law

Georgia's Workers' Compensation law provides for payment of compensation, including rehabilitation benefits.[1] The employer and insurer have 48 hours after a determination that the injury is compensable to appoint a rehabilitation supplier or give a reason why rehabilitation is not necessary. If it is determined that rehabilitation is required, the employer must select a rehabilitation supplier within 15 days from notification of the determination.[2]

In the event of a catastrophic injury, including paralysis, loss of a limb, severe brain damage, extensive burns, or total blindness, an employer must furnish the employee with reasonable and necessary rehabilitation services.[3]

Upon the refusal of the employee to accept rehabilitation, the Workers' Compensation Board is entitled, in its discretion, to suspend and reduce the payments otherwise payable to the employee. The Workers' Compensation Board may recommend review by a panel of specialists to determine whether or not suspension or reduction of compensation is justified.[4] The fees of suppliers and the reasonableness and necessity of their services are subject to the approval of the Board. Suppliers must file with the Board required forms and a copy of the statement of fees charged. Without the filing of such information, no fees may be collected. The Workers' Compensation Board may also require recommendations from a panel of appropriate peers of the reha-

---

1. O.C.G.A. §§ 34-9-200 and 34-9-207.
2. O.C.G.A. § 34-9-200.1(a).
3. O.C.G.A. § 34-9-200.1.
4. O.C.G.A. § 34-9-200.1(c).

bilitation supplier in determining whether the fees submitted and necessity of services rendered were reasonable.[5]

A rehabilitation supplier must hold one of the following certifications:

1. certified rehabilitation counselor;
2. certified insurance rehabilitation specialist;
3. certified rehabilitation registered nurse;
4. work adjustment and vocational evaluation specialist; or
5. licensed professional counselor;

and must be registered with the Workers' Compensation Board. Failure to comply with the registration requirements, may result in revocation of registration of the rehabilitation supplier's registration.[6]

For purposes of the Workers' Compensation Act, the term *physician* includes individuals licensed to practice a healing art and any remedial treatment and care in the state of Georgia. Provision is made for maintaining a list of four physicians or professional associations or corporations of physicians who are reasonably accessible to employees with the employee having the right to select the physician for treatment. Provision is made also for change of physician.[7] Physician and hospital fees are required to be approved under schedules of usual, customary, and reasonable charges.[8]

(A) Diagnostic Studies

1. The employer or the insurer must assess the injured party's need for rehabilitation within 90 days of notification of injury. The employer or its insurer has the exclusive right within a 90-day period to appoint a rehabilitation supplier or give reason why rehabilitation is not necessary and must notify the injured employee and the Workers' Compensation Board on forms prescribed by the Workers' Compensation Board.

2. If the employer or its insurer has not appointed a rehabilitation supplier within the 90-day period, any party may petition the Workers' Compensation Board for an assessment of the rehabilitation needs of the injured employee and, if appropriate,

---

5. O.C.G.A. § 34-9-200.1(d).
6. O.C.G.A. § 34-9-200.1(f).
7. O.C.G.A. § 34-9-201.
8. O.C.G.A. § 34-9-205.

the appointment of a rehabilitation supplier to restore the employee to a suitable employment.

3. The Workers' Compensation Board may order at any time an assessment of the need for rehabilitation services. If the Workers' Compensation Board on its own determines that a rehabilitation supplier is needed, it will appoint a supplier.

4. A change in the designated rehabilitation supplier may be made only with the approval of the Workers' Compensation Board. Any party to the case may request the Board to change the rehabilitation supplier.

Rehabilitation suppliers have the sole responsibility for the management and treatment of each individual case. The Workers' Compensation Board's recognized principal supplier must complete, with the injured employee, the initial rehabilitation evaluation within 30 days of appointment to the case. An appropriate plan for services is reported on forms for both noncatastrophic and catastrophic medical care. Coordination services should be completed within 60 days of appointment to the case. The rehabilitation supplier must provide direct service delivery and close the rehabilitation case when appropriate.

A board-recognized principal supplier may obtain specific services from another qualified individual, facility, or agency for direct services outside the scope of expertise of the approved supplier upon Board approval of a plan that specifies such service. The principal supplier is charged with the duty of completing, signing, and filing all reports with the Workers' Compensation Board and serving copies on the employer and insurer. The initial evaluation consists of a personal interview between the employee and the principal supplier and includes a review of medical and other records to determine the employee's need for rehabilitation services and the feasibility of providing rehabilitation services. The written evaluation report must include at least the following:

1. a summary of current medical status, secondary conditions affecting recovery, treatment, prognosis, and estimate of time frames, if possible;

2. employer contacts regarding return to work, including whether at the same job, a modified job, a different job, a graduated return to work, or termination of employment;

3. social history;

4. educational background;

5. employment history;

6. financial status as applicable to the rehabilitation process;

7. transportation ability;

8. summary of positive and negative indicators for return to work; and

9. statement of the supplier's conclusion regarding the employee's need for rehabilitation service and the likelihood that the employee will benefit from further rehabilitation service.

After the individualized rehabilitation plan is completed, the supplier provides all parties and the Board with a copy within 60 days of the appointment. Rehabilitation commences with the approval of the plan, which includes goals, justification for goals, objectives to achieve the goals, dates for completion of objectives, delineation of responsibilities of the parties involved, and estimated rehabilitation cost to complete the plan.

Absent written objections to the Workers' Compensation Board, which are to be served on all parties within 15 days, the plan will be approved and no further correspondence will be necessary.

The types of rehabilitation plans include

1. medical care coordination to obtain maximum medical improvement and independence in activities of daily living;

2. independent living, including the necessary home and vehicle modifications, home care in order that a catastrophically injured employee can return to a less restricted lifestyle and a life care plan;

3. extended evaluation to establish an appropriate vocational goal;

4. return to work and assistance with job placement in order to return to suitable employment, including on-the-job training in the same or different work setting leading to employment;

5. training that is feasible and necessary to obtain suitable vocational goals; and

6. self-employment plan, when return to work plans and training plans are not feasible and reasonable probability of success in self-employment can be documented.

Rehabilitation suppliers are required to comply with a code of ethics, which requires adherence to normative standards designed to promote the welfare of the patient. The supplier should explain the purpose of the relationship and the injured employee's role, demonstrate honesty and objectivity in interactions provide written reports, and help the injured employee identify appropriate rehabilitation goals. The list of duties and obligations owed the injured employee include confidentiality, the identification of parties who will receive information and reports, the preparation of professional files and reports, and respect for the privacy of the injured worker.

A peer review committee is established to provide procedures for rehabilitation suppliers to evaluate, request, and make recommendations to the Workers' Compensation Board regarding disputes concerning the necessity of services, reasonableness of fees, and violation of ethical standards. Rehabilitation expenses are limited to the usual and customary charges prevailing in the state.

(B) Fees

Payment of medical expenses or rehabilitation services are fixed as usual and customary charges as determined by the Workers' Compensation Board.[9] Employers and insureds may automatically conform charges according to fee schedules adopted by the Workers' Compensation Board, and charges listed in the fee schedule are presumed to be the usual and customary and must be paid within 60 days from the date of receipt. Any health service provider whose fee is reduced to conform to the fee schedule may request a hearing and present evidence as to the reasonableness of charges. For charges that are not contained in the fee schedule and are disputed within 60 days as not being reasonable, usual, and customary, the aggrieved party is allowed to settle the dispute through a peer review committee established by the Workers' Compensation Board. Peer review committees include those established by the Metropolitan Atlanta Foundation for Care, Inc.; Georgia Medical Care Foundation; Georgia Psychological Association; Georgia Chiropractic Association, Inc.; and Georgia Dental Association.[10]

(C) Certification of Health Care Providers

A health care provider may make written application to the Workers' Compensation Board to become certified to provide managed care to injured employees.[11] The Board shall prescribe a

---

9. O.C.G.A. § 34-9-205(b) and (c).
10. O.C.G.A. § 34-9-205(b).
11. O.C.G.A. § 34-9-208(a).

reasonable fee for each application as well as the period of validity for each certificate issued.[12]

The application, in a form prescribed by the Board, shall include

1. a list of the names of all individuals who will provide services under a managed care plan with evidence of compliance with any licensing or certification requirements for those individuals to practice in Georgia;
2. a description of the times, places, and manner of providing services under the plan;
3. a description of the times, places, and manner of providing any other related optional services that the applicant wishes to provide; and
4. satisfactory evidence of the ability to comply with any financial requirements to ensure delivery of services in accordance with the plan.[13]

The Board will certify the health care provider if the Board finds that the plan meets the Board's treatment standards; provides appropriate financial incentives; reduces service costs without sacrificing quality; provides adequate methods of peer review and dispute resolution; provides for cooperative efforts by employees, employer, and the health care provider; provides for a method of reporting to the Board concerning the medical and health care service costs; and complies with such other requirements as the Board determines necessary.[14]

---

12. O.C.G.A. § 34-9-208(b).
13. O.C.G.A. § 34-9-208(c).
14. O.C.G.A. § 34-9-208(d).

Emotional Distress as a Basis for Civil Liability

Emotional distress, mental pain and suffering, and mental anguish may, in certain circumstances, form the basis for an independent tort action. These items can also constitute a recoverable element of damage in a tort claim. MHPs may be asked to evaluate the person who claims to have sustained emotional distress and to testify as to its origin and existence, severity, duration, and prognosis.

(A) Intentional Infliction of Emotional Distress

Although there is no statute creating an independent tort action for intentional infliction of emotional distress, Georgia judicial decisions recognize such a tort.[1] "To recover for emotional distress, it must be demonstrated that the defendant committed a 'wanton, voluntary or intentional wrong the natural result of which is the causation of mental suffering.'"[2] "Thus, actual intent

---

1. Pierson v. News Group Publications, Inc., 549 F. Supp. 635 (S.D. Ga. 1982); Georgia Power Co. v. Johnson, 155 Ga. App. 862, 274 S.E.2d 17 (1980). The Georgia Court of Appeals has left open the question of whether a plaintiff may assert a claim for intentional infliction of emotional distress under the Federal Employees' Liability Act (FELA). *See* Bowers v. Estep, 204 Ga. App., 420 S.E.2d 336 (1992).

2. Pierson, *supra* note 1, at 643 (quoting Whitmire v. Woodbury, 154 Ga. App. 159, 267 S.E.2d 783 (1980), *rev'd* on other grounds, 246 Ga. 349, 271 S.E.2d 491 (1980)). *See* Coleman v. Housing Authority of Americus, 191 Ga. App. 166, 381 S.E.2d 303 (1989) in which the Court of Appeals held that sexual harassment by an employer states a claim for intentional infliction of emotional distress.

on the part of the defendant to produce such distress is not essential to recovery. A reckless and willful disregard of the consequences of one's actions, coupled with knowledge of the probable results, also form a basis for recovery."[3] "The acts of the defendant must be 'so terrifying or insulting as naturally to humiliate, [or] embarrass . . . the plaintiff.' "[4] "The behavior must amount to 'egregious, physically intimidating conduct.' "[5] It is not necessary to prove physical injury to recover for emotional distress when the claim is based on intentional or reckless misconduct.[6]

(B) Negligent Infliction of Emotional Distress

Georgia, like most jurisdictions, does not recognize negligent infliction of emotional distress as an independent cause of action.[7] Damages for mental anguish can be awarded on a negligence theory only if there is an accompanying physical injury[8] or pecuniary loss.[9] Thus, when negligence is the basis of the action and when the plaintiff has sustained a physical injury or a monetary loss, mental pain and suffering, fright, shock, and emotional distress are recoverable elements of damage. Recovery may also be had for future mental pain and suffering when accompanied by physical injury. All damages must, of course, be proven through competent evidence. This evidence can include testimony from the injured party, from individuals who have observed the injured party, and from expert witnesses who have examined the injured party.

---

3. *Id.* (quoting Delta Finance Co. v. Ganakas, 93 Ga. App. 297, 91 S.E.2d 383 (1956)).
4. *Id.* (quoting Georgia Power Co. v. Johnson, 155 Ga. App. 862, 863, 274 S.E.2d 17, (1980)).
5. *Id.* (quoting Young v. Colonial Oil Co., 451 F. Supp. 360, 361 (M.D. Ga. 1978)).
6. Hamilton v. Powell, Goldstein, Frazer & Murphy, 252 Ga. 149, 311 S.E.2d 818 (1984).
7. *See* W. Keeton, *Prosser and Keeton on Torts*, § 54 (5th ed. 1984). For an argument that Georgia should recognize an action for damages for emotional distress even without accompanying physical injury or impact, *see* Hamilton, 252 Ga. at 151, 311 S.E.2d at 820 (Smith, J., dissenting).
8. Hamilton, 252 Ga. 149, 311 S.E.2d 818 (1984).
9. Floyd v. Stevens-Davenport Funeral Home, 110 Ga. App. 271, 138 S.E.2d 333 (1964) (citing Pollard v. Phelps, 56 Ga. App. 408, 193 S.E. 102 (1937)).

(C) Emotional Distress as an Element of Damages

When the defendant's conduct is willful, wanton, or intentional, as opposed to merely negligent, the plaintiff may recover for mental suffering, emotional distress, and humiliation even though there has been no physical injury.[10] As with any element of damage, mental suffering must be proven. The measure of damages is the "enlightened conscience of impartial jurors." As a result of changes made in 1987 as part of so-called "tort reform" legislation, when the entire injury is in the nature of mental suffering ("the peace, happiness, or feelings of the plaintiff") punitive damages are not permitted.[11]

The 1987 Georgia General Assembly made other significant changes in the law governing punitive damages. The prior law, applicable to claims arising before July 1, 1987, provides that when there are aggravating circumstances in the act or intention, the jury may award additional damages as a deterrent or as compensation for the wounded feelings of the plaintiff.[12] In all cases arising on or after July 1, 1987, punitive damages may not be awarded as compensation to the plaintiff but only to punish, penalize, or deter a defendant.[13] Therefore, when the entire injury is mental in nature, no punitive damages may be awarded and when punitive damages are authorized, they cannot be awarded to compensate for mental suffering.[14] Of course, mental pain and suffering may be recovered as an element of general damage as discussed earlier.

---

10. Westview Cemetery v. Blanchard, 234 Ga. 540, 216 S.E.2d 776 (1975).
11. O.C.G.A. § 51-12-6.
12. *See* Hale v. Hale, 199 Ga. 150, 33 S.E.2d 441 (1945) (quoting Jacobus v. Congregation of the Children of Israel, 107 Ga. 518, 33 S.E. 853 (1899), ("In a suit for damages for wrongfully disinterring a dead body, if the injury has been wanton and malicious, or is the result of gross negligence or a reckless disregard of the rights of others, equivalent to an intentional violation of them, exemplary damages may be awarded, in estimating which the injury to the natural feelings of the plaintiff may be taken into consideration.").
13. O.C.G.A. § 51-12-5.1.
14. Stepperson, Inc. v. Long, 256 Ga. 838, 353 S.E.2d 461 (1987). Awarding damages under both code sections for the same injury would violate the prohibition against double damages.

Insanity of Wrongdoers and Civil Liability

A person's mental status may affect his civil liability for intentional harm inflicted on another. An individual's mental status may also determine whether his acts are covered or excluded from coverage under a liability insurance policy. An MHP may be asked to examine the individual and to testify as to his mental state at the time of the alleged conduct.

(A) Insanity as a Defense to Civil Liability

The common law rule, and the rule of the Restatement (Second) of Torts,[1] is that a mentally disabled person is liable for his torts whether based on intent or negligence.[2] Georgia courts have modified this rule, holding that "an insane person is liable for his torts the same as a sane person, except for those torts in which malice, and therefore intention, is a necessary ingredient."[3] Thus, insanity is a defense to an intentional tort, but not to a tort based on negligence.[4] A mentally disabled person must adhere to the

---

1. Restatement (Second) of Torts, § 283B (1965).
2. *See* W. Keeton, *Prosser and Keeton on Torts*, § 135 (5th ed. 1984).
3. State Farm Fire & Casualty Co. v. Morgan, 185 Ga. App. 377, 380, 364 S.E.2d 62, 65 (1987), *aff'd*, 258 Ga. 276, 368 S.E.2d 509 (1988), *modifying* Continental Cas. Co. v. Parker, 167 Ga. App. 859, 307 S.E.2d 744 (1983).
4. *Id.* For a discussion of insanity as a defense to a criminal action, *see infra* chapter 7.9. *Insanity* is, of course, a legal and not a psychological or medical term. In addition, the legal concept of insanity varies depending on the particular context.

same standard of care as the "ordinarily prudent person"[5] in conducting his affairs to avoid civil liability.

(B) Mental State and Insurance Coverage

A tortfeasor's mental state may also become an issue in determining whether there is insurance coverage for his tortious conduct. Many homeowner's insurance policies contain an exclusion for bodily injury or property damage "which is expected or intended by the insured." In *State Farm Fire & Casualty Company v. Morgan*, the Georgia Supreme Court affirmed the Court of Appeals' holding that voluntary intoxication, which rendered an insured incapable of forming the intent or expectation of causing injury, would place the insured's conduct outside the policy's intentional conduct exclusion.[6] The court noted that the issue was one of contract law, not tort or statutory law, because the insurance policy is a contract.[7] Thus, the rule in criminal cases that voluntary intoxication is not a defense is inapplicable in the contract law situation.

In determining whether an insured's mental state would preclude application of the policy exclusion, the test is whether the mental disorder affected the insured's capacity to intend the consequences of his acts.[8] Even if an insured met the legal test of insanity (inability to distinguish right from wrong or suffering from a delusional compulsion), this would not avoid the application of the policy exclusion unless the mental disorder undermined the individual's ability to intend the consequences of his actions.[9]

However, in *Allstate Insurance Company v. Jarvis*, a case of first impression, the Court of Appeals held that a psychologist's testimony cannot rebut the presumption that a child molester intended to injure his victim.[10] A child who was sexually molested filed a damages action against Jarvis. Jarvis sought coverage from

---

5. O.C.G.A. § 51-1-2.
6. Hamilton v. Powell, Goldstein, Frazer, & Murphy, 252 Ga. 149, 311 S.E.2d 818 (1984).
7. Because the insurance policy is a contract, the insurance company is free to expand the scope of the exclusion in subsequent policies.
8. Roe v. State Farm Fire & Casualty Co., 188 Ga. App. 368, 373 S.E.2d 23, 25 (1988).
9. State Automobile Insurance Company v. Gross, 188 Ga. App. 542, 373 S.E.2d 789 (1988).
10. Allstate Insurance Company v. Jarvis, 393 S.E.2d 489, 195 Ga. App. 335 (1990).

Allstate, which filed a declaratory judgment action contending that the policy excluded coverage for injury "which may reasonably be expected to result from the intentional or criminal acts of an insured or which are in fact intended by the insured." A psychologist testified that Jarvis was a pedophile and incapable of forming the intent to injure the child. The court held that this testimony was not admissible to rebut the presumption that the offense of child molestation carries with it a presumption of intent to inflict injury.

There is some confusion in the cases as to whether the intent test is applicable generally in the civil liability context. That is, are criminal law concepts of insanity a defense to a tort suit, or is mental incapacity a defense only when it affects the individual's intent-forming capacity? The latter would appear to be the better view and is consistent with the Georgia courts' interpretation of exclusion clauses in insurance policies.[11]

---

11. *See* Judge Beasley's dissent in Roe, *supra* note 8, and special concurrence in State Automobile Insurance, *supra* note 9.

Competency to Contract

A party's lack of the mental capacity to contract may be a basis for rendering the contract unenforceable, void, or voidable. A common example of such an occurrence is the case of a decedent's legal representative or heirs wishing to disaffirm a conveyance of property made while the person was believed to be suffering from a mental disability.[1] In cases in which the competency of an individual to contract is at issue, an MHP may become involved either to evaluate the individual's current mental capacity or to testify as to the individual's mental capacity at the time of the contract.

(A) Legal Test of Competency to Contract

The legal test for capacity to contract is a cognitive or understanding test.[2] This subjective test, often difficult to apply, essentially asks whether the party lacked the capacity to understand the nature and consequences of the transaction in question.[3] The Georgia Code states that the test is to determine whether the individual is "insane, mentally ill, mentally retarded, or mentally incompetent to the extent that he is incapable of managing his

---

1. *See, e.g.*, Warren v. Federal Land Bank, 157 Ga. 464, 122 S.E. 40 (1924); Eagan v. Conway, 115 Ga. 130, 41 S.E. 493 (1903).
2. The *cognitive test* is the traditional test for mental capacity to contract at common law and is the majority rule in American courts. E. Farnsworth, *Contracts*, Section 4.6 (1982).
3. *Id.*; Ison v. Geiger, 179 Ga. 798, 177 S.E. 596 (1934).

estate."[4] In *Slaughter v. Heath*, the court referred to a condition of *non compos mentis* or the total deprivation of reason as rendering a person incapable of entering into a valid contract.[5] In *Eagan v. Conway*, the court stated:

> Extreme old age, accompanied by loss of memory and will and impaired mental faculties, resulting in an incapacity to transact business or to make a voluntary and intelligent disposition of property, necessarily implies a mental condition incompatible with the ability to make a valid contract. . . .[6]

The party seeking relief from the contract bears the burden of persuasion.[7] The trier of fact may consider the circumstances surrounding the contract, the opinions of lay persons who have observed the party's behavior, the opinion of experts, past records of treatment or hospitalization, and previous adjudications of mental illness.[8] If the contract was entered into while the person was in a so-called "lucid interval," the contract is valid.[9] Additionally, even if the party was mentally incompetent at the time the contract was entered into, he may subsequently ratify the contract, either expressly or implied, during a lucid interval.[10]

(B) Effect of Mental Incompetence

A contract of a mentally incompetent person may be either voidable or void.[11] A voidable contract is one that can be disaffirmed in court by the contracting party, by his legal representative, his executor, or by his heirs at law.[12] Under Georgia law, the contract of a mentally incompetent person who has never been adjudged insane, mentally ill, mentally retarded, or mentally incompetent is, at his or his representative's instance, merely voidable.[13] Such a contract, if subsequently ratified by the incom-

---

4. O.C.G.A. § 13-3-24. Note that the capacity to contract and the capacity to make a will are not identical. *See* chapter 5.7.
5. 127 Ga. 747, 57 S.E. 69 (1907).
6. 115 Ga. 130, 133, 41 S.E. 493, 495 (1903).
7. E. Farnsworth, *supra* note 2.
8. *Id.*
9. O.C.G.A. § 13-3-24(a).
10. *Id.*; Georgia Power Co. v. Roper, 201 Ga. 760, 41 S.E.2d 226 (1947); Bunn v. Postell, 107 Ga. 490, 33 S.E. 707 (1899). His personal representative might also affirm the contract.
11. O.C.G.A. § 13-3-24. The contract of a minor and of an intoxicated person are also voidable. O.C.G.A. §§ 13-3-20 and 13-3-25.
12. E. Farnsworth, *supra* note 2, Section 4.7.
13. O.C.G.A. § 13-3-24(a); Holcomb v. Garcia, 221 Ga. 115, 143 S.E.2d 184 (1965); Morris v. Mobley, 171 Ga. 224, 155 S.E. 8 (1930); Warren v. Federal Land Bank, 157 Ga. 464, 122 S.E. 40 (1924).

petent in a so-called "lucid" interval, is binding.[14] Additionally, if not ratified, the general rule is that the incompetent must make restitution of benefits received under the agreement if the other party was unaware of the mental impairment.[15]

Any contract entered into by a party who has been formally adjudicated insane, mentally ill, mentally retarded, or mentally incompetent and for whom a guardian has been appointed to manage his affairs is considered void rather than merely "voidable."[16] Such contracts are absolutely null and void, and the person is deemed, conclusively, to lack the ability to contract.[17] One may, however, recover for "necessaries" provided to the incompetent under the contract.[18] If an individual is adjudicated insane, but no guardian has been appointed, the contract entered into is merely voidable.[19]

---

14. Georgia Power Co. v. Roper, 201 Ga. 760, 41 S.E.2d 226 (1947); Bunn v. Postell, 107 Ga. 490, 33 S.E. 707 (1899).
15. Georgia Power Co. v. Roper, 201 Ga. 760, 41 S.E.2d 226 (1947); Dean v. Goings, 184 Ga. 698, 192 S.E.2d 826 (1937).
16. O.C.G.A. § 13-3-24(b).
17. American Trust & Banking Co. v. Boone, 102 Ga. 202, 29 S.E. 182 (1897).
18. O.C.G.A. § 13-3-24(b). To recover for "necessaries," the party must prove that the legal guardian of the incompetent has failed or refused to supply sufficient necessaries. See O.C.G.A. § 13-3-20(b) (requirement to recover for necessaries provided to minors).
19. Georgia Power Co. v. Roper, 201 Ga. 760, 41 S.E.2d 226 (1947).

Competency to Execute a Will

A certain minimum mental capacity is required for an individual to execute a valid will. If challenged, and if it is proven that the testator lacked the requisite mental capacity, a will can be declared void, and the property in question would likely pass under the laws of intestacy. The laws of intestacy provide for the disposition of the property of a person who dies without a valid will.

The law of testamentary capacity uses a number of legal terms that have little relation to modern concepts of psychology and psychiatry. These include "the ravings of a madman," "the silly pratings of an idiot," "the childish whims of imbecility," "insanity," and "monomania." All of these phrases reduce to the question of whether the testator (the deceased who made the will) had sufficient mental capacity to make a rational decision as to the disposition of his property at the time he signed the will. An MHP who previously treated or evaluated the deceased may be asked to testify as to the mental status of the deceased at the time that the will was signed. An MHP may also be called upon to render an expert opinion based on medical and treatment records, the testimony of other witnesses, and other relevant information.

(A) Legal Test of Testamentary Capacity

Georgia law provides that "[e]very person may make a will unless he is laboring under some legal disability arising either from a want of capacity or from a want of perfect liberty of action."[1] The law states the following:

> The amount of intellect necessary to constitute testamentary capacity is that which is necessary to enable the testator to have a decided and rational desire regarding the disposition of his property. The testator's desire must be decided, as distinguished from the wavering, vacillating fancies of a distempered intellect, and rational, as distinguished from the ravings of a madman, the silly pratings of an idiot, the childish whims of imbecility, or the excited vagaries of a drunkard.[2]

In *Morgan v. Bell*, the court stated the test as follows:

> A person has testamentary capacity who understands the nature of a testament or will, viz., that it is a disposition of property to take effect after death, and who is capable of remembering generally the property subject to disposition and the persons related to him by the ties of blood and of affection, and also of conceiving and expressing by words, written or spoken, or by signs, or by both, any intelligible scheme of disposition. If the testator has sufficient intellect to enable him to have a decided and rational desire as to the disposition of his property, this will suffice.[3]

Although evidence of mental capacity either prior to or subsequent to the execution of the will may be considered, the controlling question is whether the testator lacked sufficient capacity at the time of execution of the will.[4] "An insane person generally may not make a will; however, during a lucid interval he may do so."[5] "A monomaniac may make a will if the will is in no way the result of or connected with his monomania."[6]

Certain Georgia statutes provide additional factors that may apply when determining whether an individual possessed the mental capacity to execute a will. For example, a child under the age of 14 years is considered to lack testamentary capacity and cannot, therefore, execute a valid will.[7] However, the fact that an individual is deaf, mute, blind, eccentric, elderly, or a convicted

---

1. O.C.G.A. § 53-2-20. In contrast, the Living Will Act provides that a living will may be revoked at any time by the declarant without regard to his or her mental state or competency. *See* O.C.G.A. § 31-32-5(a).
2. O.C.G.A. § 53-2-21(b).
3. Morgan v. Bell, 189 Ga. 432, 5 S.E.2d 897 (1939) (quoting Slaughter v. Heath, 127 Ga. 747, 57 S.E. 69 (1907)); *see also* Spivey v. Spivey, 202 Ga. 644, 44 S.E.2d 224 (1947).
4. Spivey, 202 Ga. 644, 44 S.E.2d 224 (1947).
5. O.C.G.A. § 53-2-23.
6. *Id.* "[M]onomania exists when one, because of partial insanity, becomes imbued with an hallucination or delusion that something extravagant exists which has no existence whatever, and is incapable of being permanently reasoned out of conception." Moreland v. Word, 209 Ga. 463, 465, 74 S.E.2d 82, 84 (1953) (quoting Stephens v. Bonner, 174 Ga. 128, 162 S.E. 383 (1931)).
7. O.C.G.A. § 53-2-22.

criminal does not deprive the individual of the power to make a will.[8]

(B) Testamentary Capacity Versus Capacity to Contract

The standard for testamentary capacity is lower than that for the capacity to make a valid contract. That is, the "incapacity to contract may coexist with a capacity to make a will."[9] It takes a higher degree of mentality or intellect to make a contract than to make a will.[10] To make a will, the testator must have a rational desire as to the disposition of his property, whereas to enter into a contract a person must be possessed of mind and reason equal to a full and clear understanding of the nature and consequence of his act in making the contract.[11]

(C) Pleading and Practice

To be validated, a will must go through the process of probate. The burden is on the person attempting to establish the validity of the will (the "propounder") to make out a *prima facie* case and to show that the testator had sufficient capacity to execute the will.[12] Although there is a presumption in favor of testamentary capacity, that alone is not enough to make out a *prima facie* case.[13] Evidence must be presented to show the existence of testamentary capacity. Once the *prima facie* case is made out, if capacity is challenged by caveat (a challenge to the validity of the will), the burden shifts to the caveator to prove that the testator lacked testamentary capacity at the time he executed the will.[14] The issue of capacity is ordinarily a question of fact for the jury to decide after hearing testimony by both sides.[15]

---

8. O.C.G.A. §§ 53-2-24 to 53-2-26.
9. O.C.G.A. § 53-2-21(a); Smith v. Davis, 203 Ga. 175, 45 S.E.2d 6009 (1947).
10. Anderson v. Anderson, 210 Ga. 464, 80 S.E.2d 807 (1954); Joiner v. Joiner, 225 Ga. 699, 171 S.E.2d 297 (1969).
11. Joiner v. Joiner, 225 Ga. 699, 171 S.E.2d 297 (1969).
12. Slaughter v. Heath, 127 Ga. 747, 57 S.E. 69 (1907); Spivey v. Spivey, 202 Ga. 644, 44 S.E.2d 224 (1947); Cornelius v. Crosby, 243 Ga. 26, 252 S.E.2d 455 (1979).
13. Franklin v. First Nat'l Bank, 187 Ga. 268, 200 S.E. 679 (1938).
14. Cornelius, 243 Ga. 26, 252 S.E.2d 455 (1979).
15. Espy v. Preston, 199 Ga. 608, 34 S.E.2d 705 (1945); Johnson v. Dodgen, 244 Ga. 422, 260 S.E.2d 332 (1979).

5.8

Competency to Vote

The right to vote may be denied on the basis of a lack of mental capacity. MHPs may be called on to conduct evaluations or to testify regarding an individual's mental capacity to vote, either in the context of a guardianship proceeding or in a special proceeding in which an individual has been denied the right to register to vote.

The Georgia Constitution grants Georgia residents who are at least 18 years of age and who meet minimum residency requirements the right to register and to vote in elections.[1] However, "[n]o person who has been judicially determined to be mentally incompetent may register, remain registered, or vote unless the disability has been removed."[2] Thus, the test for depriving a person of the right to vote based on mental capacity is a more rigorous one than the test for capacity to write a will or to contract since the right to vote is a fundamental right guaranteed under the U.S. Constitution.[3] Presumably, an adjudication of incompetency is conclusive proof of lack of competency to vote.[4]

---

1. Ga. Const., art. II, § 1, ¶ 2.
2. Ga. Const., art. II, § 1,¶. 3 and O.C.G.A. § 21-2-219 (a.1)(2); *See* 1985 Op. Att'y Gen. No. 85-48 (judge of probate court may, in the course of a proceeding for the appointment of a guardian for an incapacitated adult, judicially determine an individual to be mentally incompetent and thereby remove the individual's right to vote).
3. *See* Harper v. Virginia Bd. of Elections, 383 U.S. 663 (1966) (the political franchise of voting is a fundamental political right); Kronlund v. Honstein, 327 F. Supp. 71 (N.D. Ga. 1971) (state has a compelling interest in preserving the integrity of the electoral process and may prohibit "idiots" and insane persons from participating in elections).
4. *Cf.* American Trust & Banking Co. v. Boone, 102 Ga. 202, 29 S.E. 182 (1897) (adjudication of incompetency and appointment of guardian is deemed conclusive proof of inability to contract).

Georgia law specifically provides that a patient in a facility for the mentally ill or mentally retarded retains his right to vote if he is otherwise eligible to vote.[5] A person committed to a facility for the mentally ill is not considered to have acquired residence for voting purposes in the county in which the facility is located.[6] A person who has been denied the right to register to vote has a right of appeal to the superior court.[7]

---

5. O.C.G.A. §§ 37-3-144 and 37-4-107. *See also* 1981 Op. Att'y Gen. No. 81-11.
6. O.C.G.A. § 21-2-241(a)(11).
7. O.C.G.A. § 21-2-224.

5.9

Competency to Obtain a Driver's License

Georgia law provides that a driver's license shall not be issued to any person

1. who is a habitual user of alcohol or any drug to a degree rendering him incapable of safely driving a motor vehicle;

2. who has previously been adjudged to be afflicted with or suffering from any mental disability or disease and who has not, at the time of application, been returned to competency; and

3. whom the commissioner of the Department of Public Safety has good cause to believe would not, by reason of mental disability, be able to operate a motor vehicle with safety upon the highway.[1]

As to the second ground, an actual adjudication of mental disability is required. Mere voluntary admission to a mental health facility would not constitute grounds for disqualification as no adjudication is involved. It should also be noted that the statute, like many other provisions of Georgia law, improperly equates incompetency with mental disability.

As to the third ground for disqualification, no further definition of mental disability is given, and broad discretion is thereby conferred on the Department of Public Safety. The Rules of the Department of Public Safety provide that whenever there is reason to believe that an applicant is physically or mentally incompetent to operate a motor vehicle, the applicant must have a medical report form completed by a physician of the applicant's choice.

---

1. O.C.G.A. §§ 40-5-22(c)(3), (4), and (6).

The medical report form is then reviewed by the Driver's License Advisory Board, which may require the applicant to submit to an examination by a medical specialist within the applicant's geographic area.[2]

In determining whether to recommend issuance or denial of a driver's license, the department has established guidelines for the Driver's License Advisory Board, which include consideration of mental capacity. Emotional disturbance as it affects the ability to operate a motor vehicle is to be considered on an individual case basis. Factors to be considered include

1. the ability to maintain a reasonably stable and realistic personality; and

2. manifestation of an emotionally erratic pattern, showing periods of irresponsibility, outward or inward aggressiveness, distorted perceptual thought, impulsiveness, suicidal tendencies, or paranoid thought.[3]

If the Advisory Board recommends disapproval of the application, there is a right of appeal within the department. There is also a right of appeal, with trial by jury, to the superior court from the department's final decision.[4]

---

2. Rule 570-17-.10 of the Rules of the Department of Public Safety. Ga. Admin. Comp. R. & Regs. r. 570-17-.10.
3. Ga. Admin. Comp. R. & Regs. r. 570-17-.05.
4. O.C.G.A. § 40-5-66.

5.10

Product Liability

Georgia law defines a tort as "the unlawful violation of a person's legal right."[1] A person claiming injuries or damages arising out of the use of a product may institute a suit against the manufacturer of the product based on claims of negligence, warranty, or strict tort liability.[2] The central idea of a product liability claim is that the product is unreasonably dangerous to the user. MHPs, who have special expertise in human factors, may be called upon to testify and evaluate the dangerousness of a product for purposes of offering their opinion in court.

(A) Elements of a Product Liability Claim

Under Georgia statutory and case law, a seller of personal property is subject to liability for physical harm to the user or the user's property if the product, when sold, is in a defective condition, is unreasonably dangerous, or performs in some way that is foreseeably dangerous to the purchaser of the product. Its use must be reasonably contemplated by the ordinary consumer who purchases it with ordinary knowledge common to the community as to its characteristics for a normal or expected use. Georgia law does not require that there be privity or direct contractual rela-

---

1. O.C.G.A. § 51-1-1.
2. O.C.G.A. § 51-1-11.

tions between the manufacturer and the ultimate consumer in order for liability to exist.[3]

(B) Defenses to a Product Liability Claim

Georgia law provides three basic defenses to product liability claims. First, the defendant may introduce evidence that the plans or designs of the product or the methods and techniques of manufacturing, inspecting, testing, and labeling the product conform with the state of the art at the time the product was first sold by the defendant.[4] The evidence may be considered in determining whether the product was defective and unreasonably dangerous. Second, the defendant is not liable for any alterations or modifications to the product, made by a person other than the defendant after the product was sold, if those modifications were not reasonably foreseen by the seller.[5] Finally, the plaintiff's use of the product must have been reasonably foreseeable and not contrary to any express and adequate instructions or warnings included with the product that the person should have known about.[6]

3. O.C.G.A. § 51-1-11(b)(1); *see also* Copeland v. Ashland Oil, Inc., 188 Ga. App. 537, 373 S.E.2d 629, *cert. denied*, 188 Ga. App. 911, 373 S.E.2d 629 (1988).
4. Firestone Tire & Rubber Co. v. Pinyan, 155 Ga. App. 343, 270 S.E.2d 883 (1980).
5. Talley v. City Tank Corp., 158 Ga. App. 130, 279 S.E.2d 264 (1981).
6. *Id.*

5.11

Unfair Competition

Business competition is encouraged throughout the state of Georgia, thus ensuring a vigorous market and low prices. Competitors, however, cannot use tactics that have been judicially declared to be unfair, such as defaming competitors or their goods, stealing trade secrets, or starting a business with an ex-employer's confidential customer list. Of interest to MHPs and particularly to psychologists is a type of marketing intended to confuse the consumer into believing that one business's products or services were produced by another. MHPs may be asked to conduct consumer surveys to determine whether the defendant's business practices resulted in confusion and to testify in court as to their findings.

(A) Legal Tests of Unfair Competition

One form of false marketing that constitutes unfair competition is the passing off of goods or services as those of another.[1] There are two elements to this test: the defendant must have taken some action to mislead or confuse purchasers as to the identity of the manufacturer or its merchandise, and consumers must have been confused.

---

1. O.C.G.A. § 10-1-372. *See also* chapter 3.14, Antitrust Limitations to Practice, which includes a discussion on the Fair Business Practice Act.

(B) Trademark Confusion

A trademark is any mark, name, symbol, or device or any combination thereof adopted by a person to designate his or her goods.[2] It must be affixed to the goods and must not be a common or generic name. Trademarks are typically registered under federal law, but may also be registered under state law. In either event, registration does not determine whether the person has established a trademark. The relevant inquiry generally turns on whether the mark is a generic term or symbol or has an established distinctiveness.[3]

A business name can also be a trademark. Georgia law provides that the essence of a trademark infringement case arising from similar names of two businesses is the confusion to the public.[4] If confusion exists, the relevant inquiry for the court is whether the name taken by the defendant had previously come to indicate the plaintiff's business and whether this confusion caused injury to the plaintiff's business reputation. Whether there is confusion depends not only on the similarity in names, but also on factors such as the type of services and the prospective clientele. The basic inquiry is whether the name causes confusion to persons using reasonable care.[5]

---

2. O.C.G.A. § 10-1-440.
3. Dolphin Homes Corp. v. Tocomc Dev. Corp., 223 Ga. 455, 156 S.E.2d 45 (1967).
4. Jellibeans, Inc. v. Skating Clubs of Ga., Inc., 716 F.2d 833 (11th Cir. 1983).
5. See Giant Mart Corp. v. Giant Discount Foods, Inc., 247 Ga. 775, 279 S.E.2d 683 (1981).

Employment Discrimination

Both federal and state law prohibit certain employers from engaging in discriminatory employment practices. An MHP who is an employer, both individually or as part of a group or professional association, may be covered by various employment discrimination laws. MHPs, generally psychologists, may also be called upon to advise employers as to personnel selection, discharge, and promotion procedures, and to develop testing instruments for those purposes. The impact of employment discrimination laws should be taken into account when giving advice as to testing and other employment-related procedures. In addition, MHPs may be called upon to testify as to the merits of an employment discrimination case (for example, does an individual have a mental condition that constitutes a disability), as well as to compensatory damages when such damages are recoverable.

(A) Federal Antidiscrimination Laws

For Georgia employees and employers, federal law is the primary source of prohibitions on unlawful discrimination in employment. These laws include Title VII of the 1964 Civil Rights Act, which prohibits discrimination by private and public employers on the basis of race, sex, national origin, and religion;[1] the Age Discrimination in Employment Act, which prohibits private and public employers from discriminating in employment on account of age;[2] the Equal Pay Act, which prohibits private and public

---

1. 42 U.S.C. § 2000e *et seq.*
2. 29 U.S.C. § 623 *et seq.*

employers from paying different wages on the basis of sex;[3] a provision of the Civil Rights Act of 1866, which prohibits discrimination on the basis of race and national origin in contracts, including employment relationships;[4] the Rehabilitation Act, which prohibits federal agencies and contractors and any other employers receiving federal financial assistance from discriminating on the basis of handicap;[5] and the Americans With Disabilities Act, which prohibits discrimination in employment against individuals with disabilities in both private and public employment.[6] In addition, public (i.e., governmental) employers, who discriminate on the basis of classifications such as race, national origin, sex, religion, or other prohibited classification, may run afoul of the Equal Protection Clause of the Fourteenth Amendment to the U.S. Constitution and can be sued under the Civil Rights Act of 1871.

(B) Georgia Antidiscrimination Laws

Georgia law prohibits employers with 10 or more employees from discriminating on the basis of sex by paying wages to employees of one sex at a lesser rate than the rate paid to employees of the opposite sex for comparable work.[7] The law is modeled after the federal Equal Pay Act. However, the Georgia law covers fewer employers than the federal law, has a shorter statute of limitations, and provides less relief than the federal law (back pay plus attorney's fees not to exceed 25% of the judgment, in contrast with federal law, which permits double the amount of the back pay plus fully compensatory attorney's fees). It is not surprising that there are no published opinions involving the Georgia law.

The Georgia Equal Employment for the Handicapped Act[8] prohibits discrimination on the basis of handicap by any private or public employer having 15 or more employees. A handicapped individual is defined as

> [a]ny person who has a physical or mental impairment which substantially limits one or more of such person's major life activities, and who has a record of such impairment. The term

---

3. 29 U.S.C. § 206.
4. 41 U.S.C. § 1981. *See* Patterson v. McLean Credit Union, 491 U.S. 164, 109 S. Ct. 2363 (1989).
5. Saint Francis College v. Majd Ghaidan Al-Khazraji, 483 U.S. 1011, 107 S. Ct. 3244 (1987); Runyon v. McCreary, 427 U.S. 160, 96 S. Ct. 2586 (1976).
6. 42 U.S.C. § 1983. The definition of handicapped individual is contained in 29 U.S.C. § 706(7).
7. 42 U.S.C. § 12101 *et seq.* For a detailed discussion of the Americans With Disabilities Act; *see* chapter 5.13.
8. O.C.G.A. § 34-5-1 *et seq.*

"handicapped individual" shall not include any person who is addicted to the use of any drug or illegal or federally controlled substance nor addiction to the use of alcohol.[9]

The law prohibits discrimination against a qualified handicapped individual in hiring, firing, pay, or any other term or condition of employment unless the handicap restricts the individual's ability to engage in the particular job or occupation.[10] It is a defense to an action based upon handicap discrimination that the employment decision was based upon an employer's good faith reliance upon a professional opinion rendered by a licensed physician, rehabilitation specialist, psychologist, physical therapist, dentist, or other similar licensed health care professional concerning that individual.[11]

As a remedy, the court may grant equitable relief, including hiring, reinstatement, and promotion, and may award as damages back pay and reasonable attorney's fees. Any action under the Handicapped Act must be brought within 180 days after the prohibited conduct occurred.[12]

The Georgia Fair Employment Practices Act[13] prohibits discrimination in employment by any state agency on the basis of race, religion, national origin, sex, handicap, and age.[14] The enforcement procedure is similar to the procedure used under Title VII before the federal Equal Employment Opportunity Commission (EEOC).[15] A charge of discrimination must be filed with the Commission on Equal Opportunity within 180 days after the discriminatory act. Within 90 days, the Commission must determine whether there is reasonable cause to believe that the employer had engaged in an unlawful practice. If the Commission finds no reasonable cause, the charge will be dismissed. The charging party may then request a right-to-sue letter from the EEOC and pursue the claim in federal court under Title VII or may seek review in superior court. If reasonable cause is found, the Commission will attempt conciliation between the parties. If conciliation fails, a special master is appointed to conduct a hearing using the procedures set forth in the Georgia Administrative Procedures Act (APA).[16] If a discriminatory practice is found to exist, the special master may order equitable relief, including hiring, reinstatement, and promotion, and may award back pay.

---

9. O.C.G.A. § 34-6A-1 *et seq.* O.C.G.A. § 34-6A-2(3).
10. O.C.G.A. § 34-6A-4.
11. O.C.G.A. § 34-6A-3(c).
12. O.C.G.A. § 34-6A-6.
13. O.C.G.A. § 45-19-20 *et seq.*
14. O.C.G.A. § 45-19-29.
15. O.C.G.A. § 45-19-31. Charges filed with OFEP, with the exception of handicap cases, are also filed with the EEOC.
16. O.C.G.A. § 45-19-37. The APA can be found at O.C.G.A. Title 50, Chapter 13.

Attorney's fees may also be awarded.[17] Appeal from both the special master and from a Commission order dismissing a charge is made to the superior court under the APA. The appeal is based on the record, unlike Title VII in which the parties receive a trial *de novo*.[18]

---

17. O.C.G.A. § 45-19-38. However, if the plaintiff's attorney was provided by the Commission, attorney's fees may not be awarded. *See* Department of Corrections v. Finney, 203 Ga. App. 445, 416 S.E.2d 805 (1992).
18. O.C.G.A. § 45-19-39. *See* Kilmark v. Board of Regents, 175 Ga. App. 857, 334 S.E.2d 890 (1985). *See also* Coleman v. Housing Authority of Americus, 191 Ga. App. 166, 381 S.E.2d 303 (1989) in which it was held that sexual harassment by an employer states a tort claim for intentional infliction of emotional distress.

5.13

The Americans With Disabilities Act

The Americans With Disabilities Act (ADA), signed into law on July 26, 1990, is one of the most comprehensive pieces of civil rights legislation ever enacted. It is composed of five sections (Titles).

Title I prohibits discrimination in employment against a qualified individual. It requires employers to make reasonable accommodation of individuals with disabilities unless undue hardship would result. Title II makes it illegal for state or local governments to discriminate against individuals with disabilities in the provision of public services. Title III makes it illegal for places of public accommodation to discriminate against individuals with disabilities in the provision of goods, services, facilities, privileges, advances, or accommodations. Title IV applies to the telecommunications industry and requires the provision of relay services, including making such services available to individuals with hearing and speech impairments. Title V contains miscellaneous provisions dealing with matters such as retaliation, attorney's fees, state immunity, and alternative dispute resolution.

Title I outlaws employment discrimination against individuals with disabilities in much the same way as Section 504 of the Rehabilitation Act forbids discrimination against handicapped individuals by government employers or by recipients of federal funds. As it affects a large percentage of private sector employers, Title I is normally the focal point of discussions about the ADA.

An understanding of its provisions is important to MHPs in two regards. First, many MHPs are themselves employers of a sufficient number of employees to make them subject to the Act. (Alternatively, some MHPs are employees with disabilities whose interests may be protected by the Act.) Second, an MHP may have patients who are individuals with disabilities as defined in the Act. It is desirable for the MHP to be aware of the Act's scope and provisions in evaluating and counseling such patients. Moreover, should a patient believe that she or he is experiencing employment discrimination based on a mental health disability, the MHP's observations may be relevant and may be useful in determining whether the individual has a covered disability and, if so, what reasonable accommodations could or should be made.

(A) General Rule

No covered entity shall discriminate against a qualified individual with a disability because of that disability.[1] This rule applies to

1. job application procedures,
2. hiring,
3. advancement or discharge,
4. employee compensation,
5. job training, and
6. other terms, conditions, and privileges of employment.

The ADA also prohibits an employer from retaliating against an applicant or employee who has asserted his or her rights under the ADA. In addition, the ADA makes it unlawful to discriminate against an employee (whether disabled or not) on the basis of his or her relationship or association with an individual with a disability.

(B) How the Rule Operates

1. Employers covered by the Act may not treat individuals with disabilities differently from anyone else in hiring, advancement, compensation, and other employment matters so long as that individual is capable of performing the essential functions of the job at issue with or without reasonable accommodation measures by the employer.
2. Employers are required to take reasonable accommodation measures to employ an individual with a disability but are not required to take steps that will result in undue hardship to the employer.

---

1. 42 U.S.C. § 12112(a).

(C) Definitions[2]

1. A *covered entity* means an employer, employment agency, labor organization, or joint labor–management committee.

2. An *employer* is an individual, engaged in an industry affecting commerce, who has 15 or more employees for each working day in each of 20 or more calendar weeks in the current or preceding calendar year (except that the minimum number will be 25 employees for the first 2 years following the effective date of the Act, that is, until July 26, 1994).

3. A *qualified individual with a disability* is one who, with or without reasonable accommodation, can perform the essential functions of the employment position that he or she holds or desires.

   a. The employer determines what the essential functions of the job are (job descriptions are primary evidence).

   b. The employer determines the requirements for the position, including education, experience, skills, and licenses.

   c. There is no obligation to hire an individual who poses "a direct threat to the health and safety of others."

4. An *individual with a disability* includes one who

   a. has a physical or mental impairment that substantially limits one or more major life activities; or

   b. has a record of such an impairment; or

   c. is regarded as having such an impairment.

   Mental impairment is defined as "[a]ny mental or psychological disorder, such as mental retardation, organic brain syndrome, emotional or mental illnesses, and specific learning disabilities."[3] Note that current drug users are not covered by the ADA. By contrast, former drug users who have been successfully rehabilitated and those who are not currently using drugs and are participating in a supervised rehabilitation program are covered. People who are erroneously regarded as being drug users are covered.

   Alcoholics and current users of alcohol are not excluded from the definition of "individual with a disability." However, employers may prohibit workers from being under the influence of alcohol in the workplace. Alcoholics may also be held to the same performance standards as other employees, even when deficiencies in performance are directly related to alcoholism.[4]

---

2. 42 U.S.C. § 12111.
3. 29 C.F.R. § 1630.2(h)(2).
4. 42 U.S.C. § 12114(c).

As defined in the ADA and the accompanying regulations, "disability"does *not* include sexual behavior disorders such as transvestism, transsexualism, pedophilia, exhibitionism, voyeurism, and gender identity disorders not resulting from physical impairments. Compulsive gambling, kleptomania, and pyromania are not considered disabilities under the ADA. Also excluded are psychoactive substance abuse disorders resulting from illegal drug use. ADA protection is not extended to individuals on the basis of these conditions.[5]

Individuals who are HIV-positive or who suffer from AIDS are covered by the ADA, as are individuals with other communicable diseases.

Reasonable accommodation includes

1. the making of existing facilities used by employees readily accessible to and usable by individuals with disabilities; and

2. job restructuring, modified work schedules, reassignment to a vacant position, acquisition or modification of equipment; appropriate adjustment of examinations, training materials, or policies; the provision of readers or interpreters; and other reasonable accommodations.

Undue hardship refers to an action requiring significant difficulty or expense when considered in light of the following factors:

1. the nature and cost of the accommodation needed;

2. the overall financial resources of the specific facility where the accommodation would be made;

3. the size, type, and financial resources of the covered employer;

4. the covered employer's type of operation, including composition, structure, and functions of its work force; and

5. the geographic, administrative, and fiscal relationship between the specific facility and the covered employer.

(D) Employer Defenses: General Rule

Employers *may* deny jobs to individuals with disabilities if such a denial can be shown to be job related and consistent with business necessity, if no reasonable accommodations can be made.

Legitimate reasons for adverse employment actions include the following:

1. The applicant was not qualified.

---

5. 29 C.F.R. § 1630.3(d).

2. The applicant could not perform essential functions of the job, even with reasonable accommodation.

3. The applicant would pose a direct threat to the health and safety of self or others in the workplace.

4. A specific exception permits an employer to deny a food-handling position to applicants with certain infectious or communicable diseases if reasonable accommodations will not eliminate transmission.

Individuals with a history of mental illness are particularly susceptible to attempts to invoke exception (3) in the preceding list. In determining whether an individual with a history of mental illness would pose a direct threat under this exception, the employer must first identify the specific behavior that would pose a direct threat. The employer should then consider

1. the duration of the risk;

2. the nature and severity of the potential harm;

3. the likelihood that the potential harm will occur; and

4. the imminence of potential harm.[6]

The exclusion may not be based on assumptions about mental illness in general or about characteristics of certain types of disorders. There must be a case-by-case examination of each individual's own history. There must also be either recent threats or overt acts, or a substantial history of such behavior. These threats or acts either must have actually caused harm or must have directly threatened such harm. Even if a substantial threat is found, there must still be a determination of whether there are reasonable accommodation measures that would reduce the risk to an acceptable level.

The ADA requires specific factual data to support this defense. Relevant evidence may include input from the individual with a disability and information about the individual's previous experience in similar positions. The opinions of psychologists, physicians, counselors, and therapists who have expertise in the disability at issue or direct knowledge of the individual with the disability may be also considered.

---

6. 29 C.F.R. § 1630.2.

(E) Permissible Hiring Practices Under the ADA

The basic principle of Title I of the ADA is that a prospective employee's disability may not be taken into account in making employment decisions *unless* the disability has the effect of preventing the employee from performing an essential function of the job *and* reasonable accommodation cannot be made to neutralize that effect. The permissible guidelines for preemployment screening flow naturally from this concept. In general, employers should not engage in any preemployment screening inquiries that may elicit information about disabilities unless such inquiries are directly tied to the applicant's ability to perform the job.

(E)(1) Interviewing

1. It is unlawful to ask an applicant whether he or she is disabled. It is also unlawful to inquire about the nature or severity of a disability, even after it is mentioned by the applicant.

2. It is permissible to ask an applicant questions about his or her ability to perform job-related functions so long as the questions are not phrased in terms of a disability. It is also permissible to ask the applicant to describe or demonstrate how he or she will perform job-related functions, with or without reasonable accommodation.

(E)(2) Medical Examinations

1. Medical examinations may be required only *after* a job offer has been made (contingent upon the medical examination) and then only if everyone working in that job category must also take the examination.

2. If an individual is not hired because a medical examination reveals a disability, the employer must be able to show that the reasons for exclusion are job related and consistent with business necessity.

3. An employer may conduct voluntary medical examinations as part of an employee health program.

4. Any information obtained from medical examinations as described in (1) and (2) above must be kept in separate and confidential files.

5. Even after an applicant is hired, it is not permissible to require a medical examination or ask an employee questions about a disability unless the inquiries are job related and consistent with business necessity.

The postoffer medical examinations permitted under the ADA may include both physical and psychological testing. The ADA recognizes that, in many industries, there are legitimate physical and psychological criteria for certain positions. However, the exclusionary criteria must not tend to screen out classes of individuals with disabilities unless they are job related and consistent with business necessity.

(E)(3) Controlled Substances and Drug Testing

1. *Drug* means a controlled substance as defined in Schedules I through IV of Section 202 of the Controlled Substances Act.[7]

2. An employer may test for illegal drugs, and that test will not be considered a medical examination as described earlier.

3. An employer may prohibit use of drugs and alcohol in the workplace; require employees to be free from the influence of drugs and alcohol in the workplace; and require that employees comply with the Drug Free Workplace Act of 1988.[8]

(F) Enforcement and Consequences of Violations

The U.S. Equal Employment Opportunity Commission (EEOC) is the enforcing agency for the ADA.[9] The EEOC enforces other federal employment discrimination claims, including Title VII (prohibiting discrimination on the basis of race, sex, religion, and national origin) and the Age Discrimination in Employment Act (ADEA). After July 26, 1992, individuals who believe that they have been discriminated against on the basis of a disability may file a charge with the EEOC. The filing of an EEOC charge is a prerequisite to further legal action. In most cases, the charge must be filed within 180 days of the discrimination.

The EEOC will investigate and make an initial attempt to resolve the charge following the same procedures it uses in handling Title VII cases. If conciliation is not obtained, the individual

---

7. 21 U.S.C. § 812.
8. 41 U.S.C. § 701.
9. The Drug Free Workplace Act applies to employers who are federal grant recipients. It requires employers to publish a statement prohibiting the use or distribution of controlled substances in the workplace; to establish "drug free awareness" programs for employees; and to require employees to abide by the published statement. The EEOC has published regulations implementing the Act; *see* 56 Fed. Reg. 35725 (1991). The regulations will be codified as 29 C.F.R. Part 1630. The EEOC has also published interpretive guidance on the Act; *see* 56 Fed. Reg. 35739.

may file an action in the appropriate U.S. District Court. The remedies available to successful complainants under the ADA are the same as those available to Title VII plaintiffs. These remedies were formerly limited to hiring, promotion, reinstatement, back pay, front pay (under some circumstances), and attorney's fees. Under the ADA, reasonable accommodation may also be ordered. Since the passage of the Civil Rights Act of 1991, however, Title VII remedies have been expanded to include compensatory and punitive damages of up to $300,000, depending on the size of the employer. These are now available under the ADA.

Civil and Criminal Trial Matters

Jury Selection

The constitutions of the state of Georgia and of the United States guarantee a trial by jury in most instances in civil cases and in all criminal cases if the accused faces the possibility of imprisonment. Although the phrase *jury selection* describes the process by which the court impanels a jury, the term is less than precise because jurors are not selected, but are actually removed from the panel by the judge or struck from the jury panel by legal counsel for each party on the basis of real or suspected bias, prejudice, disqualification, and counsel's assessment of the juror's attitude toward the case. If not initially disqualified as the result of financial interest in the matter or relationship to the parties, the jurors are put through a *voir dire* examination. This is a questioning process that is designed to remove from the jury those persons who may be biased against a party in ways that are not specifically considered to be disqualifying. *Voir dire* is the process by which the lawyers gain information about the jurors and seek, at the same time, to educate the prospective jurors about the case.

Potential jurors are eliminated from the jury pool by a motion to strike for cause or by the use of peremptory strikes following *voir dire* examination. Thus, jury selection is actually a process of elimination. MHPs may be involved in this process by assisting the trial attorney in the selection process. MHPs are employed to perform pretrial surveys designed to uncover attitudes concerning the case or its issues; formulate questions to ask potential jurors designed to reveal bias, interest, prejudice, or attitude; evaluate jurors based on the results of pretrial surveys; or perform in-court observations and convey to counsel impressions of the jurors.

(A) Juror Qualifications

In Georgia, jury lists are compiled using the voter registration rolls of each county.[1] The selection process begins with the random selection of names from the voter registration rolls. Persons selected must complete a juror eligibility questionnaire. The jurors are required to be at least 18 years of age, citizens of the United States, and residents of the state of Georgia for at least 6 months. Individuals who are suffering from a mental disability or who have been convicted of a felony are disqualified from service. Those who have served as elected officials in the preceding 2 years may not serve on a grand jury, but may serve on a trial jury.

Length of jury service varies from county to county, depending on the system of jury service adopted. Some counties have a one day, one trial system that permits the juror to report only for one day. If the juror is not selected for a jury during that day, jury service is deemed to have been completed on the basis of attendance for the single day. If selected for a jury, the juror must serve until discharged, regardless of the number of days that are required. Other counties have formulated similar systems that attempt to shorten jury service by permitting prospective jurors to be dismissed after 1, 2, or 3 days of jury service.

(B) Criminal Trials

The Georgia Constitution provides that, in criminal cases, the defendant shall have a public and speedy trial by an impartial jury.[2] Trial by jury is a right that may be waived by the defendant.[3] The defendant must expressly and intelligently waive the right to a trial by jury,[4] but there is no requirement that the waiver be done in open court.[5]

---

1. O.C.G.A. § 15-12-40.
2. Ga. Const. of 1983, art. I, § 1, ¶ 11.
3. Clarke v. Cobb, 195 Ga. 633, 24 S.E.2d 782 (1943); Little v. Stynchcombe, 227 Ga. 311, 180 S.E.2d 541 (1971).
4. Johnson v. State, 157 Ga. App. 155, 276 S.E.2d 667 (1981).
5. Sims v. State, 167 Ga. App. 479, 306 S.E.2d 732 (1983).

(C) Jury Size

Criminal defendants in Georgia courts are tried by 12-person juries for felonies[6] and 6-person juries for misdemeanors.[7] In federal courts, criminal defendants are tried before a 12-person jury. The parties may, with the consent of the court, agree to try the case with a fewer number of jurors or without a jury.[8] Civil juries in federal court may be between 6 and 12 jurors, and all jurors participate in the verdict. Civil juries in the Georgia superior courts consist of 12 individuals. In Georgia state courts, a jury consists of 6 individuals unless a demand for a 12-person jury is made.[9] The former practice of using alternate jurors has been abolished.[10]

(D) Unanimity Requirement

The jury must reach a unanimous verdict, unless the parties and the court stipulate otherwise.

(E) Change of Venue

Generally, civil defendants are entitled by the Georgia Constitution to be tried in the county of their residence or, for corporate defendants, either in the county of incorporation or in the county in which the principal place of business is located. Upon a proper showing to the trial judge of prejudice in the jury panel, civil parties are entitled to a change of the place of trial (known as the *venue of the action*) to ensure impartiality.[11] Criminal defendants are normally tried in the county in which the crime occurred. Criminal defendants and, in some instances, the prosecution are entitled to have the place of trial moved to another county within the state if the defendant cannot receive a fair and impartial trial in the original county.

If a request to change venue is based on pretrial publicity, the party must prove that the jury's exposure to the prejudicial material will probably result in the denial of a fair trial. Only when the publicity is overwhelming and outrageous, however, will un-

---

6. O.C.G.A. § 15-12-160 (Supp. 1992).
7. O.C.G.A. § 15-12-125 (1990).
8. Fed. R. Crim. P. 23.
9. O.C.G.A. § 15-12-122.
10. Fed. R. Civ. P. 48.
11. O.C.G.A. § 9-10-50.

fairness be presumed. Otherwise, the defendant must show that specific publicity is prejudicial to the defendant and that the prejudice has affected prospective jurors. MHPs may be involved in designing and undertaking surveys to sample the attitudes of potential jurors within the forum county to determine the level of prejudice or bias toward the parties, the type of case, the attorneys, or the issues to be presented. The trial attorney may then use the results in a pretrial motion for a change of venue. In addition, MHPs may testify in a pretrial hearing on the matter when there is a challenge to the *array* (the entire jury panel and selection process) or a challenge to the selection process or the composition of the jury. Usually, the MHP's role, beyond challenges to the process and procedure, is limited to advising the lawyer in the selection–rejection process of *voir dire* examination.

(F) *Voir Dire*

In legal parlance, *voir dire* means "to speak the truth." *Voir dire* is the process by which an attorney attempts to gather information about a juror to assist in eliminating jurors with unfavorable attitudes toward a party or the case, and to attempt to influence favorably the jurors who will ultimately try the case. In Georgia, this process is performed by lawyers under the supervision of the court.[12] Jury panels are assembled randomly from the group of jurors who have been summoned to jury duty that day. Jury panels are then escorted to the courtroom in numbers usually at least double the size of the final jury that will try the case. Accordingly, for a 6-person jury, no fewer than 12 jurors will be summoned for the selection, or *drawing*, of a jury. Occasionally, alternate jurors are selected to ensure that a juror's illness or inability to serve during trial will not result in a mistrial. (There are no alternates in federal civil trials.) If an alternate is to be selected, then at least two additional jurors are summoned and report to the courtroom for *voir dire* examination. In death penalty trials, the number of prospective jurors is usually increased to accommodate the disqualification of some jurors as a result of their opposition to the death penalty and to deal with the greater likelihood of bias or prejudice.

Questions to the jury panels are presented in two forms: questions to the entire panel concerning general topics and personal questions to each prospective juror. Questions relating to occupation, place of residence, education, membership in organi-

---

12. O.C.G.A. § 15-12-133 (1990). In contrast, in the federal courts, *voir dire* is generally controlled by the judge.

zations, family relationships, and personal interests are examples of personal questions, responses to which are sometimes supplied to the attorneys before trial in the form of a questionnaire. The use of a questionnaire is designed to shorten the *voir dire* process. Examples of general questions are whether or not any member of the panel is acquainted with the parties or the attorneys, is familiar with the case, has been charged with a crime, or has been a party or witness in any litigation.

On the basis of the response to the questions, the attorney first determines whether there is any basis for a challenge to the juror for cause. Cause exists if, for example, a prospective juror is related by blood or marriage to any party, has personal knowledge of the facts of the case, or has a bias or prejudice for or against a party.[13] At the conclusion of the general questions, particular questions are directed to individual jurors. If the responses raise the potential for bias or prejudice, the attorney may challenge the individual juror for cause. After further examination by the court and the parties, the court may dismiss the juror from the jury panel.

The entire exercise of impaneling a jury is designed to permit the attorney to ask questions of the potential juror in such a fashion as to gain information that may assist the attorney in making a determination concerning whether the potential juror will be fair and impartial.[14] Although the type and manner of questions directed to the juror are matters of judicial discretion, the Georgia courts have traditionally allowed wide latitude in the exercise of this valuable right.[15] The trend, however, is to restrict this process, particularly in federal courts. Some courts require that questions for *voir dire* examination be submitted in advance. In most federal courts, the judge actually performs the *voir dire* examination based on written questions that have been submitted to the court prior to the *voir dire* process.

After the *voir dire* examination, the attorneys representing the opposing parties alternately strike a juror from the panel. Such strikes are referred to as peremptory challenges or strikes. In criminal cases, the defendant has double the number of strikes as the prosecution;[16] in civil cases, both parties have an equal number of strikes. In the event of multiple defendants or plaintiffs, the strikes are usually shared by each of the principal parties on each side of the case.

When making peremptory strikes from a jury panel, the lawyers do not normally have to show any cause or reason for the

---

13. O.C.G.A. §§ 15-12-124 (1990) and 15-12-135 (1990).
14. McKinney v. State, 155 Ga. App. 930, 273 S.E.2d 888 (1980).
15. Haston v. Hightower, 111 Ga. App. 87, 140 S.E.2d 525 (1965).
16. O.C.G.A. § 15-12-165.

strikes. However, if the parties can show the court that the opposing side has used the peremptory strikes to exclude persons from the jury on the basis of race or gender, then the party accused of making the discriminatory strikes must show the court a neutral, nondiscriminatory reason for the selection.[17]

The MHP may perform an important consulting role in the peremptory challenge process and may be valuable in formulating a juror profile of the type of juror that the client may desire. The MHP may also assist in explaining the basis for the exercise of a peremptory challenge should that become an issue.

(G) Civil Trials

A defendant is not entitled to a trial by jury in every civil suit. Although the right to a trial by jury is broad in Georgia, the right to a jury trial depends on whether the action is at law or in equity.[18] Actions at law generally seek a remedy that is restricted to monetary damages. Cases in equity usually seek the direction of the court to require an individual to do or refrain from doing a specific act. A restraining order or injunction to prohibit a person from, for example, polluting a river or building a wall on the plaintiff's property is a form of relief granted in a case in equity. Jury trials are permitted in cases at law, but are permitted in equity cases only when the court requires an advisory verdict from the jury.[19] In such cases, the jury, in returning its verdict, answers questions put to it in interrogatory form rather than making a determination as to which side should prevail. Unanimity is required in all cases, both civil and criminal.

---

17. Edmondson v. Leesville Concrete Company, 111 S. Ct. 2077 (1991); Powers v. Ohio, 111 S. Ct. 1364 (1991); Baison v. Kentucky, 476 U.S. 79, 106 S. Ct. 1712 (1986).
18. Williams v. Overstreet, 230 Ga. 112, 195 S.E.2d 906 (1973); Duncan v. First Nat'l Bank, 597 F.2d 51 (5th Cir. 1979).
19. O.C.G.A. § 9-11-49.

Expert Witnesses

MHPs are frequently asked to offer opinions as expert witnesses in both criminal and civil cases on matters that are beyond the knowledge of the average person and that will assist the trier of fact to decide more intelligently the case before it. MHPs are frequently called to testify as expert witnesses in domestic relations and child custody cases, in personal injury litigation, in cases in which mental state is at issue, and in criminal cases on the issues of competency and sanity.

(A) Qualifying as an Expert Witness

Witnesses may be qualified (allowed by the court to testify) as experts if they have knowledge, skill, experience, training, or education concerning an issue that is beyond an average lay person's competence and if the testimony will be helpful to the trier of fact.[1] Generally, an expert must have been educated in a particular trade or profession or have special knowledge derived from either experience or education.[2] The determination of whether to qualify a witness as an expert lies solely within the discretion of the court.[3]

Under Georgia law, a witness offered as an expert may be cross-examined on his or her qualifications by a request by oppos-

---

1. O.C.G.A. § 24-9-67 (1982); *see also* Smith v. State, 247 Ga. 612, 277 S.E.2d 678 (1981).
2. Brown v. State, 245 Ga. 588, 266 S.E.2d 198 (1980).
3. Hicks v. State, 157 Ga. App. 69, 276 S.E.2d 129 (1981).

ing counsel to *voir dire* the expert before the witness is qualified and accepted as an expert. It is incumbent upon both the offering attorney and the court to restrict the expert's testimony to those issues that are within the expert's area of competence and training. Qualification as an expert does not entitle the expert to testify on any subject matter to which a litigant directs a question. The expert's testimony must be focused on and directed to the area of the expert's declared expertise.

In spite of the expert's qualifications and declared expertise, the jury is instructed that it is not required to accept the testimony of any witness, expert or otherwise, and that the testimony of an expert, like that of all witnesses, is to be given only the weight and credit to which the jury thinks it is properly entitled.[4]

Expert testimony on issues to be decided by the jury is admissible when the conclusion of the expert is one that jurors would not ordinarily be able to draw for themselves.[5] Expert opinions are offered to aid the jury's effort to determine the facts, but cannot substitute for the jury's ultimate determination. The jury is free to weigh the expert's credibility and to reconcile conflicting testimony. However, unlike a fact witness, an expert witness may offer an opinion on the ultimate fact to be decided by the jury (e.g., that a person was or was not competent at the time of executing a will).

(B) Form and Content of Testimony

An expert witness may testify in the form of an opinion or inference regarding the ultimate issue for the trier of fact to decide. It is important to remember that an expert may give opinions regarding only the area in which he or she is an expert.[6] In one case, the Georgia Supreme Court upheld a trial judge's ruling that a psychologist did not have the requisite medical expertise to give an opinion as to whether chemical exposure was the cause of the plaintiff's brain damage.[7] An expert may also be asked to assume facts, in the form of a hypothetical question, even when the facts have not been admitted in evidence, so long as the facts are and will be offered in evidence during the trial. The effect

---

4. Georgia Pattern Jury Charges.

5. Smith v. State, 247 Ga. 612, 277 S.E.2d 678 (1981).

6. Hammond v. State, 156 Ga. 880, 120 S.E.2d 539 (1923).

7. Chandler Exterminators, Inc. v. Morris, 262 Ga. 257 (1992). The holding in the Chandler case was subsequently overruled by the Georgia General Assembly. *See* O.C.G.A. § 43-39-1(1), as amended by 1993 Ga. Laws, p. 355, § 1.

of the rule is that expert witnesses may offer an opinion based on facts of which the expert has no personal knowledge, but is relying on facts revealed to him from another source. The primary reason for the rule is to avoid problems with hearsay testimony.[8]

In federal court, although not in Georgia state courts, expert witnesses can offer their opinion based on facts or data of a type reasonably relied on by experts in this field. The facts or data need not be admissible in evidence.[9] The expert can also testify in the form of an opinion without initially disclosing the facts or data on which the opinion is based. An opposing party, however, has the right to a thorough cross-examination of the expert and may require that the expert reveal this information.[10]

The trial lawyer through cross-examination may attempt to impeach (discredit) the expert's testimony by referring to passages from a treatise that are inconsistent with the testimony so long as the expert relied on the treatise or is willing to concede that it is authoritative. An expert is also subject to the techniques commonly used in any cross-examination, such as use of prior inconsistent statements, differing opinion in the professional community, or facts demonstrating bias or an interest in the outcome of the trial, such as the fee being paid.

A party may call an expert to offer an opinion or inference concerning the ultimate factual issue if the opinion or inference assists the court or jury in understanding the evidence and does not merely permit the jury to adopt the opinion of the expert as the legal conclusion in the case.

"Although it is permissible for the expert to give his opinion to facts in issue or even the ultimate issue when such question is a proper one for opinion evidence, the expert is not permitted to state a legal conclusion as to the ultimate matter in issue."[11] For example, an expert in a malpractice action may testify about the appropriate standard of care (see chapter 3.10) and whether the defendant's conduct deviated from that standard, but cannot conclude that the defendant is "liable" for the injury. In a criminal case, the expert can give an opinion as to the existence of a factual element, but not the legal conclusion that the defendant is guilty of the crime charged. Thus, a physician may testify that there was

---

8. Hearsay is an out-of-court statement or assertion by a declarant that is repeated by a witness to prove the truth of the matter asserted in the statement. For instance, a witness to an automobile accident cannot testify concerning another person's statement at the accident scene. The hearsay rule, however, has numerous exceptions that may permit MHPs to use testimony, such as a patient's medical history or statements that explain conduct.

9. Fed. R. Evid. 704.

10. Fed. R. Evid. 705.

11. Nichols v. State, 177 Ga. App. 689, 340 S.E.2d 654 (1986).

forcible entry, but not that it was rape. An MHP may, however, if properly qualified, offer an opinion concerning whether the defendant is competent to stand trial (see chapter 7.5) or was insane at the time of the offense (see chapter 7.9).

6.3

Admissibility of Polygraph Examinations[1]

Polygraph examinations are inadmissible in any case in the state of Georgia unless the parties specifically stipulate and agree to the admissibility of the results of the test.[2] The objection to polygraph results is generally based on the grounds that such tests are not scientifically reliable and are too often intended to frighten or intimidate rather than to induce truthful responses. Another objection is that polygraph evidence is irrelevant because it does not relate to the guilt or innocence of the accused, but merely to the polygraph examiner's opinion of the defendant's veracity in answering out-of-court questions.[3] The examiner's testimony expresses only the examiner's opinion of whether the person examined believed that he or she was telling the truth at the time of the examination.[4] Evidence that the defendant was willing or unwilling to submit to a polygraph test is completely irrelevant and inadmissible at trial.[5]

---

1. As discussed in chapter 1.10, the laws governing licensure and regulation of polygraph examiners in Georgia were repealed in 1992.
2. Chambers v. State, 240 Ga. 76 (1977).
3. *Agnor's Georgia Evidence* § 10-14 (3d ed.).
4. Harris v. State, 168 Ga. App. 458 (1983).
5. Browne v. State, 175 Ga. App. 246 (1985).

Competency to Testify

As a general rule, a witness is presumed to be competent to testify at a hearing or trial. Questions regarding competency deal with mental capacity, special status (e.g., an attorney is deemed to be not competent to testify as to confidential communications with a client), or particular circumstances that raise questions as to the witness's ability to understand the oath. If an objection is made, the determination of competency is made by the trial judge.[1] Georgia law excludes from trial the testimony of individuals who do not have the "use of reason" or who do not understand the nature of an oath.[2] Although there is no rule that categorically excludes testimony from a witness who is mentally ill or from a child under a specific age, the court may make an independent determination concerning whether to hear from the witness and whether the witness is impressed with a duty to tell the truth. MHPs may be asked to aid the court in the assessment of whether a person is incompetent to testify by reason of either mental incapacity or immaturity.

(A) Legal Tests of Competency to Testify

A potential witness is competent to testify if he

> ... know[s] and appreciate[s] the fact that as a witness he assumes a solemn and binding obligation to tell the truth relative

---

1. O.C.G.A. § 24-9-7 (1982).
2. O.C.G.A. § 24-9-5 (Supp. 1992).

to the case and concerning such matters as he may be interrogated on, and that if he violates the obligation he is subject to be punished by the court.[3]

Although the witness must be able to understand the nature of an oath, the fact that the witness does not understand the meaning of the word "oath" is not determinative.[4]

It is noteworthy that a person's ability to testify is determined at the time of the legal proceeding, rather than the time when the person observed the event in question. When witnesses testify at hearings and in depositions (a pretrial proceeding in which witnesses are questioned under oath by the attorneys in the same manner in which they would be questioned at trial), the issue becomes one of competency at the time at which the testimony is rendered, rather than at the time at which the testimony is offered.

(B) Determination of Witness Competency

The determination of whether a witness is competent to testify is a matter that is addressed to the sound discretion of the trial court. An appellate court will not disturb the trial court's decision unless the trial court abused its discretion.[5] The witness must, however, be able to communicate his or her testimony to the jury in some fashion. The use of interpreters for foreign languages or sign language can render a witness's testimony competent. The court again makes its determination of competency after an examination. Likewise, a witness's intoxication and drunken condition when attempting to testify or at the time of the occasion about which he or she testifies affects the witness's credibility and not competency.[6] The same provision of law is applied to individuals under the influence of a drug or medication.[7]

If the question of competency is raised at trial, the court makes an initial determination of the witness's competency to testify. The court may also permit additional testimony by an MHP as to a witness's mental status.

---

3. Smith v. State, 247 Ga. 511, 277 S.E.2d 53 (1981).
4. Lashley v. State, 132 Ga. App. 427, 208 S.E.2d 200 (1974).
5. Porter v. State, 237 Ga. 580, 229 S.E.2d 384 (1976), *cert. denied*, 430 U.S. 956 (1977).
6. O.C.G.A. § 24-9-6 (1982).
7. Geter v. State, 231 Ga. 615, 203 S.E.2d 195 (1974).

6.5

Psychological Autopsy

A psychological autopsy is a process by which a deceased person's state of mind or mental condition is analyzed to form the basis of expert testimony as to motivation, intention, or mental capacity. The mental state, including motivation and capacity, of an individual prior to death can be a central issue in litigation. For example, whether an individual was subject to undue influence at the time of the execution of a will may determine the will's validity. Similarly, whether a death was the result of an accident or of a suicide may determine whether there is insurance coverage.

As a separate evidentiary device, psychological autopsies are unknown to the law of Georgia. However, the term "psychological autopsy" is merely shorthand for the process by which an expert MHP renders an opinion regarding the mental state of the deceased at the time in question. Expert testimony is admissible under the standards discussed in chapter 6.2. The fact that the subject of the testimony may be dead does not otherwise affect the admissibility of the testimony.

6.6

The Battered Woman Syndrome

The Battered Woman Syndrome refers to personality characteristics and behavior that are frequently found in women who are physically abused by their mates over a prolonged period of time.[1] The Georgia courts have held that expert opinion as to the battered woman syndrome is admissible to assist the jury in evaluating the battered woman's claim of self-defense.[2]

In *Smith v. State*, the Georgia Supreme Court dealt first with the general question of the admissibility of expert testimony on factual issues to be decided by the jury. The court stated the rule as follows:

> Expert opinion testimony on issues to be decided by the jury, even the ultimate issue, is admissible when the conclusion of the expert is one which jurors would not ordinarily be able to draw for themselves; i.e., the conclusion is beyond the ken of the average layman.[3]

The court then held that expert testimony as to the battered woman syndrome was admissible when the testimony went to the nature of the syndrome and ways that it could affect the defendant's behavior. The court found that

---

1. The syndrome is sometimes referred to as the battered wives syndrome. However, in Georgia, the defense is available to any woman involved in an established relationship with a man. *See* Smith v. State, 247 Ga. 612, 277 S.E.2d 678 (1981).
2. For a complete discussion of the syndrome and its application to the law of self-defense, *see* Mather, *The Skeleton in the Closet: The Battered Woman Syndrome, Self-Defense, and Expert Testimony*, 39 Mercer L. Rev. 545, 546 (1988). A person is justified in using a reasonable amount of force to protect herself from an attack if she reasonably believes that: (a) she is in immediate danger of bodily harm; (b) the force is necessary to avoid the danger; and (c) she is not the aggressor. *Id.* at 563.
3. Smith v. State, 277 S.E.2d at 683.

the expert's testimony explaining why a person suffering from battered woman's syndrome would not leave her mate, would not inform police or friends, and would fear increased aggression against herself, would be such conclusions that jurors could not ordinarily draw for themselves. Hence we find that the expert's opinion in this case was improperly excluded from the jury's consideration.[4]

The courts have permitted licensed psychologists, as well as a nurse trained in psychology and employed by a community shelter for battered women, to testify that the defendant's personality fit the characteristics of the battered woman syndrome.[5] The court will not, however, permit an expert to give an opinion as to whether the defendant was, in fact, in reasonable fear for her life, as this is a matter that the average person can determine without expert assistance.[6]

---

4. *Id.*
5. *See* Chapman v. State, 258 Ga. 208, 367 S.E.2d 541, 543 (1988).
6. Mullis v. State, 248 Ga. 338, 282 S.E.2d 334 (1981).

Rape Trauma Syndrome

Rape trauma syndrome (RTS) is a posttraumatic stress disorder caused by sexual assault.[1] The symptoms include "fear of offender retaliation, fear of being raped again, fear of being out alone, sleep disturbance, change in eating habits, and sense of shame."[2] The prosecution may wish to introduce expert testimony about RTS to rebut the defendant's claim that the victim consented to sexual intercourse.[3] Alternatively, a rape victim who kills the rapist might also claim the presence of RTS as a defense to charges of murder, claiming that she was unable to form the necessary intent to commit murder.[4]

The Georgia courts have not yet addressed the question of the admissibility of expert testimony concerning RTS. The jurisdictions that have addressed RTS are split on the issue of its admissibility.[5] The general test for the admissibility of expert testimony, in Georgia is the following:

> Expert opinion testimony on issues to be decided by the jury, even the ultimate issue, is admissible where the conclusion of the expert is one which jurors would not ordinarily be able to draw for themselves; i.e., the conclusion is beyond the ken of the average layman.[6]

---

1. Massaro, *Experts, Psychology, Credibility, and Rape: The Rape Trauma Syndrome Issue and Its Implications for Expert Psychological Testimony, 69* Minn. L. Rev. 395, 396 (1985).
2. *Id.* (quoting State v. Marks, 231 Kan. 645, 653, 647 P.2d 1292, 1299 (1982)).
3. *Id.*
4. *See* Massaro, *supra* note 1, at 436–437.
5. The Kansas Supreme Court held that expert testimony concerning RTS is admissible when offered to prove nonconsent to intercourse. The supreme courts of California, Minnesota, and Missouri have held that such testimony is inadmissible.
6. Smith v. State, 247 Ga. 612, 277 S.E.2d 678, 683 (1981).

In other words, for expert testimony to be admissible it must relate to evidence that is difficult for the average juror to understand.[7] Thus, the Georgia courts may rule in favor of the admissibility of expert opinion on RTS in a proper case in which the state offers such testimony to rebut common myths surrounding the nature of rape, the psychological consequences of rape, or whether or not a rape victim has consented to sexual relations with the accused.[8]

---

7. Mullis v. State, 248 Ga. 338, 282 S.E.2d 334 (1981). In Smith, the court found that the expert's testimony explained why an individual suffering from the battered woman syndrome would not leave her mate, would not inform the police or friends, and would fear increased aggression against herself, and would thus aid the jurors in drawing conclusions that they could not ordinarily draw for themselves. Smith, 247 Ga. at 619, 277 S.E.2d at 683. In Mullis, the court held that expert testimony on the issue of whether the defendant was in fact in fear for her own safety was not admissible since this was a conclusion that could be reached by the jury without expert assistance. Mullis, 248 Ga. at 339, 282 S.E.2d at 337.

8. See, e.g., Massaro, supra note 1, at 402 for a discussion of the mythology of rape. It should also be noted that Georgia has a rape shield statute that places limitations on the admissibility of evidence of a rape victim's prior sexual relations. See O.C.G.A. § 24-2-3; see also Note, Can Georgia's Rape Shield Statute Withstand a Constitutional Challenge?, 36 Mercer L. Rev. 991 (1985).

6.8

Hypnosis of Witnesses

Hypnosis by trained physicians and psychologists is recognized as a valid therapeutic technique. However, the role of hypnosis in criminal investigations and in courtroom testimony is controversial, and the rules governing its use differ from jurisdiction to jurisdiction.

One of the difficulties with the use of hypnosis is that individual responses vary greatly. Although hypnosis is generally used to enhance the recall of an event, the actual response to hypnosis may be quite different. Hypnosis may produce recollections that are substantially similar to prehypnotic recollection, or it may yield recollections that are more inaccurate than prehypnotic memory. Most frequently, hypnosis increases the reporting of both accurate and inaccurate recollections.[1]

There are three primary risks inherent in the use of hypnotically refreshed testimony. The first is that the witness may become suggestible and provide answers that the subject believes will meet with the hypnotist's approval. Second, the witness may confabulate, that is, the witness may fill in gaps in his memory or embellish details based on fantasy, exaggeration, or memories from other events. Third, the witness may experience cementing or memory hardening in which the witness develops extreme confidence in the memories, whether they are true or false. Cementing gives the witness confidence in his testimony and makes cross-examination more difficult.[2]

---

1. Council on Scientific Affairs, *Scientific Status of Refreshing Recollection by the Use of Hypnosis*, 253 J.A.M.A. 1918, 1921 (1985); *See* Rock v. Arkansas, 483 U.S. 44, 107 S. Ct. 2704 (1987).
2. *See* Walraven v. State, 255 Ga. 276, 281 (1985); Rock v. Arkansas, 483 U.S. at 60.

In reviewing the use of hypnotically refreshed testimony, the Georgia courts have applied the general rule used to determine the admissibility of evidence based on scientific principles. This rule requires proof that the technique has reached a scientific stage of verifiable certainty.[3]

In *Walraven v. State*,[4] the court applied this standard to the question of the admissibility of the testimony of a previously hypnotized witness. The court reviewed the scientific literature and decisions from various jurisdictions that have noted the dangers inherent in the use of hypnosis to refresh memory or to prompt recall. The court held that a witness who has been previously hypnotized may testify only "as to the specific content of recorded statements that he has made prior to hypnosis, or as to events occurring after the hypnosis session."

To demonstrate that the courtroom testimony is the same as the prehypnosis testimony, the prehypnotic statements must be recorded and preserved with sufficient reliability. The Georgia rule that permits testimony as to the content of prehypnotic recorded statements differs from the rule in some jurisdictions in which the testimony of a previously hypnotized witness is totally inadmissible.[5]

In addition, the Georgia courts will permit testimony as to events that have occurred after the hypnosis session. Thus, a posthypnotic identification is admissible if the party wishing to introduce the identification demonstrates by clear and convincing evidence that the identification is not only reliable, but that it did not arise from nor was it cemented during the hypnosis session. To avoid any question of impermissible suggestion, all hypnosis sessions should be recorded. The hypnotist should be alone with the subject during the session. At the beginning of the session, prior to hypnosis, the hypnotist should ask the witness to relate the facts as remembered.[6]

---

3. Harper v. State, 249 Ga. 519, 292 S.E. 389 (1982).
4. 255 Ga. 276, 336 S.E.2d 798 (1985).
5. In Rock v. Arkansas, 483 U.S. 44 (1987), the Supreme Court held that a *per se* rule of inadmissibility of hypnotically refreshed testimony could not be applied to bar the testimony of a defendant who had been hypnotized.
6. *Id.* at 281–282.

6.9

Eyewitness Identification

One of the most effective methods of persuading a jury as to the identity of a person who allegedly committed a crime is through the testimony of an eyewitness. There are several legal and factual problems associated with such testimony. The major constitutional issues involved in eyewitness identification are whether the eyewitness identification was tainted by a suggestive lineup or showup[1] and whether the defendant was represented by counsel at a pretrial lineup or showup.[2] Questions may also arise as to whether or not a witness can testify about his after-the-fact, pretrial identification of the defendant. Georgia permits such testimony,[3] whereas some states exclude it on hearsay grounds or because it unduly reinforces the in-court identification.[4]

The jury, as the fact finder, is always free to evaluate the credibility of an eyewitness.[5] The question has arisen as to whether or not the court will permit expert testimony on the reliability of eyewitness identification generally as a basis for impeaching the credibility of the specific eyewitness. Studies have shown that even though juries tend to give great weight to eyewitness identification, the reliability of eyewitness testimony is

---

1. *See* Manson v. Brathwaite, 432 U.S. 98, 97 S. Ct. 2243 (1977).
2. *See* Gilbert v. California, 388 U.S. 263, 87 S. Ct. 1951 (1967).
3. *See* Thomas v. State, 128 Ga. App. 538, 197 S.E.2d 452 (1973).
4. W. Daniel, *Georgia Criminal Trial Practice*, § 6-2 (1988).
5. O.C.G.A. § 24-4-4: "In determining where the preponderance of evidence lies, the jury may consider all the facts and circumstances of the case, the witnesses' manner of testifying, their intelligence, their means and opportunity for knowing the facts to which they testified, the nature of the facts to which they testified, the probability or improbability of their testimony, their interest or want of interest, and their personal credibility so far as the same may legitimately appear from the trial."

suspect.[6] Psychological and perceptual phenomena, such as unconscious transference, memory loss, and the effect of stress on perception and memory, can all affect eyewitness identification. The question is whether expert testimony on these phenomena will be permitted to impeach the credibility of the witness.[7] The Georgia Supreme Court addressed this issue in *Jones v. State*:[8]

> Generally, expert testimony as to the credibility of a witness is admissible if the subject matter involves organic or mental disorders, such as insanity, hallucinations, nymphomania, retrograde amnesia, and testimony concerning physical maladies which tend to impair mental or physical faculties. If, however, the characteristic attacked does not involve some organic or mental disorder or some impairment of the mental or physical faculties by injury, disease or physical faculties by injury, disease or otherwise, expert testimony is usually excluded. Expert testimony is usually excluded also when the question is whether the subject matter is within the scope of the ordinary layman's knowledge and experience.[9]

Thus, the court has ruled that determinations as to the credibility of eyewitnesses are within the scope of the ordinary layman's knowledge and are exclusively within the province of the jury.[10] In the absence of a contention that the eyewitness suffers from some mental or physical disability, the court will not permit expert testimony on the reliability of eyewitness identification to impeach the witness's credibility.[11] Georgia courts feel that the best way to attack the credibility of an eyewitness's identification is by vigorous cross-examination.[12]

---

6. *See* E. Loftus & J. Doyle, *Eyewitness Testimony: Civil and Criminal* (1987); United States v. Wade, 388 U.S. 218 (1967) (stating that eyewitness identification is particularly riddled with dangers that may prevent a fair trial and is a major cause of miscarriages of justice because of mistaken identification).

7. E. Loftus & J. Doyle, *supra* note 6.

8. 232 Ga. 762, 208 S.E.2d 850 (1974).

9. *Id.* at 765, 208 S.E.2d at 853.

10. *Id.*

11. *Id.* However, in the case of Askew v. State, 185 Ga. App. 282, 363 S.E.2d 844 (1987), the court permitted a police detective to testify as an expert on the ability of witnesses to give accurate descriptions of crime perpetrators.

12. *Id. Contra,* E. Loftus & J. Doyle, *supra* note 6, § 11.06 (1987) (discussing strategies for offering expert testimony to impeach eyewitness identification); E. Cleary, *McCormick on Evidence* § 203 (3d ed., 1984): "Any relevant conclusions supported by a qualified expert witness should be received unless there are distinct reasons for exclusion"; "Probably the limits and weaknesses of human powers of perception should be studied more widely by judges and lawyers in the interest of a more accurate and objective administration of justice." *Id.* at § 45.

Criminal Matters

7.1

Screening of Peace Officers

Any person employed or appointed as a peace officer[1] in Georgia must be certified by the Georgia Peace Officer Standards and Training Council.[2] To be certified, the prospective peace officer must be at least 18 years of age, be a U.S. citizen, have a high school diploma or its equivalent, not possess a criminal record, and successfully complete a basic training course. In addition, the peace officer must be examined "by a licensed physician or surgeon [and] found to be free from any physical, emotional or mental conditions which might adversely effect his exercising the powers or duties of a peace officer."[3] Neither the law nor the Council's regulations contain standards for determining when a mental condition might adversely affect a peace officer's performance of his or her duties. A prospective peace officer who has been denied certification has the right to an administrative hearing.[4]

---

1. A peace officer is any person employed or hired by any instrumentality of government or railroad who has the authority to enforce the laws through arrest. *See* O.C.G.A. § 35-8-2(8).
2. O.C.G.A. § 35-8-1 *et seq.*
3. O.C.G.A. § 35-8-8.
4. O.C.G.A. § 35-8-7.2.

Competency to Waive the Rights to Silence, Counsel, and a Jury Trial

Persons taken into custody by the police for a criminal offense have the right to remain silent[1] and the right to an attorney,[2] including a court-appointed attorney if they are indigent. A defendant charged with a criminal offense has the right to counsel and the right to a trial by jury.[3] These rights are guaranteed under both the United States and the Georgia constitutions. Criminal defendants may waive these rights if they are competent to do so. The courts may ask MHPs to examine criminal defendants and to testify whether they were competent to waive these rights at the time of the arrest or other pretrial proceedings and whether they are presently competent to waive these rights at the time of trial.

(A) The Right to Remain Silent

In 1966, the U.S. Supreme Court ruled in *Miranda v. Arizona* that when a criminal suspect is taken into custody, he must be warned of his right to remain silent prior to any questioning.[4] He may, however, waive the right to remain silent if such a waiver is made

---

1. U.S. Const. amend. V ("nor shall he be compelled in any criminal case to be a witness against himself...."); Ga. Const. art. I, § 1, ¶ 16 ("No person shall be compelled to give testimony tending in any manner to be self-incriminating.").
2. U.S. Const. amend. VI ("In all criminal prosecutions, the accused shall enjoy the right ... to have the Assistance of Counsel for his defense."); Ga. Const. art. I, § 1, ¶ 14 ("Every person charged with an offense against the laws of this state shall have the privilege and benefit of counsel....").
3. U.S. Const. amend. VI ("In all criminal prosecutions, the accused shall enjoy the right to a speedy and public trial, by an impartial jury...."); Ga. Const. art. I, § 1, ¶ 11 ("In criminal cases, the defendant shall have a public and speedy trial by an impartial jury....").
4. 384 U.S. 436 at 444, 86 S. Ct. 1602 (1966).

"knowingly and intelligently."[5] An in-custody suspect must clearly and affirmatively waive his right to silence.[6] A waiver cannot be implied from the silence of the suspect nor from the fact that he made a confession.[7] There is no presumption that the defendant knowingly and intelligently waived his *Miranda* rights.[8]

The Supreme Court has held that a defendant's mental state alone is insufficient to prove that a confession was involuntary. There must be some evidence of police coercion in obtaining the confession or in the waiver of *Miranda* rights.[9] It is, therefore, unusual for a waiver of *Miranda* rights to be held invalid. For example, a waiver by a suspect with a mental age of 6 and an IQ of 60 has been upheld.[10] The fact that a defendant is illiterate and was in a special education class when he was in school does not mean that he is incapable of understanding his *Miranda* rights when they are read to him.[11] A waiver may also be valid even though the defendant is suffering from a mental illness or is moderately retarded.[12] Moreover, the court is not required to accept expert testimony that an individual was incapable of knowingly and intelligently waiving his rights. For example, in *Nelms v. State*, experts testified that the defendant was schizophrenic and psychotic. The Georgia Supreme Court affirmed as not clearly erroneous the trial court's finding that the defendant's confession was made voluntarily and competently.[13]

(B) The Right to Counsel

The *Miranda* case also held that an in-custody suspect must be warned that he has the right to talk to an attorney and to have the attorney present while he is being questioned, and that if he cannot afford an attorney, one will be appointed for him prior to

---

5. *Id.* at 475; Johnson v. State, 186 Ga. App. 801, 368 S.E.2d 562 (1988).
6. Colbert v. State, 124 Ga. App. 283, 183 S.E.2d 476 (1971).
7. *Supra* Miranda, note 4, at 475.
8. Tague v. Louisiana, 444 U.S. 469, 100 S. Ct. 652 (1980).
9. Rachals v. State, 258 Ga. 48, 364 S.E.2d 867 (1988); Colorado v. Connelly, 479 U.S. 157, 107 S. Ct. 515 (1986).
10. United States v. Bush, 466 F.2d 236 (5th Cir. 1972); *see also* Gates v. State, 244 Ga. 587, 261 S.E.2d 349 (1979), *cert. denied*, 445 U.S. 938 (1980) (the fact that a defendant was 21 years old with a 6th grade education does not mean he was incapable of knowingly and intelligently waiving his constitutional rights).
11. Donaldson v. State, 249 Ga. 186, 289 S.E.2d 242 (1982).
12. Parker v. State, 161 Ga. App. 478, 288 S.E.2d 297 (1982). *See also* Cunningham v. State, 255 Ga. 727, 342 S.E.2d 299 (1986) (a .30 blood-alcohol level did not prevent a valid waiver).
13. 255 Ga. 473, 340 S.E.2d 1 (1986). *Also see* Marlowe v. State, 187 Ga. App. 255, 370 S.E.2d 20 (1988).

any questioning.[14] As is the case of the right to remain silent, a criminal suspect may knowingly and intelligently waive his right to have an attorney present at the time of the interrogation.[15] However, even when there is a valid waiver of counsel and a suspect begins to answer questions, he may at any time change his mind and exercise his right to remain silent. If he exercises this right, questioning must cease immediately. When a suspect makes an ambiguous or equivocal request for counsel during interrogation (e.g., "maybe I should call a lawyer"), the request must be clarified by the police before proceeding with further interrogation.[16]

In *Edwards v. Arizona*, the court held that waivers of counsel must not only be made voluntarily, but also must constitute a "knowing and intelligent relinquishment or abandonment of a known right or privilege."[17] Furthermore, the court has held that when a defendant requests counsel at arraignment, the police may not thereafter initiate any interrogation with the defendant.[18]

In *Sanders v. State*, the Georgia Court of Appeals held that when an in-custody defendant requests a lawyer, an analysis of whether he has later waived that right proceeds in two steps. First, a determination must be made as to whether the defendant initiated further talks with the police after the request. If so, the question is whether his waiver was shown to be voluntary under the totality of the circumstances.[19]

(C) The Right to a Jury Trial

The test for waiver of the right to a jury trial in a criminal case is essentially the same as the test for waiver of the rights to silence and counsel. The state has the burden of showing that the defendant knowingly and intelligently waived his right to a jury trial.[20] However, a defendant may revoke the waiver, provided he acts in a timely manner and does not substantially "delay or impede the cause of justice."[21]

---

14. Miranda, *supra* note 4, at 479.
15. *Id.* at 475; Brown v. State, 122 Ga. App. 570, 177 S.E.2d 801 (1970); Roger v. State, 156 Ga. App. 466, 274 S.E.2d 815 (1980).
16. Miranda, *supra* note 4, at 473.
17. Hall v. State, 255 Ga. 267, 336 S.E.2d 872 (1985).
18. 451 U.S. 477, 101 S. Ct. 1880 (1981).
19. Michigan v. Jackson, 475 U.S. 625, 106 S. Ct. 1404 (1986).
20. Sanders v. State, 182 Ga. App. 581, 582, 356 S.E.2d 537 (1987).
21. Hill v. State, 181 Ga. App. 473, 352 S.E.2d 651 (1987). In a civil case, the failure to request a trial by jury may constitute a waiver. *See* Green v. Austin, 222 Ga. 409, 150 S.E.2d 346 (1966). *See also* Fed. R. Civ. P. 38(b); Goss v. Bayer, 184 Ga. App. 730, 362 S.E.2d 768 (1987) (right to a jury trial is impliedly waived by participating in a bench trial and by failing to protest or object to a bench trial).

Precharging and Pretrial Evaluations

In some states, the prosecutor may request a mental health evaluation to determine whether to charge a person with a criminal offense or to divert him or her to the mental health system or to some other social services program. Georgia, however, does not have any provision of this type for adult offenders. There are procedures in juvenile court for the diversion of children to mental health or social services agencies.[1] In addition, a peace officer may take a person who has committed a criminal offense and who appears to be mentally ill directly to an emergency receiving facility for evaluation.[2]

---

1. *See* chapters 4.15 and 4.19.
2. O.C.G.A. § 37-3-42. *See* chapter 8.4, Involuntary Civil Commitment of Mentally Ill Adults.

7.4

Bail Determinations

Most persons charged with a crime have the right to secure their release from jail pending trial by posting bail.[1] Even those persons convicted of less serious offenses and sentenced to serve less than 7 years may be granted an appeal bond.[2] In determining whether to set bail and at what amount, the primary consideration is to ensure that the defendant appears at trial or to ensure that he begins serving his sentence.[3] As a general rule, the amount of the bail cannot be excessive.[4] There is no provision in Georgia law requiring that a defendant be evaluated by an MHP to assist in the bail determination. However, an MHP may be called upon, generally by defense counsel, to conduct an evaluation and to testify at a bail hearing representing the individual's risk of fleeing, his potential dangerousness, his ties to the community, and his ability to comply with court-imposed conditions of release.[5]

---

1. O.C.G.A. § 17-6-1. The right to bail in the federal courts is determined by 18 U.S.C. §§ 3142 and 3143 and pursuant to the requirements of the Eighth Amendment.
2. O.C.G.A. § 17-6-1(g).
3. *See* Spence v. State, 252 Ga. 338, 313 S.E.2d 475 (1984); Jones v. Grimes, 210 Ga. 585, 134 S.E.2d 790 (1964).
4. U.S. Const. amend. VIII; Ga. Const. art. I, § 1, ¶ 17; *See* Reid v. Perkerson, 207 Ga. 27, 60 S.E.2d 151 (1950) ("Excessive bail is the equivalent of a refusal to grant bail, and in such a case habeas corpus is an available and appropriate remedy for relief.").
5. *See* Uniform Sup. Ct. R. 27; O.C.G.A. § 17-6-1(b).

(A) Determining Whether Bail Is Appropriate

A person charged with a misdemeanor may not be refused bail, either before trial, after indictment, after a motion for new trial, or while an appeal is pending. A person charged with certain serious felonies and certain repeat offenders may be granted bail only by a judge of the superior court.[6] A person charged with all other offenses may be granted bail before a court of inquiry, such as a magistrate's court.[7] Each person who is entitled to bail shall be permitted one bail for the same offense as a matter of right, while subsequent bails are in the discretion of the court.[8] Bail for a defendant who has been convicted and has filed an appeal shall not be granted to any person convicted of certain serious offenses, or to any person sentenced to serve a period of incarceration of 7 years or more.[9] Whether or not to grant an appeal bond to a person convicted of any crime not specified in the statute is within the discretion of the judge.[10]

The court may release a person on bail if the court finds that the person

1. poses no significant risk of fleeing from the jurisdiction of the court or of failing to appear in court when required;
2. poses no significant threat or danger to any person, to the community, or to any property in the community;
3. poses no significant risk of committing any felony pending trial; and
4. poses no significant risk of intimidating witnesses or otherwise obstructing the administration of justice.[11]

(B) Setting the Amount of Bail

The amount of bail to be assessed is left to the sound discretion of the trial judge.[12] The issue confronting the judge is to place the amount high enough to ensure, reasonably, the presence of the defendant when it is required, while at the same time avoiding an amount higher than that reasonably necessary, which would

---

6. O.C.G.A. § 17-6-1(a).
7. O.C.G.A. § 17-6-1(b).
8. O.C.G.A. § 17-6-13.
9. O.C.G.A. § 17-6-1(g).
10. *Id. See* Birge v. State, 240 Ga. 501, 241 S.E.2d 213 (1978).
11. O.C.G.A. § 17-6-1(e).
12. Jones v. Grimes, 219 Ga. 585, 134 S.E.2d 790 (1964).

result in the bail being excessive.[13] The court also has the discretion to authorize the release of a defendant upon his own recognizance, that is, without the need for money, property, or a surety.[14]

Factors that are considered in fixing bail include the ability of the defendant to pay, the seriousness of the offense, the penalty, the character and reputation of the accused, the defendant's health, the probability of the defendant appearing for trial or to serve the sentence, prior forfeiture of other bonds, and whether the defendant is a fugitive.[15] The principal factor considered is the probability of the appearance of the accused or of his flight to avoid punishment.[16] In appeal bond cases, the court will also take into account whether or not the appeal is frivolous or taken for purposes of delay.[17] While other states have also dealt with the insanity of the accused as a factor affecting the right to bail,[18] Georgia courts have not addressed this as a factor.

In cases involving family violence, the court is authorized to impose specific conditions along with a money bail. These include prohibiting the defendant from having any contact with the victim and requiring the immediate enrollment in domestic violence counseling, substance abuse treatment, or other therapeutic requirements.[19]

---

13. *Id.*
14. O.C.G.A. § 17-6-12.
15. Jones, *supra* note 12.
16. *Id. See also* Spence, *supra* note 3.
17. Shaw v. State, 178 Ga. App. 67, 341 S.E.2d 919 (1986); Birge v. State, 240 Ga. 501, 241 S.E.2d 213 (1978).
18. *See* Annotation, Insanity of Accused As Affecting Rights to Bail in Criminal Case, 11 A.L.R.3d 1385 (1967).
19. O.C.G.A. §§ 17-6-1(f)(2) and (3).

Competency to Stand Trial

Georgia courts, commentators, and lawyers frequently confuse and misuse the various mental states recognized in the law. This is particularly true in the criminal law field where the legal concepts of insanity, incompetency, and mental illness are often used interchangeably and frequently inappropriately.[1] The proper definitions of these terms are as follows:

1. Insanity refers to the defendant's mental state at the time of the offense and relates to the defendant's responsibility for the criminal act. Generally, a person shall not be found guilty of a crime if, at the time of the act, he did not have the mental capacity to distinguish between right and wrong in relation to the act or, if because of mental disease, injury, or congenital deficiency, he acted because of a delusional compulsion that overmastered his will to resist committing the act.[2] The term "insanity" is also frequently used in the civil context where it can have a number of different meanings.[3]

2. Mental incompetency to stand trial refers to the defendant's mental state at the time of trial. It has no bearing on the defendant's criminal responsibility (i.e., guilt or innocence), but rather is concerned with whether he has the mental capacity and ability to understand the charges and the proceedings and to assist in his defense.[4] Incompetency to stand trial is sometimes referred to as a "special plea of insanity" even though it is based on a different standard and concerns the

---

1. These are, of course, legal and not psychological or medical terms.
2. O.C.G.A. §§ 16-3-2 and 16-3-3. *See also* O.C.G.A. § 16-3-4.
3. *See* Section 5, Other Civil Matters.
4. O.C.G.A. § 17-7-130.

present as opposed to the past. Incompetency also has a number of meanings in the civil context.[5]

3. Mentally ill means having a disorder of thought or mood that significantly impairs judgment, behavior, capacity to recognize reality, or to cope with the ordinary demands of life. This is the same definition employed in the civil commitment context. Guilty but mentally ill refers to the defendant's mental state at the time of the commission of the crime and encompasses those individuals who were not "insane," but were "mentally ill."[6]

The question of competency to stand trial is concerned neither with the defendant's criminal responsibility for the acts alleged nor with his ability to distinguish right from wrong, but rather with his ability to participate in the proceedings in a meaningful way.[7] Thus, the defendant who enters a special plea of incompetency to stand trial has the right to have the question of his mental condition at the time of the trial inquired into before being required to plead to the indictment.[8] MHPs will normally be called upon to testify at a special proceeding before a specially impaneled jury regarding the defendant's competency to stand trial.[9] Additionally, if the jury finds the defendant to be incompetent, the court will transfer the defendant to the Department of Human Resources for an evaluation to determine whether the defendant can attain competency to stand trial at a later date or whether he should be committed under the civil commitment laws of the state.[10]

(A) Legal Determination of Competency to Stand Trial

Mental competence relates only to the ability of the defendant, at the time of the trial, to intelligently participate in the trial.[11] The most commonly cited test for competency is that announced by the U.S. Supreme Court in *Dusky v. United States*:[12]

---

5. *See* chapters 4.1 to 4.3 and chapters 5.6 to 5.9.
6. O.C.G.A. §§ 17-7-131(b)(3) and (c).
7. W. Lafave & A. Scott, *Handbook on Criminal Law*, § 39 (1972); *see* Echols v. State, 149 Ga. App. 620, 255 S.E.2d 92 (1979).
8. Martin v. State, 147 Ga. App. 173, 248 S.E.2d 235 (1978).
9. *See* O.C.G.A. § 17-7-130.
10. *Id.*
11. Echols, *supra* note 7.
12. 362 U.S. 402, 80 S. Ct. 788 (1960).

[I]t is not enough for the ... judge to find that "the defendant [is] oriented to time and place and [has] some recollection of events," but that the "test must be whether he has sufficient present ability to consult with his lawyer with a reasonable degree of rational understanding—and whether he has a rational as well as factual understanding of the proceedings against him."[13]

Under this test, there are two distinct issues to be determined: (1) whether the defendant is sufficiently coherent to provide his counsel with information necessary or relevant to constructing a defense; and (2) whether he is able to comprehend the significance of the trial and his relation to it.[14]

The Georgia Supreme Court has stated the test for competency as follows:

[T]he issue raised by a special plea of insanity at the time of the trial "is not, whether the defendant can distinguish between right and wrong, but is, whether he is capable at the time of the trial of understanding the nature and object of the proceedings going on against him and rightly comprehends his own condition in reference to such proceedings, and is capable of rendering his attorneys such assistance as a proper defense to the indictment preferred against him demands."[15]

A defendant has a constitutional right under the Due Process Clause of the Fourteenth Amendment to the U.S. Constitution to not be put on trial while incompetent.[16] Procedural due process also requires that the trial court afford the accused an adequate hearing on the issue of competency.[17] The Georgia statute, as well as the rules of court, require the defendant to file a written plea of mental incompetency.[18] The Georgia Supreme Court has held that in the absence of a special plea, a trial judge is under no mandatory duty to impanel a special jury to determine the issue of mental incompetency.[19] However, the defendant cannot constitutionally be tried if he is incompetent. Thus, in *Baker v. State*,[20] the court held that constitutional guarantees required that a trial court inquire into competency, even where the special plea proce-

---

13. *Id.*
14. Lafave & Scott, *supra* note 7.
15. Crawford v. State, 240 Ga. 321, 326, 240 S.E.2d 824, 827 (1977) (quoting Brown v. State, 215 Ga. 784, 787, 113 S.E.2d 618, 620 (1960)).
16. Baker v. State, 250 Ga. 187, 297 S.E.2d 9 (1982); *see also* Bishop v. United States, 350 U.S. 961, 76 S. Ct. 440 (1956).
17. Baker, *supra* note 16.
18. O.C.G.A. § 17-7-130 (1982); *see also* Uniform Sup. Ct. R. 31.4.
19. Ricks v. State, 240 Ga. 853, 242 S.E.2d 604 (1978).
20. 250 Ga. 187, 297 S.E.2d 9 (1982). *Also see* Christenson v. State, 261 Ga. 80, 402 S.E.2d 41 (1991).

dures for raising competency were not followed, if evidence of incompetence comes to the court's attention.[21]

In *Holloway v. State*, the defendant attempted to abort his trial and change his plea to guilty. He had an IQ of 49 and was found by the trial court to be mentally incompetent to enter a plea of guilty and was, therefore, required to proceed to trial. He was found guilty and sentenced to death. The Georgia Supreme Court held that the trial court erred in not ordering a hearing on his competency to proceed once evidence of incompetency was introduced.[22] Thus, the failure to properly raise the issue of incompetency to stand trial by pretrial plea does not automatically constitute a waiver of the due process right not to be tried when incompetent because "it is contradictory to argue that a defendant may be incompetent, and yet knowingly or intelligently 'waive' his right to have the court determine his capacity to stand trial."[23]

Whatever the judgment on a plea of incompetency to stand trial, it is an interlocutory judgment not subject to direct appeal without a certificate for immediate review from the trial judge.[24]

(B) Procedures for Raising the Competency Issue

The issue of the defendant's competency to stand trial is usually raised by pretrial motion (sometimes referred to as a special plea of insanity) at the time of arraignment, when the defendant is called upon to plead to the charges against him. In addition, and as described earlier, the issue of the defendant's incompetency may be raised at any time during the course of the trial.[25] If the defendant enters a plea of incompetency to stand trial, the court must impanel a special jury to determine whether the defendant is, in fact, incompetent under the legal test stated.[26]

Georgia law concerning the examination and evaluation of defendants raising the plea of mental incompetency is unclear. The statutory provision on pleas of mental incompetency states that

---

21. Baker, *supra* note 16. *Also see* Harris v. State, 256 Ga. 350, 349 S.E.2d 374 (1986).
22. 257 Ga. 620, 361 S.E.2d 794 (1987).
23. Pate v. Robinson, 383 U.S. 375 at 384, 86 S. Ct. 836 (1966).
24. Spell v. State, 120 Ga. App. 398, 170 S.E.2d 701 (1969).
25. Lafave & Scott, *supra* note 7; *see also* O.C.G.A. § 17-7-130 (1982).
26. O.C.G.A. § 17-7-130 (1982). A plea of mental incompetency to stand trial was previously referred to as a special plea of insanity. For a history of the Georgia plea of incompetency, *see* Echols, *supra* note 7.

Whenever a plea is filed that a defendant in a criminal case is mentally incompetent to stand trial, it shall be the duty of the court to cause the issue of the defendant's mental competency to stand trial to be tried first by a special jury. If the special jury finds the defendant mentally incompetent to stand trial, the court shall retain jurisdiction over the defendant but shall transfer the defendant to the Department of Human Resources.[27]

The law makes no explicit provision regarding pretrial psychological or psychiatric examination. The very next section of the law, which deals with the insanity defense (i.e., the defendant's mental state at the time of the offense) does provide for a court-appointed psychiatrist or psychologist to examine the defendant and to testify at trial.[28] The Uniform Superior Court Rules, adopted by the Georgia Supreme Court, treat the pleas of insanity and incompetency as procedurally the same. The rules require the filing of a written notice of the plea and provide for the entry of an order requiring evaluation of the defendant's condition for the purpose of determining competency to stand trial.[29]

In *Motes v. State*,[30] a decision dealing with the insanity defense, the court held that if the defendant wants to introduce expert testimony, the state must be allowed to have a psychiatrist examine the defendant who, in light of the partial waiver of the right to remain silent, must cooperate by talking to the court-appointed expert.[31] However, if the defendant chooses to prove his incompetency by means other than expert testimony, then the defendant can elect whether or not to talk to the court-appointed expert. Any statement made by the defendant to a court-appointed psychiatrist/psychologist is not covered by the psychiatrist/psychologist–patient privilege.[32] Moreover, a psychiatrist or psychologist may testify regarding a defendant's competency to stand trial and his understanding of *Miranda* rights without violating the defendant's Fifth Amendment privilege against self-incrimination.[33]

The trial on a plea of mental incompetency is civil in nature, with the burden of proof on the defendant, or movant, to prove by a preponderance of the evidence that he is not mentally compe-

---

27. O.C.G.A. § 17-7-130.
28. O.C.G.A. § 17-7-130.1.
29. Uniform Sup. Ct. R. 31.4 and 31.5. The rules also provide model forms for mental evaluations. They improperly use the term "competency" to refer to both the special plea of competency at the time of trial and the plea of not guilty by reason of insanity. *See* Rule 31.5, Specimen Order No. 1 & 2.
30. 256 Ga. 831, 353 S.E.2d 348 (1987).
31. *Id.*
32. Harris, *supra* note 21.
33. Marlowe v. State, 187 Ga. App. 255, 370 S.E.2d 20 (1988).

tent to stand trial.[34] However, the defendant has the constitutional right to the effective assistance of counsel at the competency hearing.[35] The defendant must overcome the statutory presumption of competence.[36] If the defendant introduces no evidence in support of his plea, the judge may direct a verdict for the state on the issue of competency.[37] Since the proceeding is regarded as civil in nature, the state may call the defendant for purposes of cross-examination, although no questions may be asked concerning the accused's guilt or innocence.[38] The guilt or innocence of the defendant is not relevant at such a proceeding, and permitting the prosecution to introduce evidence of guilt on a special plea would constitute error.[39] However, the defendant's statements made during the commission of the crime may be admitted if they shed light on competency.[40] If the plea of incompetency is not sustained, the state is free to proceed with the trial on the merits.[41]

(C) Disposition of Defendants Found Incompetent to Stand Trial

If the special jury finds the defendant incompetent to stand trial, the court will retain jurisdiction over the defendant and transfer him to the Department of Human Resources (DHR) for an evaluation.[42] Within 90 days after receiving actual custody of the defendant, DHR will conduct an evaluation and make a determination as to whether or not the defendant is presently mentally incompetent to stand trial and, if so, whether or not there is a substantial probability that he will attain mental competency to stand trial in the foreseeable future.[43] If the person is found to be mentally competent to stand trial, the department will report that finding, and the reasons for the finding, to the committing courts, and the defendant will be returned to the court for further proceedings.[44]

---

34. Banks v. State, 246 Ga. 178, 269 S.E.2d 450 (1980); Henderson v. State, 157 Ga. App. 621, 278 S.E.2d 164 (1981); Partridge v. State, 256 Ga. 602, 351 S.E.2d 635 (1987).
35. Almond v. State, 180 Ga. App. 475, 349 S.E.2d 482 (1986).
36. Banks v. State, 269 S.E.2d at 453.
37. Williams v. State, 238 Ga. 298, 232 S.E.2d 535 (1977).
38. Brown, *supra* note 15.
39. Crawford, *supra* note 15.
40. Brown v. State, 256 Ga. 387, 349 S.E.2d 452 (1986).
41. Spell, *supra* note 24; Watson v. State, 229 Ga. 787, 194 S.E.2d 407 (1972).
42. O.C.G.A. § 17-7-130(a).
43. O.C.G.A. § 17-7-130(b).
44. Id.

If the defendant is found by DHR to be mentally incompetent to stand trial, and there is no substantial probability that he will attain competency in the foreseeable future, the DHR will report that finding to the court.[45] If the defendant meets the criteria for civil commitment under the civil commitment statutes, he will then be civilly committed to a state institution by the appropriate court using the general civil commitment procedures.[46] If the defendant does not meet the criteria for civil commitment, or if he becomes competent after having been committed, the committing court will be notified, and the defendant will be returned to the court for further proceedings.[47]

If the defendant is found to be mentally incompetent to stand trial, but there is a substantial probability that he will attain competency in the foreseeable future, DHR will retain custody over the defendant for the purpose of continued treatment for an additional period that cannot exceed 9 months.[48] At the end of the 9-month period, if the defendant continues to be incompetent to stand trial, he will be civilly committed if he meets the civil commitment criteria.[49] If the defendant does not meet the commitment criteria, or if he becomes mentally competent after having been committed, the committing court will be notified and the defendant will be returned to the court for further proceedings.[50]

When a person is returned to court, the court may dismiss the charges, or if the person is presently competent, it may proceed to try the case.[51] Any person who is returned for trial is entitled to file another special plea of incompetency, thereby commencing the process anew.[52]

---

45. O.C.G.A. § 17-7-130(c).

46. *Id.*

47. *Id.*

48. O.C.G.A. § 17-7-130(d).

49. *Id.* The U.S. Supreme Court has ruled that a person charged by a state with a criminal offense who is transferred to a mental institution on account of his incompetency to proceed at trial cannot be held more than a reasonable time necessary to determine if there is substantial probability that he will attain competency in the foreseeable future. If there is no substantial probability that he will attain competency in the foreseeable future, the state must either release him or institute the customary civil commitment proceedings that would be required to commit indefinitely any other citizen. Jackson v. Indiana, 406 U.S. 715, 92 S. Ct. 1845 (1972).

50. O.C.G.A. § 17-7-130(d).

51. O.C.G.A. § 17-7-130(e).

52. O.C.G.A. § 17-7-130(f).

Provocation (Voluntary Manslaughter)

Voluntary manslaughter is the intentional killing of a human being prompted by serious provocation. A person commits murder "when he unlawfully and with malice aforethought, either express or implied, causes the death of another human being."[1] A person commits voluntary manslaughter "when he causes the death of another human being under circumstances which would otherwise be murder and if he acts solely as the result of a sudden, violent, and irresistible passion resulting from serious provocation sufficient to excite such passion in a reasonable person. . . ."[2] Both offenses involve an intentional and unlawful act. Sufficient provocation, however, negates the malice element of murder and reduces the crime to voluntary manslaughter.[3] This is because the so-called "hot blood" aspect of voluntary manslaughter is inconsistent with the notion of malice required for murder.[4]

To justify a jury charge on voluntary manslaughter, the evidence must show not only an act of violent passion, but it must also show some serious provocation "sufficient to excite such passion in a reasonable person," not just the particular defen-

---

1. O.C.G.A. § 15-5-1.
2. O.C.G.A. § 16-5-2.
3. *See* Holloway v. McElroy, 632 F.2d 605 (5th Cir. 1980). Malice is the unlawful, deliberate intention to kill a person without excuse, justification, or mitigation. Mason v. Balkcom, 487 F. Supp. 554 (M.D. Ga. 1980), *rev'd on other grounds*, 669 F.2d 222 (5th Cir. 1982), *cert. denied*, 460 U.S. 1016 (1983). Georgia law does not require premeditation or a preconceived intention to kill. Malice may be formed in an instant and immediately result in a fatal blow or shot. Wright v. State, 255 Ga. 109, 335 S.E.2d 857 (1985). A homicide may be ruled justifiable if the defendant acts in self-defense rather than acting out of sudden anger or provocation. Murff v. State, 251 Ga. 478, 306 S.E.2d 267 (1983).
4. Holloway, *supra* note 3, at 629.

dant.[5] In other words, the test of provocation is an objective rather than a subjective test. Therefore, expert testimony from an MHP regarding a particular defendant's susceptibility to provocation would probably not be admissible.

Georgia courts have ruled also as a matter of law that insulting words alone will not justify the excitement of passion that will reduce a crime from murder to manslaughter.[6] However, words may be sufficient provocation if the content relates to conduct that is provocative. For example, if one spouse taunts the other with prior acts of adultery, this may constitute sufficient provocation if it is the adulterous conduct, not the words alone, that provoked the sudden violent and irresistible passion leading to homicide.[7]

The Georgia statute also provides that if there was an interval between the provocation and the killing "sufficient for the voice of reason and humanity to be heard," the killing will constitute murder, not voluntary manslaughter.[8] In other words, if there is a sufficient "cooling off" period between the provocation and the homicide, it cannot constitute voluntary manslaughter.[9]

Whether the provocation was sufficient to arouse the passion of a reasonable man and the question of the cooling off period are questions of fact for the jury.[10] There are no Georgia cases dealing directly with the question of whether expert testimony is admissible to prove provocation. However, the courts will not permit a psychiatrist or psychologist to give expert opinion testimony on the question of whether the defendant possessed criminal in-

5. Swett v. State, 242 Ga. 228, 248 S.E.2d 629 (1978); Partridge v. State, 256 Ga. 602, 351 S.E.2d 635 (1987).
6. Pare v. State, 258 Ga. 225, 367 S.E.2d 803 (1988).
7. Cash v. State, 258 Ga. 460, 368 S.E.2d 756 (1988). *Also see* Strickland v. State, 257 Ga. 230, 357 S.E.2d 85 (1987).
8. O.C.G.A. § 16-5-2; Keye v. State, 136 Ga. 707, 222 S.E.2d 172 (1975) (defendant left the scene of an argument, purchased a knife, and returned to continue the fray, thus having an opportunity for the "voice of reason" to be heard).
9. Brooks v. State, 249 Ga. 583, 292 S.E.2d 694 (1982). *But see* Strickland, *supra* note 7. In contrast, use of abusive language may be considered justification for simple assault or simple battery. *See* O.C.G.A. § 16-5-25; Mitchell v. State, 41 Ga. 527 (1871).
10. Ward v. State, 151 Ga. App. 36, 258 S.E.2d 699 (1979) (knocking defendant down and choking are sufficient provocation); Ellis v. State, 168 Ga. App. 757, 309 S.E.2d 924 (1983) (beating and kicking are sufficient provocation); Parks v. State, 234 Ga. 579, 216 S.E.2d 804 (1975) (finding old girlfriend and new boyfriend on sofa is insufficient provocation); Davis v. State, 140 Ga. App. 890, 232 S.E.2d 164 (1977) (5 to 15 minutes is not sufficient "cooling off" period as a matter of law).

tent.[11] The general rule in Georgia is that expert testimony, even when it concerns the ultimate issue to be decided, is admissible only when the conclusion is "beyond the ken of the average layman."[12] It is likely that the Georgia courts would find that the issue of the degree of provocation and whether or not there has been sufficient "cooling off" to be within the average person's understanding and, therefore, not a proper subject for expert opinion.

---

11. *See* chapter 7.7, Mens Rea. *See, generally,* Jones v. State, 232 Ga. 762, 208 S.E.2d 850 (1974) (expert opinion is not permitted to determine credibility of eyewitness's identification of defendant); Nichols v. State, 177 Ga. App. 689, 340 S.E.2d 654 (1986) (doctor's testimony, "this is rape," addressed a question of law and fact and is not a proper one for expert opinion testimony). *But see* Askew v. State, 185 Ga. App. 282, 363 S.E.2d 844 (1987), in which a police officer was permitted to give expert testimony as to the ability of witnesses to give accurate descriptions of crime perpetrators.

12. *See* Smith v. State, 247 Ga. 612, 277 S.E.2d 678 (1981), *rev'g* Smith v. State, 156 Ga. App. 419, 274 S.E.2d 703 (1980).

7.7

Mens Rea

In general terms, a crime consists of at least two elements: an act or omission to act, and a specified state of mind.[1] The state of mind element is commonly referred to as *mens rea* (guilty mind), *scienter*, or *criminal intent*. The state of mind requirement varies from one criminal offense to another.[2] At common law, the words and phrases used by judges to express the state of mind requirement included "maliciously," "fraudulently," "feloniously," "willfully and corruptly," and "with intent to."[3] Today, most crimes are codified in statutes, and the statutes embody a state of mind requirement as an element of each crime.[4]

(A) Culpable Mental States in Georgia

Georgia law defines a crime as "a violation of a statute of this state in which there is a joint operation of an act or omission to act and intention or criminal negligence."[5] The purpose of the intent

---

1. W. Lafave & A. Scott, *Handbook on Criminal Law*, § 27 (1972). Many crimes also require that a specified result flow from the act or omission.
2. *Id.*
3. *Id.*
4. *Id.*
5. O.C.G.A. § 16-2-1; *see* Mallette v. State, 119 Ga. App. 24, 165 S.E.2d 870 (1969) (stating that every crime consists of union or joint operation of act and intention).

requirement is to distinguish accidental acts from those in which the person acted with a "bad mind."[6]

The statutory presumption that the voluntary acts of a person of sound mind are intentional, but the presumption may be rebutted by evidence, has been declared unconstitutional as improperly shifting the burden of proof on the element of intent to the defendant.[7] While a person is not presumed to act with criminal intent, the fact finder may consider the circumstances surrounding the act in determining whether those circumstances manifest criminal intention.[8] However, a person who is too young, too "feeble-minded," or otherwise mentally incapable of forming the requisite criminal intent cannot commit a crime.[9]

Most crimes contain, as an element of the offense, a requisite general intent.[10] General intent means that one intends the "natural and probable consequences of his acts."[11] The requirement of intent to commit a crime can be inferred from the surrounding circumstances. In addition, a person can, in some instances, be guilty of a crime through criminal negligence even without a showing of general intent.[12] Criminal negligence is more than the ordinary negligence that is the basis of civil damage suits. It involves a "reckless and wanton negligence and [must be] of such a character as to show an utter disregard for the safety of others who might reasonably be expected to be injured thereby."[13]

The Georgia statutes, although they include an element of intent in each crime, do not usually define the terms that specify the necessary degree of intent. For example, such terms as "knowingly," "intentionally," "maliciously," and "willfully" are not defined by statute, and their definitions are left to the courts.[14] In

---

6. "A person shall not be found guilty of any crime committed by misfortune or accident...." O.C.G.A. § 16-2-2.
7. O.C.G.A. § 16-2-4. As to the constitutionality of this burden-shifting presumption, *see* Francis v. Franklin, 471 U.S. 307, 105 S. Ct. 1965 (1985), *rev'g* Franklin v. State, 245 Ga. 141 (1980).
8. O.C.G.A. § 16-2-6. Burden v. State, 187 Ga. App. 778, 371 S.E.2d 410 (1988).
9. Miley v. State, 118 Ga. 274, 45 S.E. 245 (1903).
10. Holloway v. McElroy, 632 F.2d 605 (5th Cir. 1980). Certain crimes also contain a specific intent element, as when one commits an assault "[w]ith intent to murder, to rape, or to rob...." O.C.G.A. § 16-5-21.
11. *Id.; see also* O.C.G.A. § 16-2-5.
12. Holloway, *supra* note 10.
13. Keye v. State, 136 Ga. App. 707, 222 S.E.2d 172 (1975) (quoting Thomas v. State, 73 Ga. App. 803, 38 S.E.2d 188 [1946]); *see also* Maltbie v. State, 139 Ga. App. 342, 228 S.E.2d 368 (1976) (term *heedless disregard* includes criminal negligence).
14. *See, e.g.,* O.C.G.A. § 16-5-23 (in which "intentionally" is not defined); O.C.G.A. § 16-5-24 (in which "maliciously" and "knowingly" are not defined).

a very few instances, certain other terms, such as "malice"[15] or "reckless"[16] are expressly defined by statute.

(B) Proof of Intent

Criminal intent is normally proved by conduct, demeanor, and other circumstances surrounding the commission of the criminal act.[17] The state is required to prove an intention to commit the act prohibited by law, not the intention to violate a criminal statute itself.[18] Intention can sometimes be proved directly, and sometimes it can be inferred by conduct or circumstances.[19] The general rule is that intention is manifested by all the circumstances connected with the perpetration of the offense.[20] Whether the required intent exists is a question of fact for the jury, or for the judge if acting as the trier of fact.[21]

Georgia law permits testimony from psychologists or psychiatrists to determine the state of mind of a defendant who raises the insanity defense.[22] Georgia law does not permit expert testimony as to whether or not the defendant acted with criminal intent, since such testimony concerns an ultimate fact and is an

---

15. See O.C.G.A. § 16-5-1 (definition of "express malice" in crime of murder).
16. See O.C.G.A. § 16-5-60 (definition of "reckless" in crime of reckless conduct).
17. Brooks v. State, 151 Ga. App. 384, 259 S.E.2d 743 (1979) (codefendants drove into parking lot, started looking in parked cars, entered the cars without authority of owner, opened one car by use of a coat hanger); Parham v. State, 166 Ga. App. 855, 305 S.E.2d 599 (1983) (appellant's presence, companionship with two other participants, and his intent to participate in one crime as look-out was enough to establish intent to commit armed robbery in which he had no direct participation); Kimbro v. State, 152 Ga. App. 893, 264 S.E.2d 327 (1980) (presence, companionship, and conduct before and after offense are circumstances relevant to intent).
18. Brown v. State, 182 Ga. App. 682, 356 S.E.2d 663 (1987); Pope v. State, 179 Ga. App. 739, 347 S.E.2d 703 (1986).
19. Mallette, supra note 5; Fussell v. State, 187 Ga. App. 134, 369 S.E.2d 511 (1988).
20. Id.
21. O.C.G.A. § 16-2-6. "A person will not be presumed to act with criminal intention but the trier of facts may find such intention upon consideration of the words, conduct, demeanor, motive, and all other circumstances connected with the act for which the accused is prosecuted." Id.; see Riddle v. State, 145 Ga. App. 328, 243 S.E.2d 607 (1978).
22. O.C.G.A. § 17-7-130.1; Moore v. State, 221 Ga. 636, 146 S.E.2d 895 (1966).

issue that can be determined by the average juror.[23] The federal courts also have held inadmissible a psychologist's opinion as to whether or not the defendant could appreciate the wrongfulness of his act on the basis that this was the ultimate legal issue in the case.[24]

---

23. *See, e.g.,* Jones v. State, 232 Ga. 762, 208 S.E.2d 850 (1974) (expert testimony is not allowed on the issue of credibility of the victim/witness; Nichols v. State, 177 Ga. App. 689, 340 S.E.2d 654 (1986) (doctor is not permitted to testify "this is rape"); *see also* O.C.G.A. § 24-9-65 ("If the issue shall be as to the existence of a fact, the opinion of witnesses shall be generally inadmissible."). *But see* Smith v. State, 247 Ga. 612, 277 S.E.2d 678 (1981), *rev'g* Smith v. State, 156 Ga. App. 419, 274 S.E.2d 703 (1980). *Also see* Miller v. State, 189 Ga. App. 587, 376 S.E.2d 901 (1988) (a clinical psychologist may testify that a child has been molested, but may not offer an expert opinion that the defendant was the perpetrator).
24. United States v. Manley, 893 F.2d 1221 (11th Cir. 1990).

7.8

Diminished Capacity

Some jurisdictions recognize the defense of diminished capacity (also known as diminished responsibility). In this defense, defendants assert that although they may have had the requisite *mens rea* (see chapter 7.7), it was severely diminished as a result of a mental disease or defect, which should reduce their guilt to that of a lesser offense. Georgia does not recognize this defense. However, a defendant's mental state, including diminished capacity, may be considered as a mitigating circumstance in the sentencing phase of a death penalty case.

Criminal Responsibility: The Insanity Defense

If a criminal defendant claims that he lacked the mental capacity at the time of the criminal act to be held responsible for his actions, he may plead the defense of insanity.[1] Unlike other defenses, acquittal by reason of insanity does not mean that the defendant will automatically go free.[2] Rather, a defendant found not guilty by reason of insanity is likely to be committed to a mental institution for a substantial period of time.[3] In addition, whenever a defendant pleads not guilty by reason of insanity, the jury must be instructed that it can find the defendant guilty but mentally ill or guilty but retarded rather than not guilty by reason of insanity. If the defendant is found guilty but mentally ill or guilty but mentally retarded, he will be sentenced like any convicted felon and will usually go to prison.[4]

The underlying purpose of the insanity defense is to separate from the criminal justice system those who, because of their lack of criminal intent, should not be punished, but should be treated for their illness.[5] Because punishment includes an element of moral culpability, the purpose of the criminal law would not be

---

1. *See* O.C.G.A. §§ 16-3-2 and 16-3-3.
2. W. Lafave & A. Scott, *Handbook on Criminal Law*, § 36 (1972); *see* O.C.G.A. § 17-7-131.
3. P. Kurtz, *Criminal Offenses and Defenses in Georgia*, 224 (2d ed. 1987). Because the defendant may be committed to a mental hospital for a longer period of time than if convicted, a defendant charged with a crime other than one punishable by death may elect to forego pleading the insanity defense. *See* Lafave & Scott, *supra* note 2, § 40.
4. *See* O.C.G.A. § 17-7-131(g)(2).
5. Lafave & Scott, *supra* note 2, § 36.

served by convicting a person who did not know what he was doing when he committed the crime.[6]

MHPs become involved in cases in which a defendant pleads insanity by conducting evaluations and providing expert testimony concerning the defendant's mental state at the time of the crime.[7] This testimony may be given on behalf of the defendant, the prosecution, or the court. MHPs are also called upon to evaluate and test insanity acquittees and those found guilty but mentally ill or mentally retarded, and to testify at commitment and release hearings for insanity acquittees.

(A) Legal Determination of Insanity

Georgia law recognizes four different mental states that relate to the insanity defense:

1. the "right-wrong" test for insanity;[8]
2. the delusional compulsion test for insanity;[9]
3. the mentally ill test;[10] and
4. the mentally retarded test.[11]

A finding of mental illness or retardation does not correspond to a finding of insanity. Thus, a defendant may be found guilty but mentally ill, but not insane.

(A)(1) Right–Wrong Test

The right–wrong test, or the M'Naghten Rule,[12] is the legal test for insanity used in the majority of jurisdictions throughout the country.[13] Georgia first recognized the rule in 1847 in *Roberts v. State*.[14] The test, as currently codified in Georgia, is: "A person

---

6. *Id*. An often cited, and insensitive and unrealistic, example of a defendant who did not know what he was doing is that of a man who strangled his wife, but believed he was squeezing lemons.
7. *See* O.C.G.A. § 17-7-130.1. Lay witnesses may also testify regarding the defendant's sanity. Chancellor v. State, 165 Ga. App. 365, 301 S.E.2d 294 (1983).
8. O.C.G.A. § 16-3-2.
9. O.C.G.A. § 16-3-3.
10. O.C.G.A. § 17-7-131(a)(2).
11. O.C.G.A. § 17-7-131(a)(3).
12. The M'Naghten Rule comes from a famous English case. In that case, Daniel M'Naghten shot and killed Edward Drummond, private secretary to Sir Robert Peel, believing that Peel was heading a conspiracy to kill M'Naghten. At the trial, M'Naghten claimed that he was insane and could not be held responsible because it was his delusions that caused him to act. The jury found M'Naghten not guilty by reason of insanity. M'Naghten's Case, 8 Eng. Rep. 718 (1843). For a more thorough discussion of the origination of the M'Naghten Rule, see Lafave & Scott, *supra* note 2, § 37.
13. Lafave & Scott, *supra* note 2, § 37.
14. 3 Ga. 310 (1847); *see* Kurtz, *also supra* note 3 at 224.

shall not be found guilty of a crime if, at the time of the act, omission, or negligence constituting the crime, the person did not have mental capacity to distinguish between right and wrong in relation to such act, omission, or negligence."[15]

The "right from wrong" component of the test is strictly applied. For example, the courts have held that the notion of "general insanity" does not constitute a valid defense to a crime.[16] Also, the mere finding that the defendant suffered from multiple personalities is not enough to relieve the defendant of criminal accountability.[17] Likewise, a finding of mental abnormality or mere weakness of the mind is no excuse unless it amounts to "imbecility" or "idiocy" that deprives the defendant of the ability to distinguish between right and wrong in relation to the particular act in question.[18] Evidence that the defendant had the mentality of a child does not relieve him from responsibility for a crime.[19] Nor does a mere showing of psychosis, such as schizophrenia, establish legal insanity.[20] A temporary condition of insanity has been recognized as an appropriate defense in Georgia.[21]

(A)(2) Delusional Compulsion Test

Like many other states, Georgia provides an alternative test for insanity in addition to the "right from wrong" test.[22] In *Roberts v. State*,[23] the court stated that even those defendants who could distinguish right from wrong would be acquitted if "in consequence of some delusion, the will is overmastered . . . [and] the act itself is connected with the peculiar delusion."[24] As currently codified, the delusional compulsion test provides:

> A person shall not be found guilty of a crime when, at the time of the act, omission, or negligence constituting the crime, the person, because of mental disease, injury, or congenital defi-

---

15. O.C.G.A. § 16-3-2. The "pure" M'Naghten Rule is stated as follows:

> The defendant cannot be convicted if, at the time he committed the act, he was laboring under such a defect of reason, from a disease of the mind, as not to know the nature and quality of the act he was doing; or, if he did know it, as not to know he was doing what was wrong.

Lafave & Scott, *supra* note 2, § 36.
16. Gould v. State, 168 Ga. App. 605, 309 S.E.2d 888 (1983).
17. Kirkland v. State, 166 Ga. App. 478, 304 S.E.2d 561 (1983).
18. Howard v. State, 166 Ga. App. 224, 303 S.E.2d 763 (1983).
19. Reece v. State, 212 Ga. 609, 94 S.E.2d 723 (1956).
20. Dennis v. State, 170 Ga. App. 630, 317 S.E.2d 874 (1984).
21. Jackson v. State, 149 Ga. App. 253, 253 S.E.2d 874 (1979).
22. *See* Lafave & Scott, *supra* note 2, § 37. The more common supplementary test is referred to as the "irresistible impulse" test, which was developed before the M'Naghten Rule.
23. 3 Ga. 310 (1847).
24. *Id.* at 331.

ciency, acted as he did because of a delusional compulsion as to such act which overmastered his will to resist committing the crime.[25]

This test is comprised of three elements. To support an acquittal, it must appear that

1. the defendant was laboring under a delusion;
2. the criminal act was connected with the delusion under which the defendant was laboring; and
3. the delusion was concerning a fact that, if true, would have justified the act.[26]

Thus, in *Stevens v. State*, when at the time the defendant killed his wife he was operating under the delusion that she was possessed by Satan and that he, the defendant, was defending himself against Satan's physical attacks and attempts to destroy him, the delusional compulsion test is met.[27] Likewise, epilepsy can be a defense to a crime if "reason is dethroned" because of a seizure.[28] The last element of the test, that the act would have been justified if the delusion were true, is an important restriction on the delusional compulsion test.[29] For example, a defendant who acted in an "insane delusion" that his estranged wife was seeing another man was not excused for his act because adultery is not a justification for homicide.[30] Nor does the insanity defense provide a defense on the basis of proof that the defendant suffered from an impulse control disorder.[31]

An act committed by an intoxicated person provides no excuse when the intoxication is the result of a voluntary act.[32] If, however, the defendant has developed an organic brain syndrome or other chronic condition constituting a "mental disease," then he may be found not guilty by reason of insanity if he meets the other elements of the test.

---

25. O.C.G.A. § 16-3-3. The delusional compulsion defense is not available as a defense in a civil action for assault or battery. *See* Continental Cas. Co. v. Parker, 167 Ga. App. 859, 307 S.E.2d 744 (1983).
26. Stevens v. State, 256 Ga. 440, 350 S.E.2d 21 (1986); Graham v. State, 236 Ga. 378, 223 S.E.2d 803 (1976).
27. Stevens, *supra* note 26 at 23.
28. Starr v. State, 134 Ga. App. 149, 213 S.E.2d 531 (1975); *see also* Murphy v. State, 132 Ga. App. 654, 209 S.E.2d 101 (1974).
29. Kurtz, *supra* note 3 at 225.
30. Freeman v. State, 132 Ga. App. 742, 209 S.E.2d 127 (1974); Salter v. State, 257 Ga. 88, 356 S.E.2d 196 (1987).
31. Hicks v. State, 256 Ga. 715, 352 S.E.2d 762 (1987).
32. Wells v. State, 247 Ga. 792, 279 S.E.2d 213 (1981); *see* O.C.G.A. § 16-3-4.

In 1982, the Georgia legislature, reacting in part to the public furor over the John Hinckley (who attempted to assassinate President Ronald Reagan) case, created the new status of "guilty but mentally ill." In 1988, the test for mental retardation was deleted from the definition of mental illness and the separate status of "guilty but mentally retarded" was created. Both defenses are available only in felony cases.

Mentally ill is defined as

> . . . having a disorder of thought or mood which significantly impairs judgment, behavior, capacity to recognize reality, or ability to cope with the ordinary demands of life. However, the term "mental illness" shall not include a mental state manifested only by repeated unlawful or antisocial conduct.[33]

Mentally retarded is defined as:

> . . . having significantly subaverage general intellectual functioning resulting in or associated with impairments in adaptive behavior which manifested during the developmental periods.[34]

Both definitions are substantially the same as the definitions contained in the Georgia Mental Health Code for purposes of civil commitment.[35]

Whenever a defendant asserts the insanity defense, the trial judge is required to charge the jury that they should find the defendant either guilty, not guilty, not guilty by reason of insanity, guilty but mentally ill at the time of the crime, or guilty but mentally retarded.[36] A defendant found guilty but mentally ill or retarded will be sentenced in the same manner as a defendant who is found guilty, except in death penalty cases when an automatic life sentence, as opposed to the death sentence, will be imposed.[37]

To find the defendant not guilty by reason of insanity, the jury must apply either the right–wrong test or the delusional compulsion test. To find the defendant guilty but mentally ill, the jury must find beyond a reasonable doubt that the defendant is guilty of the crime and that his or her mental condition met the statutory definition of mental illness at the time of the crime.[38] To find the defendant guilty but mentally retarded, the jury must

---

33. O.C.G.A. 17-7-131(a)(2).
34. O.C.G.A. § 17-7-131(a)(3).
35. *See* O.C.G.A. §§ 37-3-1(11) and 37-4-2(11).
36. O.C.G.A. §§ 17-7-131(b)(1) and (c).
37. O.C.G.A. §§ 17-7-131(g)(1) and (2); 17-7-131(j). *See* Zant v. Foster, 261 Ga. 450, 406 S.E.2d 74 (1991).
38. O.C.G.A. § 17-7-131(c)(2).

find beyond a reasonable doubt that the defendant is guilty of the crime and is mentally retarded.[39]

As discussed in the following, the burden of proof is on the defendant to establish insanity by a preponderance of the evidence. On the other hand, the burden is on the prosecution to prove mental illness or retardation beyond a reasonable doubt. Thus, for a defendant to be found guilty but mentally ill or retarded, the jury must be persuaded beyond a reasonable doubt that the defendant was mentally ill or retarded at the time of the act, but that he was not insane. The Georgia Supreme Court has held that the distinction between mental illness and insanity is sufficiently clear that the statutory provision does not violate the defendant's right to due process of law.[40]

Thus, a finding of guilty but mentally ill is appropriate in a case in which the defendant is suffering from a multiple personality disorder, even though he would not be considered "insane" under either of the two traditional tests.[41] If a defendant knows the difference between right and wrong at the time of the crime, even if he is determined to be suffering from some form of mental illness, the jury can reject a verdict of not guilty by reason of insanity and find the defendant guilty but mentally ill.[42]

(B) Burden of Proof

In every criminal case, the burden is on the prosecution to establish the defendant's guilt beyond a reasonable doubt. However, insanity is an affirmative defense, and the burden is on the defendant to prove by a preponderance of the evidence that he was legally insane at the time of the commission of the crime. This shifting of the burden of proof has been held to be constitutional.[43]

In addition, Georgia law provides that "every person is presumed to be of sound mind and discretion, but the presumption may be rebutted." The defendant must overcome the presumption by presenting evidence of insanity. Evidence of insanity may be presented by both lay and expert witnesses. However, the jury

---

39. O.C.G.A. § 17-7-131(c)(3).
40. Wilson v. State, 257 Ga. 444, 359 S.E.2d 891 (1987); Worthy v. State, 253 Ga. 661, 324 S.E.2d 431 (1985); Keener v. State, 254 Ga. 699, 334 S.E.2d 173 (1985); Dimauro v. State, 185 Ga. App. 524, 364 S.E.2d 900 (1988).
41. See Kirkland, supra note 17.
42. See Jackson v. State, 166 Ga. App. 477, 304 S.E.2d 560 (1983); Awtrey v. State, 175 Ga. App. 148, 332 S.E.2d 896 (1985).
43. Keener, supra note 40.

is free to reject uncontradicted testimony, including expert testimony, as to lack of sanity and to rely solely on the presumption.

While the defendant bears the burden of persuasion as to insanity, the prosecution bears the burden of proving, beyond a reasonable doubt, that the defendant was guilty but mentally ill at the time of the commission of the offense. Although this may appear to be logically inconsistent, the Georgia courts have upheld the constitutionality of the verdict of guilty but mentally ill and of the allocation of the burdens of proof.[44]

(C) Procedures for Raising the Insanity Defense

According to the Georgia statute and the Uniform Superior Court Rules, if a defendant intends to interpose the defense of insanity, he must file in advance of trial a "Notice of Intent of Defense to Raise Issue of Insanity or Mental Incompetency" as a prerequisite to raising the defense at the trial on the merits.[45] When the notice of an insanity defense is filed, the court must appoint at least one psychiatrist or licensed psychologist to examine the defendant and to testify at trial.[46]

In addition to being examined by a court-appointed expert, the defendant has the right, if indigent, to a court-appointed psychiatrist or psychologist to examine him, assist counsel in the cross-examination of the prosecution's expert witnesses, and to testify.[47] In *Ake v. Oklahoma*,[48] the U.S. Supreme Court held that an indigent defendant who makes a preliminary showing that his sanity at the time of the crime will likely be a significant factor at trial is entitled to an expert provided at state expense to assist in the preparation and presentation of his defense. The Georgia Supreme Court has followed this line of reasoning and has held that when the defendant's sanity is likely to be a significant factor at trial, the state must appoint an expert to assist the indigent

---

44. *See* cases cited at note 40.
45. O.C.G.A. § 17-7-130.1; Uniform Sup. Ct. R. 31.4. Hodges v. State, 257 Ga. 818, 364 S.E.2d 275 (1988) (failure to file notice requires exclusion of defense). In most jurisdictions, the prevailing rule is that the defendant may respond to the charge against him simply by pleading not guilty, and he need not disclose in advance his intent to raise the insanity defense. *See* Lafave & Scott, *supra* note 2, § 40.
46. O.C.G.A. § 17-7-130.1. The court has no discretion and must appoint an expert if the Rule 31.4 notice is filed. Strickland v. State, 257 Ga. 230, 357 S.E.2d 85 (1987).
47. *See, generally,* W. Daniel, *Georgia Criminal Trial Practice*, § 21-9 (1988).
48. 470 U.S. 68, 105 S. Ct. 1087 (1985).

defendant with the preparation of his defense.[49] This requirement of a court-appointed expert probably applies even if there was no advance notice of intent to raise the insanity plea filed with the court.[50]

At trial, in addition to testimony being presented regarding guilt or innocence, both the prosecution and the defense may introduce expert testimony regarding the mental condition of the defendant.[51] Lay opinions also may be admitted for purposes of determining the defendant's sanity.[52] Following the testimony of experts for the prosecution and defense, the expert appointed by the court may testify.[53] This expert may be cross-examined by both the prosecution and the defense, and each side may introduce evidence in rebuttal.[54]

The defendant, by presenting expert testimony concerning his mental condition, is deemed to have partially waived the right to remain silent and must cooperate with the court-appointed expert.[55] If the defendant refuses to cooperate, he can be prohibited from introducing expert testimony on the insanity issue. The defendant cannot, however, be prohibited from raising the insanity defense as a penalty for refusing to talk with the court-appointed expert. If the defendant chooses to prove insanity by means other than expert testimony, the defendant may invoke his right to remain silent and refuse to talk to the expert.[56] If the defendant talks to the court-appointed expert, the patient–psychiatrist/psychologist privilege does not apply.[57] However, when defense counsel has a psychiatrist or psychologist examine the defendant, the state may be barred by the attorney–client privilege from compelling the MHP to testify for the state.[58]

---

49. *See* Lindsey v. State, 254 Ga. 444, 330 S.E.2d 563 (1985); Harris v. State, 181 Ga. App. 358, 352 S.E.2d 226 (1986); Holloway v. State, 257 Ga. 620, 361 S.E.2d 794 (1987).
50. Daniel, *supra* note 47, § 21-9; Morgan v. State, 135 Ga. App. 139, 217 S.E.2d 175, *rev'd on other grounds*, 235 Ga. 632, 211 S.E.2d 47, *overruled on other grounds*; Dent v. State, 136 Ga. App. 366, 221 S.E.2d 228, *overruled on other grounds*; Davis v. State, 136 Ga. App. 749, 222 S.E.2d 188 (1975) (court may grant continuance to procure further psychiatric examination based on evidence that reasonably indicates mental instability on part of the defendant even when no special plea of insanity has been filed).
51. O.C.G.A. § 17-7-130.1.
52. Chancellor v. State, 165 Ga. App. 365, 301 S.E.2d 294 (1983); Briard v. State, 188 Ga. App. 490, 373 S.E.2d 239 (1988).
53. O.C.G.A. § 17-7-130.1.
54. *Id.*
55. Motes v. State, 256 Ga. 831, 353 S.E.2d 348 (1987).
56. *Id.*
57. Harris v. State, 256 Ga. 350, 349 S.E.2d 374 (1986); Christenson v. State, 261 Ga. 80, 402 S.E.2d 41 (1991).
58. Pratt v. State, 387 A.2d 779 (Md. 1978).

(D) Jury Instruction and Consequences of the Verdict

Georgia law pertaining to jury instructions on the question of insanity is complicated because of the various possible verdicts in such a case.[59] In cases in which the defense of insanity is interposed, there are five possible verdicts: (a) guilty; (b) not guilty; (c) not guilty by reason of insanity; (d) guilty but mentally ill, but only in felony cases; and (e) guilty but mentally retarded, also only in felony cases.[60] The judge must charge the jury on all of these verdicts when the accused contends that he was insane at the time of the crime.[61]

The judge must also instruct the jury of the consequences of each verdict:[62]

1. If the defendant is found not guilty by reason of insanity, the defendant will be committed to a state mental health facility until such time, if ever, that the court is satisfied that he or she should be released pursuant to law;

2. If the defendant is found guilty but mentally ill, he or she will be given over to the Department of Corrections or the Department of Human Resources, as the defendant's mental condition may warrant; and

3. If the defendant is found guilty but mentally retarded, he or she will be given over to the Department of Corrections or the Department of Human Resources, as the defendant's mental condition may warrant.[63]

If the defendant is found not guilty by reason of insanity, he is committed to a state mental health facility for up to 30 days where his condition will be evaluated to determine whether it meets the statutory civil commitment criteria. If the evaluation report indicates that the defendant's condition does not meet the civil commitment criteria, he may be discharged by order of the court.[64] Otherwise, the court will order a hearing to determine if the defendant should be committed to the Department of Human Resources under the civil commitment standards.[65] If his condi-

---

59. For a thorough discussion of jury charges, *see* Daniel, *supra* note 47, § 21-11.
60. O.C.G.A. § 17-7-131(b)(1).
61. O.C.G.A. § 17-7-131(c). The failure to instruct the jury as to the consequences of a verdict of not guilty by reason of insanity is reversible error. *See* Guilford v. State, 258 Ga. 253, 368 S.E.2d 116 (1988).
62. O.C.G.A. § 17-7-131(b)(3).
63. O.C.G.A. §§ 17-7-131(b)(3)(A) to (C).
64. O.C.G.A. §§ 17-7-131(d) and (e)(1).
65. O.C.G.A. § 17-7-131(e).

tion does not meet the commitment criteria, the defendant will be discharged from custody. A defendant who is committed to the Department of Human Resources may be discharged from such commitment only by order of the committing court based on an application for release filed by the defendant or the hospital. Release applications may be brought annually. The defendant bears the burden of proving at the release hearing that his condition does not meet the civil commitment criteria.[66]

When a defendant is found guilty but mentally ill or guilty but mentally retarded, the court will sentence him in the same manner as a defendant found guilty of the offense, except that if the death penalty is sought, and the defendant is found to be mentally retarded, the court may only impose a life sentence.[67] A defendant who is found guilty but mentally ill or retarded must be examined by a psychiatrist or psychologist prior to transfer to the Department of Corrections.[68] If the defendant is found not to be in need of immediate hospitalization, he will be committed to a penal facility where he will undergo further evaluation and treatment, as is clinically indicated, up to the limits of state funds appropriated therefore.[69] The defendant may be subsequently transferred to a Department of Human Resources facility at any time under regulations adopted by the Department of Corrections and the Department of Human Resources.

Because the treatment offered to mentally ill persons is often limited, and because those found guilty but mentally ill are sentenced like any convicted felon, defense counsel should carefully assess the benefits and risks to the client of a plea of guilty but mentally ill or retarded.[70]

---

66. O.C.G.A. § 17-7-131(f). The procedure for the commitment and release of insanity acquittees has been the subject of substantial litigation. The present Georgia procedures have been held to be constitutional. *See* Benham v. Edwards, 501 F. Supp. 1050 (N.D. Ga. 1980), *aff'd in part, vacated in part,* 678 F.2d 511 (5th Cir. 1982), *vacated sub nom,* Ledbetter v. Benham, 463 U.S. 1222 (1983), *on remand,* 719 F. Supp. 125 (N.D. Ga. 1985), *aff'd,* 785 F.2d 1480 (11th Cir. 1980). The Georgia Supreme Court has comprehensively addressed the release procedures in Nagel v. State, 262 Ga. 888, 427 S.E.2d 490 (1993); *after remand* 442 S.E.2d 446 (1994).

67. O.C.G.A. §§ 17-7-131(g)(1) and (j).

68. O.C.G.A. § 17-7-131(g)(1).

69. O.C.G.A. § 17-7-131(g)(2).

70. *See, e.g.,* Waldrop v. Evans, 681 F. Supp 840 (M.D. Ga. 1988), *aff'd,* 871 F.2d 1030 (11th Cir. 1989) and Greason v. Kemp, 891 F.2d 829 (11th Cir. 1990).

7.10

Competency to Be Sentenced

With the exception of the mentally retarded defendant in a death penalty case, there is no provision in Georgia law concerning the competency of a defendant to be sentenced. Since the presentence hearing is clearly a critical stage in the proceedings, the defendant must have the mental capacity to understand the nature of the proceedings and to assist counsel in his defense. It is, therefore, likely that, if confronted with the issue, the courts would hold that a defendant who is mentally incompetent cannot be sentenced, at least if there is a reasonable likelihood that the defendant can regain competency in the near future. There is, however, no statutory procedure for dealing with a defendant who becomes incompetent after the guilty verdict, but before sentencing.

In 1988, following the execution of a defendant many considered to be mentally retarded, the Georgia legislature amended the law governing pleas of insanity and incompetency to provide that a defendant found guilty but mentally retarded may not be sentenced to death.[1] Mentally retarded is defined as "having significantly subaverage general intellectual functioning resulting in or associated with impairments in adaptive behavior which manifested during the developmental period."[2] Subsequently, in *Fleming v. Zant*,[3] the Georgia Supreme Court held that the execution of the mentally retarded constitutes cruel and unusual punishment under the Georgia Constitution. Therefore, no one who is mentally retarded may be executed in Georgia, regardless of

---

1. O.C.G.A. § 17-7-131(j).
2. O.C.G.A. § 17-7-131(a)(3).
3. 257 Ga. 687, 386 S.E.2d 339 (1989). In addition, a defendant sentenced to death cannot be executed while incompetent. *See* chapter 7.19.

when they were sentenced. Georgia is one of only two states that explicitly prohibit the execution of the mentally retarded.[4]

In the *Fleming* case, the U.S. Supreme Court set forth a procedure for determining whether an individual sentenced before the statutory change is mentally retarded and, therefore, not subject to execution. The defendant must file a petition for *habeas corpus* alleging that he is mentally retarded. The defendant must present sufficient credible evidence of retardation, which must include at least one expert diagnosis of retardation. If the court finds that there is a genuine issue as to the existence of retardation, the court will issue a writ for the limited purpose of conducting a trial on the retardation issue. As with a case brought after the statutory change, the issue of retardation is tried before a jury. The defendant bears the burden of proof by a preponderance of the evidence. The jury is not bound by the opinion testimony of experts or by test results, but may consider all evidence bearing on the issue of retardation. If the jury returns a verdict of retardation, the defendant shall receive a life sentence.[5]

---

4. *See* Penry v. Lynaugh, 492 U.S. 302, 109 S. Ct. 2934, (1989) in which the Supreme Court held that the Eighth Amendment's prohibition on cruel and unusual punishment did not forbid the execution of the mentally retarded.
5. *Id. See also* Zant v. Foster, 261 Ga. 450, 406 S.E.2d 74 (1991).

7.11

Sentencing

Criminal proceedings generally involve three steps:

1. the decision to charge or indict;
2. the determination of guilt; and
3. the determination and imposition of the appropriate sentence.

Therefore, after a verdict of guilty or after the entry of a plea of guilty, the court will proceed to the sentencing phase.[1] One of the central features of the bifurcation of the determination of guilt and the appropriate sentence to be imposed is the restriction of character and background evidence to the sentencing phase.[2] The MHP may be called upon to conduct an evaluation of the defendant's condition for sentencing purposes and to testify in a presentence hearing regarding factors to be considered in aggravation or mitigation of the appropriate punishment.[3]

---

1. O.C.G.A. § 17-10-1.
2. G. Mueller, *Sentencing Process and Purpose* 3 (1977).
3. *See* Godfrey v. Francis, 251 Ga. 652, 308 S.E.2d 806 (1983), *cert. denied,* 466 U.S. 945 (1984) (permitting presentencing testimony of psychiatrist concerning aggravating circumstances of murder); 1985 Op. Att'y Gen. No. U85-29 (a superior court judge may order a psychological evaluation of criminal defendants prior to sentencing and at county expense).

(A) Presentence Hearing: Misdemeanors and Noncapital Felonies

Except in cases in which the death penalty may be imposed, upon the return of a verdict of guilty by the jury, the judge will dismiss the jury and conduct a presentence hearing.[4] The only issue to be resolved in this hearing is the determination of the punishment to be imposed.[5] In misdemeanors and noncapital felony cases, it is the judge, not the jury, who sets the sentence after a determination of guilt.[6] If the defendant pleads guilty, thus avoiding a trial, the judge will simply proceed to the sentencing phase.[7]

The sentence must be determined for a specific number of months or years and must be within the minimum and maximum periods prescribed by the statute for the particular crime for which the defendant is convicted.[8] The judge has the power to suspend or probate the sentence and to impose a fine, which may be satisfied through community service.[9]

In the presentence hearing in noncapital felony cases, the judge will hear additional evidence in extenuation, mitigation, and aggravation of punishment, including the record of any prior criminal convictions, and any pleas of guilty or of *nolo contendere*.[10] The statutes do not define what circumstances may be included as mitigating or aggravating circumstances in noncapital cases, except that victim impact statements are expressly permitted if the defendant, in committing a felony, caused physical, psychological, or economic injury to the victim, or in committing a misdemeanor, the defendant caused serious physical injury or death to the victim.[11] The court may permit the victim, a family member, or other persons with knowledge of the impact of the crime on the victim, the victim's family, or the community to testify.

Generally, the court may consider matters in aggravation or mitigation in a presentence hearing that would be inadmissible at

---

4. O.C.G.A. § 17-10-2.
5. *Id.*
6. Huff v. State, 135 Ga. App. 134, 217 S.E.2d 187 (1975). A misdemeanor is a crime punishable by a fine of not more than $1,000 and/or by confinement in a county jail or county correctional institution for not more than 12 months; *see* O.C.G.A. § 17-10-3. *See also* O.C.G.A. § 17-20-4.
7. O.C.G.A. § 17-10-1 (Supp. 1988).
8. *Id.*
9. *Id.*
10. O.C.G.A. § 17-10-2.
11. O.C.G.A. §§ 17-10-1.1 and 17-10-1.2.

trial.[12] However, the prosecution must give advance notice to the defense of the evidence in aggravation that it intends to introduce.[13] The defense must object to the lack of notice, or the requirement is deemed waived.[14] In addition to this general limitation, the court may not admit a presentence probation report as evidence in aggravation or mitigation in fixing the length of a sentence,[15] but such a report may be considered in deciding whether to suspend or probate a sentence.[16]

Although there are no statutory provisions nor any judicial decisions on the question of the court's authority to order psychological evaluations prior to sentencing, the Georgia attorney general has issued an unofficial opinion on the question.[17] The attorney general states that "where a court is persuaded that competent sentencing requires the availability of certain psychological information, . . . such would certainly be within the inherent power of the court to order."[18]

In any case in which a sentence of 5 years or more has been imposed, except in death penalty cases, the defendant has the right to have the sentence reviewed by a panel of three superior court judges to determine if the sentence is excessively harsh.[19] If, in the opinion of the sentencing review panel, the sentence is too harsh or severe in light of the circumstances of the case and the defendant, the panel has the authority to reduce the sentence. It may not, however, reduce a sentence to probation or suspend a sentence.[20]

(B) Sentencing in Death Penalty Cases

Although the judge alone decides the sentence in a misdemeanor or noncapital felony case, in cases tried by a jury in which the death penalty may be imposed, the jury determines whether the death sentence or a sentence of life imprisonment should be imposed.[21] This determination is made by the same jury that determined guilt in a bifurcated sentencing trial that immediately

---

12. *See* Dorsen v. Willis, 242 Ga. 316, 249 S.E.2d 28 (1978).
13. *Id.*; O.C.G.A. § 17-10-2.
14. Mitchell v. State, 136 Ga. App. 390, 221 S.E.2d 465 (1975).
15. Benefield v. State, 140 Ga. App. 727, 232 S.E.2d 89 (1976).
16. Mills v. State, 244 Ga. 186, 259 S.E.2d 445 (1979).
17. 1985 Op. Att'y Gen. No. U85-29.
18. *Id.* at 200.
19. O.C.G.A. § 17-10-6(a).
20. O.C.G.A. § 17-10-6(c).
21. O.C.G.A. §§ 17-10-2(c) and 17-10-31. The U.S. Supreme Court has upheld the constitutionality of Georgia's death penalty statute. *See* Gregg v. Georgia, 428 U.S. 153, 96 S. Ct. 2909 (1976); Zant v. Stephens, 462 U.S. 235, 103 S. Ct. 2733 (1983); McClesky v. Kemp, 481 U.S. 279, 107 S. Ct. 1756 (1987).

follows the guilt–innocence portion of the trial. Although the statute refers to the jury's verdict as a recommendation, the trial judge is bound to impose the sentence "recommended" by the jury.[22] If the jury cannot unanimously agree on a sentence, the judge must impose a sentence of life imprisonment.[23] In cases tried without a jury, the judge will impose sentence after the presentence hearing.[24]

The law lists 10 statutory aggravating circumstances that may be considered by the jury deciding on the appropriate penalty in a death penalty case.[25] Except in cases of treason or aircraft hijacking, the jury must find the existence of at least one statutory aggravating circumstance to return a verdict imposing the death penalty.[26] The state has the burden of proving, beyond a reasonable doubt, the existence of at least one statutory aggravating circumstance.[27] The state is not limited to just the statutory aggravating circumstances. Any lawful evidence that tends to show the motive of the defendant, his lack of remorse, his general moral character, and his predisposition to commit other crimes is admissible in aggravation, subject to the notice provisions of the statute.[28]

Prior to July 1993, evidence concerning the psychological effect on the victim, the victim's personal characteristics, and the psychological, emotional, and physical impact of the crime on the victim's family and community was inadmissible.[29] Following the U.S. Supreme Court's decision in *Payne v. Tennessee* holding that victim impact testimony was not a *per se* violation of the Eighth Amendment, the Georgia General Assembly adopted a victim impact statute. In death penalty cases, the court may permit evidence from the family of the victim or from other

22. O.C.G.A. § 17-10-31; Gregg, *supra* note 21.
23. Miller v. State, 237 Ga. 557, 229 S.E.2d 376 (1976).
24. O.C.G.A. § 17-10-30.
25. *Id.* For example, one such aggravating circumstance is if "[t]he offense of murder, rape, armed robbery, or kidnapping was outrageously or wantonly vile, horrible, or inhuman in that it involved torture, depravity of mind, or an aggravated battery to the victim;" *see* O.C.G.A. § 17-10-30(b)(7). One of the most frequently used aggravating circumstances is that the murder was committed during the course of the commission of another capital felony (rape, armed robbery, or kidnapping), an aggravated battery, arson, or burglary in the first degree; *see* O.C.G.A. § 17-10-30(b)(2).
26. O.C.G.A. §§ 17-10-30 and 17-10-31; Fleming v. State, 240 Ga. 142, 240 S.E.2d 37 (1977). In cases tried without a jury, or if the defendant pleads guilty, the judge also must find at least one statutory aggravating circumstance before imposing the death penalty, except in cases of treason or aircraft hijacking. *See* O.C.G.A. § 17-10-32 (1982).
27. Fleming, *supra* note 26.
28. Fair v. State, 245 Ga. 868, 268 S.E.2d 316 (1980).
29. Sermons v. State, 417 S.E.2d 144 (1992). The U.S. Supreme Court has held that the introduction of such evidence does not violate the Eighth Amendment. *See* Payne v. Tennessee, 111 S. Ct. 2597 (1991).

witnesses with knowledge of the victim's personal characteristics and of the emotional impact of the crime on the victim, the victim's family, and the community. The admissibility of such evidence is in the discretion of the judge and may not be used to "inflame or unduly prejudice the jury."[30] The Georgia Supreme Court upheld the law in *Livingston v. State*, but required that, as additional safeguards, the prosecution notify the defense of the victim impact testimony it intends to offer. The trial court must hold a pretrial hearing on the admissibility of the evidence.[31]

If the jury finds the existence of a statutory aggravating circumstance, it must then consider the relevant mitigating and aggravating circumstances before finding whether the death penalty is appropriate. The defendant must be offered wide latitude to proffer any aspect of his character or record as evidence in mitigation,[32] even if the evidence would be inadmissible under the normal rules of evidence.[33] The state must furnish the services of a psychologist or psychiatrist in capital cases if required by an indigent defendant.[34] The jury is not required to find any mitigating circumstances to make a recommendation of mercy that is binding on the trial court.[35]

---

30. O.C.G.A. § 17-10-1.2(a)(1).
31. Livingston v. State, No. S94A0277; Waldrip v. State, No. S94A0279; and Waldrip v. State, No. S94A0280 (1994).
32. Westbrook v. Zant, 704 F.2d 1487 (11th Cir. 1983), *overruled on other grounds;* Peek v. Kemp, 784 F.2d 1479 (11th Cir. 1986); Franklin v. State, 245 Ga. 141, 263 S.E.2d 666 (1980). A grandfather's testimony that he does not wish to see his grandson die is admissible in mitigation at the sentencing phase of a death penalty case. Romine v. State, 251 Ga. 208, 305 S.E.2d 93 (1983), *cert. denied,* 481 U.S. 1024 (1987).
33. Collier v. State, 244 Ga. 553, 261 S.E.2d 364 (1979).
34. Westbrook, *supra* note 32.
35. Gregg, *supra* note 21.

Probation

(A) General Nature of Probation and Suspended Sentences

Once guilt has been determined, the trial judge may impose a sentence consisting of imprisonment and/or a fine; may sentence the defendant to incarceration followed by a term of probation; may sentence the defendant to probation, which can include various conditions; or may impose sentence, but suspend its execution. Probation is a type of sentence that does not involve incarceration, but places the defendant under the continuing authority of the court to ensure compliance with specified conditions.[1] The court may also impose compliance with specified conditions or rules as a condition of a suspended sentence. There is, therefore, no meaningful difference between probation and a suspended sentence with conditions.[2] According to the U.S. Supreme Court, the purported purpose of probation is

> [t]o provide an individualized program offering a young or unhardened offender an opportunity to rehabilitate himself without institutional confinement under the tutelage of a probation official and under the continuing power of the court to

---

1. O.C.G.A. §§ 17-10-1 and 42-8-34. W. Lafave & J. Israel, *Criminal Procedure,* § 25.3 (1985). Probation should be distinguished from parole, which is "the conditional release from the penitentiary of a person who has served a part of his term of imprisonment and who can be imprisoned to serve the remainder of his sentence should he violate any of the terms of his release."
2. *See* W. Daniel, *Georgia Criminal Trial Practice,* § 26-17 (1987).

impose institutional punishment for his original offense in the event that he abuse this opportunity.[3]

Probation, which is an outgrowth of the traditional practice of judges "suspending" sentences, is now authorized by statute in every jurisdiction.[4]

Georgia statutes authorize both probation and suspended sentences, granting a judge broad power and authority "to suspend or probate the sentence under such rules and regulations as he deems proper."[5] Georgia judges have traditionally used both probated and suspended sentences as tools of rehabilitation and as alternatives to confinement.[6] As discussed in the following, the sentencing power of Georgia judges was severely restricted as of January 1, 1995, as the result of an amendment to the Georgia Constitution.

The statutes do not define the term "probation" or "suspended sentence," nor do they distinguish clearly the two types of sentences; they merely list them as alternative forms of disposition.[7] Technically, a judge may not both probate and suspend a sentence.[8] Thus, when a defendant is convicted, the judge may "suspend the execution of the sentence or any portion thereof or may place him on probation under the supervision and control of the probation supervisor for the duration of the probation."[9] However, because conditions may be attached to a suspended sentence, it can be the functional equivalent of probation. Although there is no requirement in the case of a suspended sentence that the defendant report to a probation officer, the judge, with his broad discretion, may require that a defendant report to a probation officer as a condition of the suspended sentence.[10]

Like probation, a suspended sentence may be subject to certain terms and conditions that the court may impose.[11] Although the courts have expressed some uncertainty concerning the precise nature of the suspended sentence, they are more certain of its effects. In *Cross v. State*,[12] the court stated:

3. Roberts v. United States, 320 U.S. 264 at 272, 64 S. Ct. 113 (1943).
4. Lafave & Israel, *supra* note 1.
5. O.C.G.A. § 17-10-1. *See also* O.C.G.A. § 42-8-34.
6. State v. Collett, 232 Ga. 668, 208 S.E.2d 472 (1974).
7. *See, e.g.,* O.C.G.A. § 17-10-1(a) (granting the judge broad power and authority to suspend or probate sentences).
8. Jones v. State, 154 Ga. App. 581, 269 S.E.2d 77 (1980).
9. O.C.G.A. § 42-8-34.
10. Daniel, *supra* note 2; *see also* O.C.G.A. § 42-8-39 (receiving a suspended sentence does "not have the effect of placing the defendant on probation. . .").
11. *See* O.C.G.A. § 17-10-1; *see also* Falkenhainer v. State, 122 Ga. App. 478, 177 S.E.2d 380 (1970) (stating that a condition that would be authorized in the case of a probated sentence would also be authorized in the case of a suspended sentence).
12. 128 Ga. App. 774, 197 S.E.2d 853 (1973).

We agree with the appellant that exactly *what* a suspended sentence is at this point is perhaps indefinite, but we are satisfied that the court may provide rules and regulations in connection therewith and may, on violation of such rules and after notice and opportunity to be heard, during the time such sentence runs in accordance with its own terms, revoke the suspension and require that the remainder be served within a penal institution.[13]

As mentioned previously, the court has broad discretion in determining whether to impose a suspended or probated sentence.[14] The court has the authority to suspend or probate a sentence in virtually any case except one in which life imprisonment or the death penalty may be imposed.[15] Though it is not clear from the wording of the statute, case law has held that the court may even probate the sentence of a fourth offender recidivist who would not be eligible for parole until the maximum sentence had been served.[16]

(B) State-Wide Probation Act

The State-Wide Probation Act[17] created a state-wide probation system administered by the Georgia Department of Corrections.[18] Prior to conducting a presentence hearing, the court may direct the appropriate probation supervisor to conduct a probation investigation and to report to the court, in writing, on the circumstances of the offense and the criminal record, social history, and present condition of the defendant.[19] The probation supervisor will make a recommendation to the court concerning the possibility of probating the defendant's sentence.[20] The purpose of the report is to provide the court with information with which to make a decision regarding suspending or probating the sentence, but the court may not use the report for determining the length of the sentence.[21] In ordering that a presentence investigation be

---

13. Cross, *supra* note 12.
14. O.C.G.A. § 17-10-1(a).
15. *Id.; see also* O.C.G.A. § 42-8-34(a); Knight v. State, 243 Ga. 770, 257 S.E.2d 182 (1979); Wallace v. State, 175 Ga. App. 685, 333 S.E.2d 874 (1985) (a trial judge has no discretion to probate or suspend any portion of a life sentence).
16. Brooks v. State, 165 Ga. App. 115, 299 S.E.2d 167 (1983); State v. Carter, 175 Ga. App. 38, 332 S.E.2d 349 (1985). The statute expressly provides that the court may probate or suspend the sentence imposed for a second offender recidivist, but is silent on the authority to probate or suspend the sentence imposed for a fourth offender recidivist. *See* O.C.G.A. § 17-10-7(a) and (b).
17. O.C.G.A. §§ 42-8-1 to 42-8-102.
18. O.C.G.A. § 42-8-22.
19. O.C.G.A. § 42-8-34.
20. *Id.*
21. Williams v. State, 165 Ga. App. 553, 301 S.E.2d 908 (1983).

conducted, the court may also order that a psychological evaluation be conducted prior to sentencing.[22]

If it appears to the court that the defendant is not likely to engage in a criminal course of conduct and that the ends of justice and the welfare of society do not require that the defendant be incarcerated, the court may either suspend the sentence or place the defendant on probation under the supervision of the probation supervisor.[23] The period of probation or suspension may not exceed the maximum sentence of confinement that could have been imposed, except in the case of suspended sentences for the offense of child abandonment.[24] In addition, an offender may not be supervised on probation for more than 2 years except for the purpose of enforcing restitution or fines or unless the sentencing court specially extends or reinstates the probation for good cause upon notice and hearing.[25] The court may require the payment of a fine or costs or both as a condition of the probation.[26]

The court will impose probation subject to certain prescribed terms and conditions, such as requiring the probationer to "[a]void injurious and vicious habits"; "[a]void persons or places of disreputable or harmful character"; "[r]eport to the probation supervisor as directed"; "[m]ake reparation or restitution"; and others.[27] The judge is not limited to the terms and conditions listed in the statute, but may impose additional terms as a condition of probation.[28] A defendant who is placed on probation after a finding of guilty but mentally ill can be required to undergo inpatient or outpatient psychiatric treatment as a condition of probation.[29] The judge may also require a probationer to serve a 90-day sentence in a "special alternative incarceration" or "shock" unit of the Department of Corrections as a condition of probation.[30] If the terms and conditions of probation are violated, the court may, after notice and a hearing, revoke suspension or probation.[31]

---

22. 1985 Op. Att'y Gen. No. U85-29.
23. O.C.G.A. § 42-8-34.
24. *Id.* In a child abandonment case, the court can suspend execution of the sentence during the minority of the child or children.
25. O.C.G.A. § 17-10-1(a)(2).
26. O.C.G.A. § 42-8-34.
27. O.C.G.A. § 42-8-35.
28. Clackler v. State, 130 Ga. App. 738, 204 S.E.2d 472 (1974). For example, according to an opinion of the attorney general, the court may require medical screening for AIDS of a convicted prostitute as a condition of probation; *see* 1986 Op. Att'y Gen. No. 86-19.
29. O.C.G.A. § 17-7-131(h).
30. O.C.G.A. § 42-8-35.1.
31. O.C.G.A. § 42-8-34.1; Simmons v. State, 96 Ga. App. 718, 101 S.E.2d 111 (1957).

The sentencing judge does not lose jurisdiction over a person placed on probation, and he may revoke the probation during the time period originally prescribed for the probated sentence to run, after a hearing and a finding of a violation of the terms of probation.[32] The court also retains jurisdiction to shorten the probation period on the defendant's or the court's own motion. Prior to shortening the probation period, the court must notify the victim or victims of all sex-related offenses or violent offenses resulting in death or bodily injury. These victims may then request an opportunity for hearing. Following this request, the court also must provide notice or an opportunity for hearing to the defendant and prosecuting attorney.[33]

Violation of the terms of probation or a suspended sentence must be established either by an admission by the probationer or by a preponderance of the evidence at a revocation hearing.[34] If the violation of a probated or suspended sentence is the commission of a felony offense or the violation of a special condition authorized by statute, the court may revoke either the balance of probation or the maximum time of the sentence authorized to be imposed for the crime constituting the violation of probation, whichever is less.[35] However, if the defendant has violated any condition of probation or suspension other than by committing a new felony offense or by violating any special provision authorized by statute, the court shall consider alternatives such as community service, intensive probation, diversion centers, probation detention centers, special alternative incarceration, or any other appropriate alternative to confinement. If the court finds that the defendant does not meet the criteria for these alternatives, then the court may revoke the balance of the probation or impose not more than 2 years in confinement, whichever is less.[36]

If the probation revocation is based on a violation other than the commission of a serious felony, a misdemeanor resulting in bodily injury to an innocent victim, or a serious infraction while assigned to an alternative probation confinement facility, then the sentence shall be served in a probation detention center, probation boot camp, diversion center, weekend lockup, or confinement in a local jail or detention facility or other community correctional alternative.[37]

---

32. O.C.G.A. § 42-8-34.1; Logan v. Lee, 247 Ga. 608, 278 S.E.2d 1 (1981).
33. O.C.G.A. § 17-10-1(a)(5)(A).
34. O.C.G.A. § 42-8-34.1(c). *See* O.C.G.A. § 42-8-35.2 (1985) for provisions relating to "special term of probation."
35. *Id.*
36. O.C.G.A. § 42-8-34.1(b).
37. O.C.G.A. § 17-10-1(a)(3)(A).

Upon the termination of the period of probation, the probationer will be released from probation and is no longer liable for any sentence for which the probation was imposed.[38] The court may discharge the probation earlier if satisfied that such action would be in the best interests of justice and the welfare of society.[39]

(C) The Sentence Reform Act of 1994

At its 1994 session, the Georgia General Assembly passed the Sentence Reform Act of 1994.[40] Commonly referred to as "two strikes and you're out," the Act provides for various mandatory minimum sentences, limits on parole eligibility, and life imprisonment without parole upon the second conviction of a violent felony. Because the Act restricts the authority of the State Board of Pardons and Paroles, it required the passage of a constitutional amendment. The Act became effective January 1, 1995. The Act was summarized by the Office of Legislative Counsel as follows:

> The Act defines the term "serious violent felony" and provides for a mandatory minimum sentence of ten years for any such conviction, provides that any sentence imposed for a first conviction of a serious violent felony shall be served in its entirety and shall not be reduced by any form of parole, early release, earned time, or by any other means, provides that a person sentenced to life imprisonment for a first conviction of a serious violent felony shall not be eligible for parole or early release until a minimum of 14 years has been served, and provides that a person sentenced to death for a first conviction of a serious violent felony, which sentence was commuted to life imprisonment, shall not be eligible for early release or parole until a minimum of 25 years has been served. The Act further provides that any person convicted of a fourth felony, other than a capital felony, shall serve the maximum time to which sentenced without possibility of parole and provides that a person convicted of a second serious violent felony shall, unless sentenced to death, be sentenced to life without parole, which sentence shall not be reduced. The Act further provides specified times at which inmates serving misdemeanor sentences or certain felony sentences shall be eligible for consideration for parole. The Act prohibits the releasing of certain inmates on parole for the purpose of regulating jail or prison populations.

---

38. *Id.*; O.C.G.A. § 42-8-37.
39. *Id.*
40. Act 1265, Senate Bill 441 (1994); O.C.G.A. § 17-10-1.

7.13

Dangerous Offenders

In some states, the law provides for the classification and sentencing of defendants as dangerous or special offenders. Georgia sentencing law does not recognize a special class of offenders known as "dangerous offenders." However, the Sentence Reform Act of 1994 creates a special class of "serious violent felonies."[1] The Act provides for various mandatory minimum sentences, limits on parole eligibility, and life imprisonment without parole upon the second conviction of a violent felony. The Act became effective January 1, 1955 following the passage of a constitutional amendment (see chapter 7.12). In general, sentences are imposed on the basis of the severity of the offenses for which the defendant is convicted along with evidence as to the defendant's prior record and background. In this regard, in the sentencing phase of a criminal trial, the prosecutor may introduce evidence of "aggravating circumstances" that the judge may consider in setting the length of imprisonment or that the jury may consider in imposing the death penalty (see chapter 7.11).

---

1. Act 1265, Senate Bill 441 (1994).

7.14

Habitual Offenders

Georgia law contains a general recidivist statute,[1] sometimes referred to as a repeat or habitual offender law, as well as several specific recidivist statutes.[2] All of these statutes provide for the imposition of longer sentences for second or subsequent felony convictions. The general statute provides specified sentences for two types of repeat offenders. First, any person convicted of a felony under the laws of Georgia, or of a crime in any other state of the United States that would be a felony in Georgia, who commits a subsequent felony punishable by imprisonment "shall be sentenced to undergo the longest period of time prescribed for the punishment of the subsequent offense of which he stands convicted. . . ."[3] The statute expressly provides that the "trial judge may, in his discretion, probate or suspend the maximum sentence prescribed for the offense."[4]

The second portion of the statute provides that any person who has been convicted of three felonies under the laws of Georgia, or of three crimes under the laws of another state of the United States that would be felonies in Georgia, and who commits a fourth felony in Georgia other than a capital felony "must, upon conviction for such fourth offense or for subsequent offenses, serve the maximum time provided in the sentence of the

---

1. O.C.G.A. § 17-10-7.
2. *See, e.g.,* O.C.G.A. § 16-8-12(a)(4) (recidivist provisions relating to automobile theft); O.C.G.A. § 16-8-41(b) (recidivist provisions relating to armed robbery convictions).
3. O.C.G.A. § 17-10-7(a). This section may be invoked whether the prior felonies were punished by prison sentences or by probation; *see* Hernandez v. State, 182 Ga. App. 797, 357 S.E.2d 131 (1987).
4. O.C.G.A. § 17-10-7(a).

judge based upon such conviction. . . ."[5] The statute also expressly provides that such an offender is not eligible for parole until the maximum sentence has been served.[6] Although there is no provision expressly allowing the judge to probate or suspend the sentence of a fourth recidivist offender, the courts have construed the statute to permit probation of such a sentence as long as the maximum time provided in the sentence is served.[7]

To invoke the statute, the previous convictions must be set out in the indictment and the defendant must be indicted as a recidivist.[8] The statute is not applicable to death penalty cases, so in capital cases, prior convictions should not be set forth in the indictment.[9]

The general recidivist statute is considered to be supplemental to other provisions relating to specified recidivist offenders.[10] For example, there are specific recidivist statutes for the offenses of theft of a motor vehicle,[11] armed robbery,[12] possession or sale of controlled substances or marijuana,[13] and burglary.[14] If the specific recidivist statute is to be used in a case, the specific recidivist statute must be set out in the indictment rather than the general statute.[15]

The issue of whether the defendant should be punished as a recidivist is a question for the judge after guilt has been determined. It is, therefore, error for the court to admit evidence of the

---

5. O.C.G.A. § 17-10-7(b).
6. *Id.*
7. *See* Brooks v. State, 165 Ga. App. 115, 299 S.E.2d 167 (1983); State v. Carter, 175 Ga. App. 38, 332 S.E.2d 349 (1985). The rationale of these cases, that the maximum time served could include a period of probation, conflicts with the 1988 revision to the State-Wide Probation Act that limits the time served on probation to 4 years. *See* O.C.G.A. § 42-8-34.1(e) (Supp. 1988), enacted by 1988 Ga. Laws 1911.
8. Brown v. State, 144 Ga. App. 509, 241 S.E.2d 621 (1978); Croker v. Smith, 225 Ga. 529, 169 S.E.2d 787 (1969).
9. O.C.G.A. § 17-10-7(b); Clemmons v. State, 233 Ga. 187, 210 S.E.2d 657 (1974).
10. O.C.G.A. § 17-10-7(d).
11. O.C.G.A. § 16-8-12(a)(4)(A).
12. O.C.G.A. § 16-8-41(b).
13. O.C.G.A. § 16-13-30.
14. O.C.G.A. § 16-7-1.
15. State v. Baldwin, 167 Ga. App. 737, 307 S.E.2d 679 (1983). For example, if O.C.G.A. § 17-10-7 is invoked, the court, on a second offense, must sentence an armed robber to "the longest period of time prescribed," which is life imprisonment; *see* O.C.G.A. §§ 17-10-7(a) and 16-8-41(b). If the court invokes the specific armed robbery recidivist statute, the same defendant must be punished by imprisonment for "not less than ten years;" *see* O.C.G.A. § 16-8-41(b). *See* State v. Baldwin. Presumably, to invoke the specific recidivist statute, the defendant must have been convicted previously of armed robbery, not just any felony. *See* § 16-8-41(b) (". . .provided, however, that, for a second or subsequent *such offense* [armed robbery], the defendant shall be punished by imprisonment for not less than ten years.") (emphasis added). Further, under § 16-8-41(b) the sentence "shall not be suspended, probated, deferred, or withheld."

previous convictions during the guilt–innocence phase of the trial.[16]

At its 1994 session, the Georgia General Assembly passed the Sentence Reform Act of 1994.[17] Commonly referred to as "two strikes and you're out," the Act provides for various mandatory minimum sentences, limits on parole eligibility, and life imprisonment without parole upon the second conviction of a violent felony. Because the Act restricts the authority of the State Board of Pardons and Paroles, it required the passage of a constitutional amendment. The Act became effective January 1, 1995, after the constitutional amendment passed. The Act is summarized by the Office of Legislative Counsel as follows:

> The Act defines the term "serious violent felony" and provides for a mandatory minimum sentence of ten years for any such conviction, provides that any sentence imposed for a first conviction of a serious violent felony shall be served in its entirety and shall not be reduced by any form of parole, early release, earned time, or by any other means, provides that a person sentenced to life imprisonment for a first conviction of a serious violent felony shall not be eligible for parole or early release until a minimum of 14 years has been served, and provides that a person sentenced to death for a first conviction of a serious violent felony, which sentence was commuted to life imprisonment, shall not be eligible for early release or parole until a minimum of 25 years has been served. The Act further provides that any person convicted of a fourth felony, other than a capital felony, shall serve the maximum time to which sentenced without possibility of parole and provides that a person convicted of a second serious violent felony shall, unless sentenced to death, be sentenced to life without parole, which sentence shall not be reduced. The Act further provides specified times at which inmates serving misdemeanor sentences or certain felony sentences shall be eligible for consideration for parole. The Act prohibits the releasing of certain inmates on parole for the purpose of regulating jail or prison populations.

---

16. Clemmons, *supra* note 9.
17. Act 1265, Senate Bill 441 (1994).

Competency to Serve a Sentence

Some state laws require that a criminal defendant be competent to serve the sentence imposed upon him. Other than the requirement that a defendant be mentally competent to be executed,[1] Georgia does not require that a defendant be competent to serve a sentence. As discussed in other chapters, a defendant may not be competent to stand trial (chapter 7.5), may be found not guilty by reason of insanity and, thus, not subject to punishment (chapter 7.8), or may be found guilty but mentally ill or mentally retarded, in which event the defendant will be sentenced as any convicted offender (chapter 7.9). A prisoner who becomes mentally ill while serving a sentence may be transferred to a mental health facility (chapter 7.17). In that instance, the prisoner would still be serving his sentence, but in a different facility.

---

1. O.C.G.A. § 17-10-61.

Mental Health Services in Jails and Prisons

Jails in Georgia are under the supervision of the county sheriff[1] and have only minimal requirements in terms of the provision of medical services, including mental health services. The sheriff is required to furnish jail inmates with "medical aid" to be reimbursed by the county treasury.[2] In addition, every inmate is required to be observed daily and a physician called "if there are indications of serious injury, wound, or illness."[3] As a practical matter, mental health services in many rural Georgia jails are frequently nonexistent.

As to state and county correctional facilities, it is the responsibility of the governmental unit or agency having physical custody of an inmate to "maintain the inmate, furnishing him food, clothing, and any needed medical and hospital attention."[4] Georgia law authorizes county governments to "purchase, rent, establish, construct, and maintain a county correctional institution for the care and detention of all inmates assigned to it by the Department of Corrections (DOC)."[5] Such county facilities are subject to rules and regulations promulgated by the DOC.[6]

---

1. O.C.G.A. § 42-4-1.
2. See O.C.G.A. § 42-4-4(a)(2); "A sheriff owes to a prisoner placed in his custody a duty to keep the prisoner safely and free from harm, to render him medical aid when necessary, and to treat him humanely and refrain from oppressing him. . . ." Kendrick v. Adamson, 51 Ga. App. 402, 402, 180 S.E. 647, 648 (1935).
3. O.C.G.A. § 42-4-32(d). There have been numerous lawsuits filed against county jails claiming inadequate medical care, including the lack of mental health care.
4. O.C.G.A. § 42-5-2.
5. O.C.G.A. § 42-5-53.
6. Id.

The DOC administers the state's correctional institutions and rehabilitative programs,[7] subject to the policy and rule-making authority of the Board of Corrections.[8] Except for misdemeanants who are sentenced to serve a sentence in a county jail, the Commissioner of Corrections has the authority to designate the place of confinement of all convicted adult misdemeanants or felons in a state or county correctional institution.[9]

The DOC is required by law to classify and separate inmates with respect to certain variables, including "mentally diseased" inmates.[10] Additionally, the Board of Corrections has promulgated rules and regulations concerning the provision of mental health services to state inmates.[11] Under these rules, when a person is committed to a correctional institution and is diagnosed as having a mental disorder, the DOC must provide "necessary" mental health care for the inmate.[12] The services should be provided on the basis of a written assessment performed by a licensed psychologist, psychiatrist, or other physician.[13] The services are administered by a Director of Mental Health appointed by the commissioner.[14] Services should be based on an individualized treatment plan.[15] The DOC must also provide mental retardation services to inmates who have remedial mental conditions or who may benefit from such services.[16]

In certain circumstances, inmates requiring treatment for mental illness or retardation may be transferred to a mental hospital operated by the Department of Human Resources.[17] If an inmate is sentenced as "guilty but mentally ill," he will be examined and treated at the correctional institution, or he may be transferred to the Department of Human Resources for treatment.[18] The right to treatment for those found guilty but mentally

---

7. O.C.G.A. § 42-2-5.
8. O.C.G.A. § 42-2-11.
9. O.C.G.A. § 42-5-51.
10. O.C.G.A. § 42-5-52.
11. Ga. Comp. R. & Regs. r. 125-4-5.
12. Ga. Comp. R. & Regs. r. 125-4-5-.01.
13. Ga. Comp. R. & Regs. r. 125-4-5-.02.
14. Ga. Comp. R. & Regs. r. 125-4-5-.01.
15. Ga. Comp. R. & Regs. r. 125-4-5-.02.
16. *Id.*
17. Ga. Comp. R. & Regs. r. 125-4-5-.03; *see infra* chapter 7.17.
18. Ga. Comp. R. & Regs. r. 125-4-5-.04; *see also* Ga. Comp. R. & Regs. r. 290-4-8 (Rules of the Department of Human Resources regarding the disposition of guilty but mentally ill defendants). The same or similar procedures should be applicable for persons sentenced as "guilty but mentally retarded," but as of this writing neither the DOC nor the Department of Human Resources had issued rules governing such treatment. *See* O.C.G.A. § 17-7-131 (Supp. 1988); *see also supra* chapter 7.9. It should also be noted that if a defendant is acquitted as "not guilty by reason of insanity," he will be committed under the civil commitment procedures to Department of Human Resources rather than to DOC. *See* O.C.G.A. § 17-7-131.

ill or mentally retarded is limited by statute to "state funds appropriated therefor."[19]

In addition to the minimal state statutory and regulatory requirements for the provision of mental health services in jails and prisons, the Eighth and Fourteenth Amendments to the U.S. Constitution require the provision of basic mental health care to jail and prison inmates.[20] Under these constitutional provisions, prison authorities may not be "deliberately indifferent" to an inmate's serious medical needs.[21] Failure to provide essential psychiatric and mental health care violates this constitutional requirement. The Georgia prison system has been the subject of numerous lawsuits asserting the lack of minimal mental health services.[22]

.

---

19. O.C.G.A. § 17-7-131(g)(2).
20. The Fourteenth Amendment provides constitutional protection to pretrial detainees, while the Eighth Amendment governs convicted prisoners. *See* Bell v. Wolfish, 441 U.S. 520, 99 S. Ct. 1861 (1979). However, the standard as to the provision of health care is essentially the same. *See* Anderson v. City of Atlanta, 778 F.2d 678 (11th Cir. 1985).
21. Rogers v. Evans, 792 F.2d 1052 (11th Cir. 1986).
22. Rogers, *supra* note 21 (the women's facility at Hardwick, Georgia); Guthrie v. Evans, 93 F.R.D. 390 (S.D. Ga. 1981) (the Georgia state prison); Waldrop v. Evans, 681 F. Supp,. 840 (M.D. Ga. 1988), *aff'd*, 871 F.2d 1030 (11th Cir. 1989) (the Georgia Diagnostic and Classification Center and the Augusta Correctional and Medical Institution); Greason v. Kemp, 891 F.2d 829 (11th Cir. 1990) (the Georgia Diagnostic and Classification Center). There are numerous unreported decisions involving other state facilities and numerous county jails.

7.17

Transfer From Penal Facilities to Mental Health Facilities

The Georgia Department of Corrections (DOC) is required by law to provide mental health services to inmates in need of such services.[1] These services are generally provided in the correctional facility. However, state law also permits the transfer of a "mentally diseased" inmate from a correctional facility to a facility operated by the Department of Human Resources (DHR).[2] An inmate who is addicted to drugs or alcohol at the time of sentencing also may be transferred to a DHR facility if his health will be injured or if his life would be endangered if immediate treatment is not provided.[3] The inmate will remain in the custody of DHR until his "sanity has been restored" or, if an alcoholic or drug addict, until he is able to serve his sentence elsewhere, at which time he will be returned to the custody of DOC.[4] If his sentence is completed while in the custody of DHR, the inmate may petition for release from the facility in accord with the procedures for the release of involuntary civil committees.[5] Prior to completion of his sentence, the patient-prisoner may not petition for release under the general civil commitment statutes.[6]

---

1. *See supra* chapter 7.16, Mental Health Services in Jails and Prisons.
2. O.C.G.A. § 42-5-52(d). Under certain conditions, a defendant may be committed directly to a DHR facility. *See* O.C.G.A. § 17-7-131 (defendants acquitted as "not guilty by reason of insanity" or sentenced as "guilty but mentally ill" or "guilty but mentally retarded"); O.C.G.A. § 17-7-130 (defendants declared incompetent to stand trial); O.C.G.A. § 17-10-62 (defendant convicted of capital crime who is declared to be incompetent to be executed).
3. O.C.G.A. § 42-5-52(e).
4. O.C.G.A. § 42-5-52(d).
5. *Id.; see, generally,* O.C.G.A. §§ 37-3-1 to 37-3-168.
6. O.C.G.A. § 42-5-52(d).

Although the law is silent on the procedures involved in the transfer of an inmate from DOC to DHR, both departments have issued official rules, regulations, and internal operating procedures governing such transfers. The determination that an inmate in a correctional facility requires hospitalization is made by a Mental Health Screening Board (Board) within DOC.[7] The Board consists of two licensed professionals, one of whom may be a physician, psychiatrist, or psychologist, while the other is a psychiatrist or psychologist designated by DHR.[8]

Before an inmate may be referred to the Board, a correctional facility staff physician or a contract physician, psychologist, or psychiatrist must certify that he has personally examined the inmate and that he recommends that the inmate be considered for psychiatric treatment.[9] The Board will personally examine the inmate and issue a written report of its findings.[10] The decision to recommend a transfer can be made only if the Board finds that the inmate is "mentally ill" and needs to be hospitalized.[11] If the Board finds that the inmate does not require transfer to a mental hospital, the inmate will be returned to his assigned facility or to another appropriate facility.[12]

If the Board finds that the inmate requires treatment in a mental hospital, the committee chairperson will provide to the inmate a written copy of the Board's evaluation and recommendation.[13] The Board must also give notice to the inmate that he has the right to a hearing held before a hearing officer in which the inmate may contest the Board's recommendation.[14] The inmate may waive the hearing, but unless the waiver is affirmatively made in writing, the hearing must be held.[15]

---

7. Ga. Comp. R. & Regs. r. 125-4-5.03; *see also* Georgia Dep't of Corrections, Hospitalization Procedures 2 (May 1, 1988) (unpublished) (the DOC procedures refer to the Board as the Psychiatric Screening Board or PSB).
8. Ga. Comp. R. & Regs. r. 125-4-5.03.
9. Georgia Dep't of Corrections, Hospitalization Procedures 1 (May 1, 1988). There are also provisions for emergency admissions and voluntary admissions. *See infra* text accompanying notes 21–24.
10. Georgia Dep't of Corrections, Hospitalization Procedures 3 (May 1, 1988).
11. *Id.* Mentally ill means having "a disorder of thought or mood which significantly impairs judgment, behavior, capacity to recognize reality, or ability to cope with the ordinary demands of life."
12. *Id.*
13. *Id.* at 3–4.
14. *Id.* at 4. The right to a due process hearing is based on the U.S. Supreme Court case of Vitek v. Jones, 445 U.S. 480, 100 S. Ct. 1254 (1980) (holding that the involuntary transfer of a prison inmate to a mental hospital implicates a liberty interest that is protected by the Due Process Clause of the Fourteenth Amendment). These hearings are commonly referred to as Vitek hearings.
15. Georgia Dep't of Corrections, Hospitalization Procedures 5 (May 1, 1988).

At the hearing, the inmate has the right to legal representation,[16] the right to a fair and impartial decision-maker, the right to reasonable notice of the hearing, the right to appear at the hearing and to present documentary evidence and witnesses, the right to cross-examine adverse witnesses, and the right to a written decision.[17] The state has the burden of proving by clear and convincing evidence that the inmate meets the criteria for transfer to a mental hospital.[18] To transfer the inmate, the hearing officer must find that the inmate is (a) mentally ill and (b) has demonstrated conduct resulting from mental illness which poses a serious threat of substantial physical harm to the inmate or others as manifested by recent overt acts or recent expressed threats of physical violence, or that the inmate is unable to care for his or her own physical health and safety so as to create a life-endangering crisis."[19] There is no provision for appeal in the DOC's procedures and the department is not governed by the Administrative Procedure Act.[20]

If a psychiatric emergency exists,[21] a DOC physician may refer an inmate directly to a hospital without a hearing.[22] The Psychiatric Screening Board will examine the inmate following admission to determine the need for hospitalization. The inmate still has the right to a due process hearing, unless waived.[23] If an inmate voluntarily seeks hospitalization, the screening and hearing procedures are deemed waived.[24]

---

16. The inmate may be represented by a third-year law student or *pro bono* attorney, or he may retain private counsel. *Id.* at 5–6. There is no requirement that the state furnish counsel at its expense. *See* Vitek, *supra* note 14, at 496.
17. Georgia Dep't of Corrections, Hospitalization Procedures 6–9 (May 1, 1988). The right to cross-examination may be limited for security reasons. *Id.* at 8.
18. *Id.*
19. *Id.*
20. *See* O.C.G.A. § 50-13-1.
21. Georgia Dep't of Corrections, Hospitalization Procedures 10 (May 1, 1988). A "psychiatric emergency" is one in which the inmate is mentally ill and "(1) presents a substantial risk of *imminent* harm to himself or others as manifested by recent overt acts or recent expressed threats of violence which present a probability of physical injury to himself or to other persons; or (2) who is so unable to care for his own physical health and safety as to create an imminently life-endangering crisis."
22. *Id.*
23. *Id.* at 10–11.
24. *Id.* at 11.

7.18

Parole Determinations

Parole is the "release of a person from imprisonment whereby, upon specified conditions, he is allowed to serve the balance of his sentence outside prison walls under supervision."[1] Unlike probation, which is granted by the court, parole is granted by the executive branch of government after some portion of the sentence has been served.[2] The parolee is released under specified conditions of parole that are intended "to assist the parolee in leading a law-abiding life."[3] The violation of the conditions of parole may result in the revocation of parole and return of the parolee to prison.[4]

(A) Authority of the Board of Pardons and Paroles

In Georgia, the exclusive authority to grant parole or a pardon is vested in the State Board of Pardons and Paroles (Board),[5] consisting of five members appointed by the governor and confirmed by

---

1. 4 C. Torcia, *Wharton's Criminal Procedure*, § 622, at 245 (12th ed. 1976). Parole should not be confused with "probation," which is granted in lieu of imprisonment. *Id.* at 246.
2. *Id.*
3. *Id.; see also* O.C.G.A. § 42-9-42. "No inmate shall be placed on parole until and unless the board shall find that there is reasonable probability that, if he is so released, he will live and conduct himself as a respectable and law-abiding person and that his release will be compatible with his own welfare and the welfare of society."
4. 4 C. Torcia, *supra* note 1, § 623, at 249–250.
5. Ga. Const. art. IV, § 2, ¶ 2; *see also* O.C.G.A. § 42-9-2.

the senate.[6] Although assigned to the Department of Corrections for administrative purposes, the Board is an independent agency established by the Georgia Constitution.[7] As discussed in the following, the authority of the Board to release certain violent felons is limited by the Sentence Reform Act of 1994, which became effective January 1, 1995 following the passage of a constitutional amendment.

The Board is authorized by law not only to grant parole to prison inmates, but also to grant pardons and reprieves; to commute penalties, including the death penalty; to remove disabilities imposed by law; and to remit any part of a sentence for any offense against the state after conviction.[8] The Board also has the authority to supervise persons placed on parole or other conditional release.[9]

The Board is never required to grant a pardon or parole; its authority is discretionary. The Eleventh Circuit Court of Appeals held in *Slocum v. Georgia State Board of Pardons and Paroles*[10] that, "[u]nder Georgia law the decision whether to release an inmate on parole is a matter committed to the discretion of the State Board of Pardons and Paroles. . . . No entitlement to or liberty interest in parole is created by the Georgia statutes."[11] However, the Georgia Constitution does place certain limits on the Board's discretion. For example, when a sentence of death is commuted to life imprisonment, the Board may not grant a pardon or parole until such person has served at least 25 years in prison.[12] The Board may not grant a pardon or parole to a convicted armed robber until such person has served at least 5 years in prison.[13]

The constitution also authorizes the legislature to place further limits on the Board's authority to grant a pardon or parole to persons incarcerated for a second life sentence and to persons receiving consecutive life sentences as the result of offenses occurring during the same series of acts.[14] The General Assembly has, in fact, placed such limits on the Board's discretion by requiring that a person convicted of murder and sentenced to life after having previously been incarcerated under a life sentence serve at least 25 years in prison before being eligible for a pardon or parole.[15] Additionally, the statute requires that a person receiving

---

6. O.C.G.A. § 42-9-2.
7. Ga. Const. art. IV, § 2, ¶ 1; O.C.G.A. §§ 42-9-1 and 42-9-2.
8. Ga. Const. art. IV, § 2, ¶ 2.
9. O.C.G.A. § 42-9-21.
10. 678 F.2d 940 (1982).
11. *Id.* at 941.
12. Ga. Const. art. IV, § 2, ¶ 2.
13. *Id.*
14. *Id.*
15. O.C.G.A. § 42-9-39.

consecutive life sentences, if any of the sentences were imposed for murder, serve consecutive 10-year periods for each such sentence up to a maximum of 30 years before being eligible for parole.[16]

Notwithstanding these, or any other statutory provisions, the Board may pardon any person convicted of a crime who is subsequently determined to be innocent of that crime.[17] Georgia's recidivism statute provides another restriction on the granting of parole. That statute provides that a person who is convicted of a fourth felony, other than a capital felony, must serve the maximum sentence given by the judge before being eligible for parole.[18]

(B) Consideration for Parole

Aside from the restrictions mentioned, the general rule is that inmates are automatically to be considered for parole, with no application being required, after they have served certain minimum portions of their sentences and periodically thereafter.[19] An inmate serving a misdemeanor sentence is eligible for automatic consideration for parole after serving 6 months or one-third of the sentence or sentences, whichever is greater.[20] An inmate serving a felony sentence is eligible for automatic consideration for parole after serving 9 months or one-third of the sentence or sentences, whichever is greater.[21] An inmate serving sentences aggregating 21 years or more is eligible for consideration for parole after

---

16. *Id.*
17. *Id.*
18. O.C.G.A. § 17-10-7. There have been challenges to "recidivist statutes" on grounds of alleged violations of due process, equal protection, and the prohibition against cruel and unusual punishment. *See, e.g.,* Landers v. Smith, 226 Ga. 274, 174 S.E.2d 427 (1970) (Georgia recidivist statute not violative of equal protection); Spencer v. Texas, 385 U.S. 554, 87 S. Ct. 648 (1967) (Texas recidivist statute not violative of Due Process Clause of Fourteenth Amendment); Rummell v. Estell, 587 F.2d 651 (5th Cir. 1978) (Texas statute not violative of Eighth Amendment ban against cruel and unusual punishment). The Georgia Court of Appeals has held that a defendant may not contest the fourth offender recidivist provision as to the restrictions on parole until such time as he claims the right of parole and the statute is asserted as a bar; *see* Ivory v. State, 160 Ga. App. 193, 286 S.E.2d 435 (1981).
19. O.C.G.A. § 42-9-45; *see also* Ga. Comp. R. & Regs. r. 475-3-.05. One exception to the "automatic consideration" rule is that persons ordered to serve consecutive county misdemeanor confinement sentences exceeding 12 months must actually make application for parole.
20. O.C.G.A. § 42-9-45.
21. *Id.* In actuality, the Board sets a tentative release date for each offender, other than those sentenced to life imprisonment, based on the Parole Decision Guidelines system.

serving 7 years.[22] The Board has the authority to consider any case for parole earlier than these automatic time frames by providing at least 10 days notice to the sentencing judge and the appropriate district attorney of such pending consideration and permitting them to express their views on the parole of such an inmate.[23]

A majority of the Board must vote to grant a pardon, parole, or other relief from sentence.[24] The decision must be in writing and must be signed by the number of Board members required for the relief granted.[25]

General subjective criteria for the grant of parole are provided by statute, although the Board is free to exercise its discretion in granting or denying parole in any particular case:

> No inmate shall be placed on parole until and unless the board shall find that there is reasonable probability that, if he is so released, he will live and conduct himself as a respectable and law-abiding person and that his release will be compatible with his own welfare and the welfare of society. Furthermore, no person shall be released on pardon or parole unless and until the board is satisfied that he will be suitably employed in self-sustaining employment or that he will not become a public charge. However, notwithstanding other provisions of this chapter, the board may, in its discretion, grant pardon or parole to any aged or disabled persons.[26]

The statute also lists general information that is to be considered by the Board in granting parole, such as a report by the prison superintendent of the inmate's prison conduct record, the result of any physical or mental examinations, the extent to which the person appears to have improved his social attitude, the inmate's prison work record and work skills, the educational programs in which the inmate has participated and the level of education of the inmate, and any other information deemed necessary by the Board.[27] Additionally, the Board may have the inmate appear before it and personally examine him.[28] Individuals, including attorneys, may also appear before the Board on behalf of an inmate who is seeking parole.[29] There is, however, no right to appear and no right to a formal hearing before the Board.

Although there is a great deal of subjectivity in the decision to grant or deny parole, the Board, in making its decision to establish

---

22. *Id.*
23. O.C.G.A. § 42-9-46; *see* Charron v. State Bd. of Pardons and Paroles, 253 Ga. 274, 319 S.E.2d 453 (1984) (upholding the constitutionality of this statute).
24. O.C.G.A. § 42-9-42.
25. *Id.*
26. *Id.*
27. O.C.G.A. § 42-9-43.
28. *Id.*
29. Ga. Comp. R. & Regs. r. 475-3-.02.

a tentative parole release month, except for persons convicted under life sentences, relies on Parole Decision Guidelines (the "grid" system). The system is designed to account for the severity of the crime and to assess the inmate's likelihood of success on parole, which is based on certain weighted factors, including the inmate's criminal and social history.[30] The Board may disregard the tentative parole date established by the Parole Decision Guidelines and deny or grant parole in contravention of such predictors.[31] The inmate may appeal the decision as to the tentative parole month within 30 days by contesting either the Crime Severity Level or Parole Success Factor scores.[32] The Board may change or modify its decision rendered under the grid system at any time and at its discretion.[33]

If parole is denied, the Board will reconsider inmates serving life sentences for parole at least every 8 years.[34] An inmate whose case is considered for parole under the Parole Decision Guidelines will be interviewed by a member of the Board if still incarcerated 3 years past the guideline recommended release date and each 3 years thereafter, provided his discharge date is at least 6 months past the scheduled interview.[35]

A special statutory provision allows the paroling of inmates because of a state of emergency created by prison overcrowding.[36] The governor may declare such an emergency if the population of the prison system has exceeded its capacity for 30 consecutive days.[37] The Board may then grant parole to a sufficient number of inmates for release to reduce the prison population to 100% of capacity.[38] The selection of inmates may be made without regard to the minimum portion of the sentences served, but no "dangerous offender" may be granted such a parole.[39] The Board is to give special consideration for early release to inmates who have participated in educational programs and who have achieved a fifth-grade level or higher education.[40]

---

30. Ga. Comp. R. & Regs. r. 475-3-.05.
31. *Id.*
32. *Id.*
33. *Id.*
34. *Id.*
35. Ga. Comp. R. & Regs. r. 475-3-.11.
36. O.C.G.A. § 42-9-60.
37. *Id.*
38. *Id.*
39. *Id.* A dangerous offender is defined as one who is convicted of murder, voluntary manslaughter, kidnapping, armed robbery, rape, aircraft hijacking, aggravated sodomy, aggravated battery, aggravated assault, incest, child molestation, child abuse, enticing a child for indecent purposes, or any felony drug offense. A person imprisoned for a second life sentence is also a dangerous offender.
40. *Id.*

(C) Conditions of Parole

Any person granted a parole is released on certain conditions of parole prescribed by the Board.[41] The Board must specify such conditions in writing, with a certified copy given the parolee.[42] The conditions may include, among other general or specific conditions, a requirement that the parolee not leave the state without the Board's consent; that the parolee contribute to the support of his dependents to the best of his ability; that he make restitution; that he abandon evil associates and ways; and that he carry out the instructions of his parole supervisor.[43]

A violation of the terms of parole may result in the parolee's arrest and return to prison to serve out the balance of his sentence.[44] The arrest may be made pursuant to a warrant issued by a Board member and based on reasonable grounds to believe that the parolee has violated the terms of parole.[45] Any parole supervisor having reasonable grounds to believe that a parolee has violated the terms of his parole is required to notify the Board so that a warrant may be issued.[46]

A parolee who is charged with a violation of the terms and conditions of parole and who has not been convicted, pleaded guilty, or entered a plea of *nolo contendere* to a subsequent offense has the right to a preliminary hearing before a parole hearing officer,[47] and a final hearing before the Board itself.[48] The parolee has a right to written notice of the hearing; the opportunity to be heard in person and to present witnesses and documentary evidence; the right to confront and cross-examine adverse witnesses; the right to subpoena witnesses and documents;[49] the right to retain counsel;[50] and the right to remain silent.[51] After the final hearing, the Board may enter an order rescinding parole and returning the parolee to serve out his sentence or reinstating the

---

41. O.C.G.A. § 42-9-42.
42. O.C.G.A. § 42-9-44.
43. *Id.*
44. *Id.*
45. O.C.G.A. § 42-9-48.
46. *Id.*
47. O.C.G.A. § 42-9-50.
48. O.C.G.A. § 42-9-51. *See* Mingo v. State, 155 Ga. App. 284, 270 S.E.2d 700 (1985) (loss of liberty involved in parole revocation is serious deprivation requiring that a parolee be afforded due process).
49. *Id.* The parolee may, of course, waive these rights, and parole may be revoked without a hearing.
50. Ga. Comp. R. & Regs. r. 475-3-.08.
51. *Id.*

parole.[52] When a parolee has been convicted of any crime, his parole will be revoked without the necessity of a hearing.[53]

The Board may discharge a person from parole after expiration of the term for which he was sentenced, or earlier under certain conditions.[54] The Board will consider early termination of parole if

1. the offender serving a determinate or indeterminate sentence has served 3 years on parole with satisfactory adjustment or 2 years with an exemplary adjustment; or

2. the offender serving a life sentence has served 4 years on parole with satisfactory adjustment or 3 years of exemplary adjustment.[55]

A person who has completed his sentence or who is eligible for early discharge or who is entering the military service may apply for restoration of his civil and political rights to vote, to hold public office, and to serve on a jury.[56] The Board automatically restores civil and political rights to a felony parolee or youthful offender parolee upon discharge from supervision if he has no other sentence to serve or no other pending criminal charges against him.[57]

(D) The Sentence Reform Act of 1994

At its 1994 session, the Georgia General Assembly passed the Sentence Reform Act of 1994.[58] Commonly referred to as "two strikes and you're out," the Act provides for various mandatory minimum sentences, limits on parole eligibility, and life imprisonment without parole upon the second conviction of a violent felony. Because the Act restricts the authority of the State Board of Pardons and Paroles, it required the passage of a constitutional amendment. The Act became effective January 1, 1995, following the passage of the constitutional amendment. The Act is summarized by the Office of Legislative Counsel as follows:

> The Act defines the term "serious violent felony" and provides for a mandatory minimum sentence of ten years for any such conviction, provides that any sentence imposed for a first con-

---

52. O.C.G.A. § 42-9-51. If the parole is revoked, the time served on parole is considered as part of the sentence.
53. O.C.G.A. § 42-9-51(c).
54. O.C.G.A. § 42-9-52.
55. Ga. Comp. R. & Regs. r. 475-3-.10.
56. Id.
57. Id.
58. Act 1265, Senate Bill 441 (1994).

viction of a serious violent felony shall be served in its entirety and shall not be reduced by any form of parole, early release, earned time, or by any other means, provides that a person sentenced to life imprisonment for a first conviction of a serious violent felony shall not be eligible for parole or early release until a minimum of 14 years has been served, and provides that a person sentenced to death for a first conviction of a serious violent felony, which sentence was commuted to life imprisonment, shall not be eligible for early release or parole until a minimum of 25 years has been served. The Act further provides that any person convicted of a fourth felony, other than a capital felony, shall serve the maximum time to which sentenced without possibility of parole and provides that a person convicted of a second serious violent felony shall, unless sentenced to death, be sentenced to life without parole, which sentence shall not be reduced. The Act further provides specified times at which inmates serving misdemeanor sentences or certain felony sentences shall be eligible for consideration for parole. The Act prohibits the releasing of certain inmates on parole for the purpose of regulating jail or prison populations.

7.19

Competency to Be Executed

Georgia law provides that a mentally incompetent person may not be put to death. The statute provides that "[a] person under sentence of death shall not be executed when it is determined . . . that the person is mentally incompetent to be executed. . . ."[1] "*Mentally incompetent to be executed* means that, because of a mental condition the person is presently unable to know why he or she is being punished and understand the nature of the punishment."[2] The code provides that an application seeking a stay of execution on the basis of mental incompetency can be filed only after an order has been entered setting an execution date.[3] The application must be filed in the superior court of the county in which the applicant is being detained.[4] By filing the application, the applicant specifically consents to submit to a state examination to assess his mental competency to be executed.[5] The applicant may also request that the court appoint a particular expert to make an examination.[6] The applicant must make a sufficient showing that his mental competency to be executed is a significant issue before the court will appoint such an expert.[7]

The burden of proof to establish incompetency is on the prisoner. If the court finds by a preponderance of the evidence that the applicant is mentally incompetent to be executed, the

---

1. O.C.G.A. § 17-10-61.
2. O.C.G.A. § 17-10-60.
3. O.C.G.A. § 17-10-67. This process is the exclusive procedure for challenging mental competency to be executed when such a challenge is made subsequent to conviction and sentence; *see* O.C.G.A. § 17-10-62.
4. O.C.G.A. § 17-10-63.
5. O.C.G.A. § 17-10-66.
6. *Id.*
7. *Id.*

court will enter an order staying the scheduled execution date.[8] If the court denies the application, the court will direct that immediate telephonic notification be given to the parties, and any stay presently entered will be dissolved.[9]

A prior adjudication of competency under this section of the Georgia Code acts as a presumption of mental competency, and the applicant must make a *prima facie* showing of a substantial change in circumstances before he would be entitled to a subsequent hearing on the question of mental competency to be executed.[10] When a person who has been found mentally incompetent subsequently regains his mental competency, the court will enter an order vacating any previously entered stay of execution.[11] This would appear to put the treating MHPs in an ethical dilemma. If they are successful in treating their patient, the patient would then be subject to execution.

---

8. O.C.G.A. § 17-10-68.
9. *Id.*
10. O.C.G.A. § 17-10-69.
11. O.C.G.A. § 17-10-71.

7.20

Pornography (Obscenity)

Georgia law regulates the general distribution and sale of obscene materials, as well as its distribution and sale to children, its display in places children are likely to frequent, and the sexual exploitation of children. MHPs may become involved as expert witnesses in this frequently controversial area of the law.

(A) Criminal Penalties

Georgia law prohibits the distribution,[1] offering to distribute, and possession with intent to distribute of obscene materials, provided that the offender does so "knowing the obscene nature thereof."[2] The knowing requirement is satisfied by either actual or constructive knowledge of the material's obscene content.[3] Although obscene material is not protected by the First Amendment and can be regulated by the state,[4] the mere possession of obscene materials in the privacy of one's home is protected by the First Amendment.[5]

Material is obscene if

1. to the average person, applying contemporary community standards, taken as a whole, it predominantly appeals to the

---

1. Distribution includes selling, lending, renting, leasing, giving, advertising, publishing, exhibiting, or otherwise disseminating obscene materials; *see* O.C.G.A. § 16-12-80.
2. *Id.*
3. *Id.*
4. Paris Adult Theatre I v. Slaton, 413 U.S. 49, 93 S. Ct. 2628 (1973).
5. Stanley v. Georgia, 394 U.S. 557, 89 S. Ct. 1243 (1968); Gable v. Jenkins, 397 U.S. 592 (1970).

prurient interest, that is, a shameful or morbid interest in nudity, sex, or excretion;

2. the material taken as a whole lacks serious literary, artistic, political, or scientific value; and

3. the material depicts or describes, in a patently offensive way, sexual conduct specifically defined below.[6]

This section of the Georgia Code also establishes an affirmative defense to the offense of distributing obscene materials if such material was disseminated to a teacher or student of a course related to such material or to a person whose receipt was authorized in writing by a medical practitioner or psychiatrist.[7] A violation of this code section is a misdemeanor of a high and aggravated nature.[8]

In *Paris Adult Theatre I v. Slaton*,[9] the U.S. Supreme Court held that the state can satisfy its burden of proof as to the obscene nature of materials simply by introducing the materials into evidence.[10] The Court reasoned that jurors need no help in determining what is or is not obscene, thus no expert testimony is required.[11] However, the Court has stated that a defendant in an obscenity case should be permitted to introduce expert evidence on the question of community standards and on the social value of the material.[12] The Georgia Supreme Court has held that a defendant may introduce testimony by a psychologist that a film is not obscene.[13]

Georgia law also provides that the unsolicited distribution of material depicting nudity or sexual conduct through the mail is

---

6. O.C.G.A. § 16-12-80(b). This definition of obscenity reflects the test articulated by the Supreme Court in Miller v. California, 413 U.S. 15 (1973). For a discussion of the issues that have been litigated under this test, *see* P. Kurtz, *Criminal Offenses and Defenses in Georgia*, 301–303 (2d ed. 1987).

   The sexual conduct specifically defined by the statute includes sexual intercourse, masturbation, excretory functions, beastiality, and sadomasochistic acts. O.C.G.A. § 16-12-80(b)(3)(A) to (E). The statute also provides that any device designed or marketed as useful primarily for the stimulation of genital organs is obscene; *see* O.C.G.A. § 16-12-80(c).

7. O.C.G.A. § 16-12-80(e). The latter defense has been referred to as the pornotherapy defense. Spillers v. State, 145 Ga. App. 809, 245 S.E.2d 54 (1978).

8. O.C.G.A. § 16-12-80(f).

9. 413 U.S. 49 (1973).

10. *Id.*

11. *Id.; see also* Dumas v. State, 131 Ga. App. 79, 205 S.E.2d 119 (1974) (unnecessary to have an expert testify on obscenity when materials are available for inspection by trier of fact).

12. Kaplan v. California, 413 U.S. 115 at 121, 93 S. Ct. 2680 (1973).

13. Dyke v. State, 232 Ga. 817, 209 S.E.2d 166 (1974), *cert. denied*, 421 U.S. 952 (1975). In another case, the Georgia Court of Appeals permitted the use of witnesses to testify that certain devices are designed primarily for stimulation of genital organs; *see* Williams v. State, 157 Ga. App. 494, 277 S.E.2d 781 (1981).

unlawful unless a special notice of the material's content is printed on the envelope containing the material.[14] The violation of this code section is a felony punishable by imprisonment from 1 to 3 years, by a fine not to exceed $10,000, or both.[15]

Under Georgia law, the use of any premises in violation of the obscenity statutes constitutes a public nuisance.[16] This provision was held to be unconstitutionally overbroad when an injunction was sought to suppress the distribution of literature on the basis of the content of previous publications.[17] The statute was also held to be an unconstitutional prior restraint on free speech when applied to authorizing the padlocking of premises on grounds that a single obscene publication rendered the premises a nuisance.[18]

The Georgia obscenity statutes also provide that any materials declared to be obscene and advertisements for obscene materials are considered contraband.[19] However, since the mere possession of obscene materials is not illegal, obscene materials are not contraband *per se*.[20]

Georgia law further provides that it is unlawful for any motion picture theater owner to show film clips of restricted material of an upcoming movie to an audience that is not similarly restricted as to viewing age unless accompanied by a parent or guardian.[21] The violation of this code section is a misdemeanor.[22]

(B) Child Obscenity Laws

Certain obscenity statutes are directed at the protection of children, when they are either the subject matter of visual media or of live sexual performances, or when children are the viewers or potential viewers of obscene materials. One provision of Georgia law provides a wide range of activities that are unlawful because they sexually exploit children.[23] This section makes it unlawful for anyone to knowingly employ or use a minor to engage in sexual conduct in the production of any visual medium; for a parent or guardian to permit the minor to engage in sexual conduct for the production of any visual medium; for anyone to

---

14. O.C.G.A. § 16-12-81.
15. *Id.*
16. O.C.G.A. § 16-12-82.
17. Sanders v. State, 231 Ga. 608, 203 S.E.2d 153 (1974).
18. 660 Lindbergh, Inc. v. City of Atlanta, 492 F. Supp. 511 (N.D. Ga. 1980).
19. O.C.G.A. § 16-12-83.
20. Warshaw v. Eastman Kodak Co., 148 Ga. App. 670, 252 S.E.2d 182 (1979).
21. O.C.G.A. § 16-12-85.
22. *Id.*
23. O.C.G.A. § 16-12-100.

employ or use, or for parents to permit such employment or use of, a minor to engage in any sexually explicit performance; for anyone to participate in the creation, selling, or distribution of a visual medium depicting a minor engaged in any sexually explicit conduct; for anyone to advertise, sell, or exchange any medium providing information as to where any visual medium depicting a minor engaged in any sexually explicit conduct can be found or purchased; and for anyone to bring into this state any material depicting a minor engaged in any sexually explicit conduct.[24] The violation of any of these provisions can result in the forfeiture of any interest in property relating to such an offense and constitutes a felony punishable by imprisonment from 1 to 20 years, a fine of up to $100,000, or both.[25]

The statute also provides misdemeanor penalties for the possession of any such material and for the failure to report to the Georgia Bureau of Investigation (GBI) one's reasonable belief that such material exists by a person who engages in processing or producing visual or printed matter.[26] Any person making such a report to the GBI in good faith is immune from civil or criminal liability.[27]

Another provision makes it unlawful to knowingly sell, loan for monetary consideration, or otherwise disseminate to a minor any picture, photograph, drawing, sculpture, motion picture, or any book, magazine, or other printed matter, that depicts sexually explicit nudity, sexual conduct, or sadomasochistic abuse and that is harmful to minors.[28] This code section also makes it unlawful for any person knowingly to exhibit, expose, or display in public at newsstands, at any other business, or at any public place frequented by minors or where minors are or may be invited, any picture, photograph, drawing, sculpture, film, book, pamphlet, magazine, or other printed or recorded matter depicting any sexually explicit nudity, sexual conduct, or sadomasochistic abuse that is harmful to minors.[29] The statute specifically exempts public libraries from this display provision.[30] The statute, including the display provisions, has been ruled constitutional.[31]

---

24. *Id.*
25. *Id.*
26. *Id.*
27. *Id.*
28. *Id.*
29. *Id.*
30. *Id.*
31. American Booksellers Ass'n v. Webb, 919 F.2d 1493 (11th Cir. 1990).

7.21

Services for Sex Offenders

In some states, the law provides for a quasi-criminal proceeding in which a sex offender may be committed to a special treatment program. MHPs may be involved in such proceedings by providing expert testimony, by conducting evaluations, and by actually providing treatment to such offenders. Although the Georgia Department of Corrections is required to provide mental health services in correctional facilities, there are no Georgia statutes creating a special category for sex offenders or requiring any specialized services for sex offenders in prison.

In its 1994 session, the Georgia General Assembly enacted a new statute imposing special parole conditions on persons convicted of a sexual offense. The State Board of Pardons and Paroles is required to adopt rules providing that, as a condition of parole, a person convicted of a sexual offense must furnish his name, address, criminal offense, and parole date to the superintendent of schools and to the sheriff of the county where the parolee resides. The information must be provided whenever the parolee changes his residence. The sheriff is required to maintain the information in a register open to the public.[1]

---

1. Act 1036, House Bill 1229 (1994), creating O.C.G.A. § 42-9-44.1.

7.22

Services for Victims of Crimes

Some states have enacted laws providing for services, including mental health services, for crime victims. Georgia law does not mandate services for crime victims, but does provide for court-ordered restitution[1] and for compensation to victims, dependent spouses or children of victims, persons injured while going to the aid of a victim, victims of family violence, and victims of individuals who operated motor vehicles while impaired by drugs, alcohol, or a combination of those substances.[2] Compensation is paid from the Georgia Crime Victims Emergency Fund[3] upon approval by the Criminal Justice Coordinating Council.[4] An award of compensation may not exceed the victim's actual expenses, such as medical expenses, mental health counseling, and lost wages, and cannot be in excess of $5,000.

An award of compensation cannot be made unless the board or director find that

1. a crime was committed;

2. the crime directly resulted in physical injury, financial hardship, or death of the victim;

3. the crime was promptly reported. If police records show that the crime was reported more than 72 hours after its occurrence, then no award can be made unless the board upon a showing of good cause finds that the delay was justified; and

---

1. O.C.G.A. §§ 17-14-1 to 17-14-16.
2. O.C.G.A. §§ 17-15-7, 19-13-1, and 40-6-391.
3. O.C.G.A. § 17-15-10.
4. O.C.G.A. §§ 17-15-3 to 17-15-4.

4. the applicant pursued restitution rights against the person who committed the crime unless the board or director determines that such action would not be feasible.

The board may also deny, reduce, or withdraw any award upon finding that the claimant has not fully cooperated with all law enforcement agencies.[5] Individuals who are injured while confined to a state or federal prison, county or municipal jail, or other correctional facility; victims of crimes that occurred prior to July 1, 1989; or individuals who are criminally responsible for the crime upon which a claim is based are not entitled to receive any award from the fund.[6] However, benefits cannot be denied to a victim who is related to the person who is criminally responsible for the crime.[7] Payments can be made directly to persons who provide services to the victim, including MHPs. Payment can also be made directly to the victim when the victim has incurred out-of-pocket losses such as lost wages.[8]

---

5. O.C.G.A. § 17-15-8(a).
6. O.C.G.A. §§ 17-15-7(c) to (e).
7. O.C.G.A. § 17-15-7(d).
8. O.C.G.A. § 17-15-4(a)(5).

Voluntary and Involuntary Receipt of State Services

8.1

Medicaid

The Department of Medical Assistance (DMA) of the State of Georgia is authorized to adopt and administer a state plan for medical assistance in accordance with Title XIX of the federal Social Security Act of 1935, as amended, also known as Medicaid, provided that the plan is administered within the appropriations made available to the department.[1] The department is authorized to establish the amount, duration, scope, and terms and conditions of eligibility to receive such medical assistance pursuant to Georgia law. Psychiatric and psychological services for children are covered under Georgia's medical plan. However, the scope and duration of such services is severly limited. The department is also authorized to establish rules and regulations that are necessary or desirable to execute the state plan and to receive the maximum amount of federal financial participation available for expenditures made pursuant to the plan. The department must establish reasonable procedures to provide to interested parties notice and an opportunity to be heard prior to the adoption, amendment, or repeal of any such rule or regulation. The department is also authorized to enter into such reciprocal and cooperative arrangements with other states, persons, and institutions, public and private, as it may deem necessary or desirable in order to execute the plan. The DMA is also required to provide notice and an opportunity for a hearing to a provider denied participation in the program or if the DMA seeks to withhold or recoup Medicaid payments.

---

1. O.C.G.A. § 49-4-142.

Health Care Cost Containment System (Georgia Public Assistance Act of 1965)

The state of Georgia provides medical services for indigent persons through the Georgia Public Assistance Act of 1965. Psychological and psychiatric service qualifications that pertain to the Georgia Public Assistance Act of 1965, as well as inpatient and outpatient treatment services for the indigent mentally ill, however, are not explicitly set forth in Georgia law.

(A) Categories of Public Assistance

The Department of Human Resources is authorized to establish any of the following categories of public assistance and to adopt plans to combine the administration of such categories of public assistance as the Department of Human Resources may elect:

1. old-age assistance;
2. aid to the blind;
3. aid to the disabled;
4. aid to families with dependent children; and
5. aid to the aged, blind, or adult disabled persons under a combined plan adopted pursuant to Title XX of the federal Social Security Act.[1]

---

1. O.C.G.A. § 49-4-3.

(B) Power of Director to Contract for Provision of Medical Evaluations

The staff and physicians of local health departments, mental health clinics, and other public agencies are required to cooperate fully with the director of human resources in the performance of his duties. The director may contract with an agency or private physician for the purpose of providing immediate accessible medical evaluations in the location that the director deems most appropriate. The Board of Human Resources is empowered to adopt regulations that ensure the effective implementation of Georgia law.[2]

(C) The Medical Assistance for the Aged Act

Medical care under the Medical Assistance for the Aged Act means essential medical, surgical, chiropractic, osteopathic, podiatric, optometric, dental, and nursing services in the home, office, clinic, or other suitable place that are provided or prescribed by physicians or dentists licensed to render such services. Medical care includes drugs and medical supplies; appliances; laboratory, diagnostic, and therapeutic services; nursing home and convalescent care; inpatient hospital care; and such other essential medical services and supplies as prescribed by law.[3] An aged public assistance recipient is a person 65 years or older who has been certified by a county department to be unable through his or her own income and resources to provide himself or herself with essential medical care without depriving himself or herself of necessary food, shelter, clothing, and other necessities of life and who is not a recipient of other programs.[4]

In Georgia, it appears that the law has been administratively interpreted to exclude long-term inpatient mental health treatment. The Board of Medical Assistance ensures that the rules and regulations promulgated pursuant to the Medical Assistance for the Aged Act exclude from eligibility any person who is an inmate of a public institution (except as a patient in a medical institution), any person who is a patient in an institution for tuberculosis or mental illness or mental retardation, or any person

---

2. O.C.G.A. § 30-5-6.
3. O.C.G.A. § 49-4-121.
4. O.C.G.A. § 49-4-121(11).

who is a patient in a medical institution as a result of a diagnosis of tuberculosis or mental illness or mental retardation with respect to any period after the person has been a patient in such an institution, as a result of such diagnosis, for 42 days.[5]

Even though the Board of Medical Assistance furnishes each recipient of medical assistance for the aged with some institutional and noninstitutional care and medical care while the recipient is sojourning out of state, long-term inpatient care for mental illness is apparently excluded.[6] The state pays the total cost of all benefits provided under the Medical Assistance for the Aged Act.[7]

(D) Scope of Medical Care Under the Medical Assistance for the Aged Act

The scope of medical care in behalf of public assistance recipients and recipients of medical care for the aged that the Department of Medical Assistance undertakes to pay is designated and limited by regulations promulgated by the Board of Medical Assistance and the requirement of Title XIX of the federal Social Security Act. The selection of the class or classes of medical care is based on, among other things, the amount of federal and state funds available, the most essential needs of public assistance recipients and recipients of medical care for the aged, and a method of meeting the need that ensures the greatest amount of medical care, as defined by law consonant with the funds available, including, but not limited to, the following categories:[8]

1. inpatient hospital services;
2. skilled nursing home services;
3. physicians' services;
4. outpatient hospital or clinic services;
5. home health care services;
6. private duty nursing services;
7. physical therapy and related services;
8. dental services;
9. laboratory and X-ray services;

---

5. O.C.G.A. § 49-4-122(b)(2)(B).
6. O.C.G.A. § 49-4-122(b)(4).
7. O.C.G.A. § 49-4-122(c).
8. O.C.G.A. § 49-4-125(a) (Supp. 1994).

10. prescribed drugs, eyeglasses, dentures, and prosthetic devices;

11. diagnostic, screening, and preventive services; and

12. any other medical care or remedial care recognized under Georgia law.

Payments for hospital care, nursing home care, and drugs or other medical and dental supplies are based on the cost of providing such services or supplies.[9] Thus, in lieu of the foregoing, it may be possible for elderly indigents to obtain some short-term as well as outpatient mental health services under the Medical Assistance for the Aged Act.

(E) Freedom to Choose Providers of Medical Care

Any person eligible to receive authorized medical care, services, and supplies as provided by law has the absolute right to select any provider who is duly authorized under Georgia law to provide such care, services, and supplies.[10]

(F) Medicaid

The Department of Medical Assistance of the State of Georgia is authorized to adopt and administer a state plan for medical assistance with Title XIX of the federal Social Security Act of 1935, as amended, also known as Medicaid, provided that the plan is administered within the appropriations made available to the department.[11] The department is authorized to establish the amount, duration, scope, and terms and conditions of eligibility to receive such medical assistance pursuant to Georgia law. Furthermore, the department is authorized to establish rules and regulations that are necessary or desirable to execute the plan and to receive the maximum amount of federal financial participation available in expenditures made pursuant to the plan. The department must establish reasonable procedures to provide to interested parties notice and an opportunity to be heard prior to the adoption, amendment, or repeal of any such rule or regulation. The department is also authorized to enter into such reciprocal

---

9. O.C.G.A. § 49-4-125(b) (Supp. 1994).
10. O.C.G.A. § 49-4-126.
11. O.C.G.A. § 49-4-142.

and cooperative arrangements with other states, persons, and institutions, public and private, as it may deem necessary or desirable in order to execute the plan.

(G) Governmental Considerations

In Georgia, counties may contract with any public authority for the care, maintenance, and hospitalization of the indigent sick. A county also may obligate itself under a hospital authority contract to pay "such sums as shall be necessary to provide adequate and necessary facilities for medical care and hospitalization of the indigent sick, including reasonable reserves necessary for expansion and necessary for the payment of the cost of the facilities. . . ."[12] In addition, furnishing medical care and hospitalization for the indigent sick may be considered governmental in nature when there is a showing that the purpose is to preserve the public health.[13]

---

12. Cheely v. State, 251 Ga. 685, 309 S.E.2d 128 (1983) (quoting O.C.G.A. § 31-7-85 (1991)).
13. *See* Hall v. Hospital Auth. of Floyd County, 93 Ga. App. 319, 91 S.E.2d 530 (1956); Knowles v. Housing Auth. of Columbus, 94 Ga. App. 852, 96 S.E.2d 534 (1957), *overruled by* Self v. City of Atlanta, 259 Ga. 78, 377 S.E.2d 674 (1989).

8.3

Voluntary Admission of Mentally Ill Adults

Georgia law governs the admission, treatment, and discharge of mentally ill adults in both state-operated and private mental health facilities.[1] MHPs are extensively involved in the evaluation, admission, diagnosis, treatment, and release of such patients.

(A) Definitions

To fully understand the laws governing the voluntary admission of mentally ill persons to mental health facilities, it is important to know the legal definitions of certain key terms.

1. *Facility* refers to "any state owned or state operated hospital, community mental health center, or other facility utilized for the diagnosis, care, treatment, or hospitalization of persons who are mentally ill; any facility operated or utilized for such purpose by the United States Department of Veterans Affairs or other federal agency; and any other hospital or facility within the State of Georgia approved for such purpose by the [D]epartment [of Human Resources]."[2] It is important to remember that the Mental Health Code governs the hospitalization of persons in private as well as public facilities.

2. *Mentally ill* means having a "disorder of thought or mood which significantly impairs judgment, behavior, capacity to

---

1. For a discussion of the admission of mentally ill minors to such facilities, *see supra* chapter 4.19.
2. O.C.G.A. § 37-3-1(7).

recognize reality, or ability to cope with the ordinary demands of life."[3]

3. *Inpatient treatment* or *hospitalization* refers to a "program of treatment for mental illness within a hospital facility setting."[4]

(B) Voluntary Admissions

The statutes do not expressly define the term "voluntary" as it relates to the admission of mentally ill persons to mental health facilities. Essentially, voluntary means that the patient or his legal guardian is applying for admission rather than someone else seeking commitment to a facility against the patient's will. There is no court involvement in the voluntary admission process. Any person 12 years of age or older may apply voluntarily for admission to a mental health facility for observation and diagnosis.[5] If the person is 18 years or older, a voluntary application for admission need not be accompanied by the consent or assistance of another person, unless the person has been declared legally incompetent, in which case his guardian may submit an application in his behalf.[6] After hospital staff conduct an evaluation and make a diagnosis, if the person is found to show evidence of mental illness and to be suitable for treatment, he may be admitted to the facility and detained until discharged.[7] Admission is not mandatory under these conditions. Rather, the law requires the chief medical officer to make a reasonable effort to provide treatment for any mental health patient in the least restrictive environment possible, closest to the patient's home community, and within the limits of available state funds.[8]

An individualized service plan, which is specifically tailored to the patient's treatment needs, must be developed as soon as possible after admission.[9] A person voluntarily admitted must be

---

3. O.C.G.A. § 37-3-1(11).
4. O.C.G.A. § 37-3-1(9.2).
5. O.C.G.A. § 37-3-20(a). For a discussion of involuntary admission of adults, *see infra* chapter 8.6.
6. *Id.*
7. *Id.* A voluntary patient may be picked up by the facility police and returned to the facility if he leaves the facility without making a proper request for discharge. *See* 1970 Op. Att'y Gen. No. U70-183.
8. O.C.G.A. §§ 37-3-1(9) and (10).
9. O.C.G.A. § 37-3-20(a).

given notice of his rights as a voluntary inpatient at the time of his admission and every 6 months thereafter.[10]

(C) Right to Discharge

A voluntary patient who is determined to have recovered from his mental illness, or to have sufficiently improved so that hospitalization is no longer necessary, must be discharged from the facility unless the discharge would be unsafe for the patient or others.[11] Additionally, a voluntary patient or his personal representative, legal guardian, parent, spouse, attorney, or adult next of kin may submit a written request for discharge at any time after admission.[12] If a patient makes an oral request for release to a staff member of the facility, the patient must be given assistance within 24 hours in preparing a written request for discharge.[13] Within 72 hours (excluding Sundays and legal holidays) of receipt of a written request for release by the chief medical officer, the patient must be discharged unless the chief medical officer finds that discharge would be unsafe for the patient or others.[14] If the chief medical officer finds that such a release would be unsafe, proceedings for involuntary treatment must be initiated.[15]

The chief medical officer may designate a physician or psychologist to make the discharge decision. If the decision of the designee is contrary to the recommendation of the treatment team, or a physician or psychologist member of the team, the chief medical officer must make the discharge decision. If there is no conflict, the decision of the designee is final.[16]

---

10. O.C.G.A. § 37-3-23. Patients' rights are outlined in the Rules and Regulations of the Department of Human Resources, Division of Mental Health, Mental Retardation and Substance Abuse and include such subjects as the type and form of treatment and use of physical restraints. *See* Ga. Comp. R. & Regs. r. 290-4-6 *et seq.*
11. O.C.G.A. § 37-3-21.
12. O.C.G.A. § 37-3-22.
13. *Id.*
14. *Id.*
15. *Id.*
16. O.C.G.A. § 37-3-21(a). *See also* Peek v. Department of Human Resources, 261 Ga. 96, 403 S.E.2d 36 (1991).

(D) Transfer of Involuntary Patient to Voluntary Status

Any involuntary patient may apply to be transferred to voluntary status and must be transferred to voluntary status unless the chief medical officer finds that this is not in the patient's best interest.[17] If the patient is transferred to voluntary status or discharged, the patient and his representative must be given notice of the change in status. In addition, notice must be given to the court, if the patient's hospitalization was ordered by the court, or to the physician or psychologist admitting the patient for evaluation. If the patient was under criminal charges, the law enforcement agency originally having custody of the patient must be given notice, and the patient can be discharged only into the physical custody of such law enforcement agency.[18]

---

17. O.C.G.A. § 37-3-24.
18. *Id.*

8.4

Involuntary Civil Commitment of Mentally Ill Adults

Georgia law provides for the involuntary civil commitment of mentally ill adults and their treatment in mental health facilities.[1] MHPs are involved in the entire commitment process from initial evaluation to final discharge.

(A) Definitions

The following terms are defined in the statutes governing the commitment process:

Court means

[i]n the case of an individual who is 17 years of age or older, the probate court of the county of residence of the patient or the county in which such patient is found. . . .[2]

Facility means

any state-owned or state-operated hospital, community mental health center, or other facility utilized for the diagnosis, care, treatment, or hospitalization of persons who are mentally ill; any facility operated or utilized for such purpose by the United States Department of Veterans Affairs or other federal agency; and any other hospital or facility within the State of Georgia approved for such purpose by the [D]epartment [of Human Resources].[3]

The Georgia Mental Health Code therefore governs the hospitalization of persons in private as well as public facilities.

---

1. *See supra* chapter 4.19 for a discussion of involuntary commitment of minors.
2. O.C.G.A. § 37-3-1(4).
3. O.C.G.A. § 37-3-1(7).

Full and fair hearing means

a proceeding before a hearing examiner or before a court in which the patient has the right to counsel, including court-appointed counsel; the right to confront and cross-examine witnesses and to offer evidence; the right to subpoena witnesses; and the right to require testimony in person or by deposition from the physician upon whose evaluation the decision may rest. The court will apply the rules of evidence applicable in civil cases. The burden of proof is on the party seeking treatment of the patient. The standard of proof is by clear and convincing evidence.[4]

Inpatient means

a person who is mentally ill and who presents a substantial risk of imminent harm to that person or others, as manifested by either recent overt acts or recent expressed threats of violence which present a probability of physical injury to that person or other persons; or is so unable to care for that person's own physical health and safety as to create an imminently life-endangering crisis; and is in need of involuntary inpatient treatment.[5]

Inpatient treatment or *hospitalization* means

a program of treatment for mental illness within a hospital facility setting.[6]

Mentally ill means

having a disorder of thought or mood which significantly impairs judgment, behavior, capacity to recognize reality, or ability to cope with the ordinary demands of life.[7]

Mentally ill person requiring involuntary treatment

[includes] a person who is an inpatient or an outpatient.[8]

Involuntary treatment means

inpatient or outpatient treatment which a patient is required to obtain pursuant to the Mental Health Code.[9]

An *outpatient* is

a mentally ill person who does not currently require inpatient care but will likely need such care if not treated, or who is unable to voluntarily comply with an outpatient treatment plan.[10]

---

4. O.C.G.A. § 37-3-1(8).
5. O.C.G.A. § 37-3-1(9.1).
6. O.C.G.A. § 37-3-1(9.2).
7. O.C.G.A. § 37-3-1(11).
8. O.C.G.A. § 37-3-1(12).
9. O.C.G.A. § 37-3-1(9.3).
10. O.C.G.A. § 37-3-1(12.1).

(B) Involuntary Civil Commitment

The involuntary commitment and confinement of a mentally ill person in a mental health facility triggers both the substantive and procedural protections guaranteed by the Fourteenth Amendment to the U.S. Constitution.[11] The Georgia statutes governing the civil commitment of adults have not been challenged on due process grounds. Given the code's stringent procedural safeguards, the Georgia civil commitment scheme would likely survive a constitutional challenge.[12]

(B)(1) Emergency Examination

A person who is suspected of being mentally ill may be involuntarily transported to an emergency receiving facility for evaluation based on a certificate executed by a physician, psychologist, clinical social worker, or clinical nurse specialist in psychiatric/mental health. The person may be delivered to a receiving facility in one of three ways:

1. Any physician, psychologist, clinical social worker, or clinical nurse specialist in psychiatric/mental health may execute a certificate stating that he has personally examined a person within the preceding 48 hours and has found that the person appears to be a mentally ill person requiring involuntary treatment.[13] The certificate expires 7 days after it is executed.[14] Any peace officer, within 72 hours after receiving such certificate, shall make a diligent effort to take such person into custody and deliver him to the nearest emergency receiving facility for purposes of examination.[15]

2. The probate court in the county in which a person may be found may issue an order commanding any peace officer to take such person into custody and deliver him to an emergency receiving facility.[16] Such an order may be based on an unexpired physician's, psychologist's, clinical social worker's, or clinical nurse specialist's certificate mentioned earlier or on the affidavits of at least two persons stating that they have seen

---

11. *See* Humphrey v. Cady, 405 U.S. 504, 92 S. Ct. 1048 (1972); Addington v. Texas, 441 U.S. 418, 99 S. Ct. 1804 (1979); Vitek v. Jones, 445 U.S. 480, 100 S. Ct. 1254 (1980). For a discussion of the constitutional limitations on the state's power to civilly commit the mentally disabled, *see* R. Remar, *An Overview of the Constitutional Rights of the Mentally Disabled: Claims and Defenses* (Georgia Center for Continuing Legal Education, 1988).
12. Remar, *supra* note 11, at 8.
13. O.C.G.A. § 37-3-41(a).
14. *Id.*
15. *Id.*
16. O.C.G.A. § 37-3-41(b).

the person in question within the preceding 48 hours and, on the basis of their observation, believe that such person is a mentally ill person requiring involuntary treatment.[17] The court order expires 7 days after it is executed.[18]

3. Any peace officer may take a person to a physician, psychologist, clinical social worker, or clinical nurse specialist for emergency examination or to any emergency receiving facility if the person is committing a penal offense and the peace officer has probable cause to believe that the person is a mentally ill person requiring involuntary treatment.[19]

A person who is admitted to an emergency receiving facility by one of the three methods listed must be examined by a physician within 48 hours of admission.[20] Immediately upon arrival at the emergency receiving facility, the patient and his representative must be given notice of the right to petition for a writ of *habeas corpus* or for a protective order.[21] The patient must be discharged unless an examining physician or psychologist concludes that there is reason to believe that the patient may be a mentally ill person requiring involuntary treatment, in which case the physician or psychologist must execute a certificate to that effect.[22] If the patient is under criminal charges and the physician or psychologist does not issue a certificate, the patient can be discharged only into the custody of the law enforcement agency having original custody.[23]

Within 24 hours of the execution of the certificate, the patient will be transported to an evaluating facility, unless the patient meets the outpatient treatment requirements.[24]

(B)(2) Court-Ordered Evaluation

An involuntary treatment evaluation may take place as a result of the emergency examination procedures previously described or as a result of a court order. The court-ordered evaluation is rare. Usually, a physician, psychologist, clinical social worker, or clinical nurse specialist issues the certificate requesting an evaluation. However, any person may file an application with the community mental health center for a court-ordered evaluation of a person alleged to be a mentally ill person requiring involuntary treat-

---

17. *Id.*
18. *Id.*
19. O.C.G.A. § 37-3-42(a).
20. O.C.G.A. § 37-3-43(a).
21. O.C.G.A. § 37-3-44.
22. O.C.G.A. § 37-3-43(a).
23. O.C.G.A. § 37-3-95.
24. O.C.G.A. § 37-3-43(b).

ment.[25] The community mental health center will make a preliminary investigation and, if the investigation shows there is probable cause to believe that the allegations are true, it will file a petition with the court in the county where the patient is located seeking an involuntary admission for evaluation.[26]

Alternatively, any person may file a petition directly with the court alleging that a person is a mentally ill person requiring involuntary treatment.[27] The petition must be accompanied by the certificate of a physician or psychologist stating that he has examined the patient within the preceding 5 days and has found that the patient may be a mentally ill person requiring involuntary treatment.[28]

In either case, the court will review the petition and, if it finds reasonable cause to believe the patient may be a mentally ill person requiring involuntary treatment, the court will hold a full and fair hearing on the petition no sooner than 10 days and no later than 15 days after the petition is filed.[29] If the court is satisfied that immediate evaluation is necessary, the court will issue an order for a peace officer to deliver the patient to an evaluating facility.[30]

(B)(3) Evaluation: Period of Detention in an Evaluation Facility

A patient who has been admitted to an evaluating facility may be detained for a period not to exceed 5 days, excluding weekends and holidays.[31] The patient will be discharged if found not to be a mentally ill person requiring involuntary treatment or if found to meet the criteria for outpatient treatment.[32]

If hospitalization appears desirable, the staff physicians or psychologists will encourage the patient to apply for voluntary hospitalization unless the patient is unable to understand the nature of voluntary hospitalization or if the patient is determined to be a mentally ill person in need of involuntary treatment. If it is determined that proceedings for involuntary treatment should be initiated, the chief medical officer (CMO) will direct that an individualized service plan be developed for the patient.[33]

---

25. O.C.G.A. § 37-3-61.
26. Id.
27. Id.
28. Id.
29. O.C.G.A. § 37-3-62.
30. Id.
31. O.C.G.A. § 37-3-64.
32. Id. See O.C.G.A. § 37-3-90 for involuntary outpatient treatment.
33. O.C.G.A. § 37-3-64.

(B)(4) Commitment Procedures

The patient may be detained at a facility beyond the 5-day evaluation period only upon the recommendation of the CMO of the evaluating facility and upon the supporting opinions of two physicians or a physician and a psychologist, each of whom has personally examined the patient.[34] A certificate containing such a recommendation will be filed, along with a petition for a hearing, in the court of the county in which the patient is being detained for evaluation.[35] The filing of the petition will authorize detention of the patient pending completion of a full and fair hearing.[36]

Copies of the certificate will be served on the patient and his representatives within 5 days after the petition is filed and will be accompanied by

1. notice that a hearing will be held and the time and place;
2. notice that the patient has a right to counsel and that counsel will be appointed if the patient cannot afford counsel;
3. a copy of the individualized service plan developed by the evaluating facility;
4. notice that the patient has the right to be examined by a physician of his choice at his own expense; and
5. notice that the patient may waive the hearing.[37]

If the hearing is waived, the certificate will serve as authorization for the patient to begin treatment under the individualized service plan.[38]

Unless waived, a full and fair hearing must be held no sooner than 7 days and no later than 12 days after the petition is filed.[39] At the hearing, the court will determine whether the patient is a mentally ill person requiring involuntary treatment and, if so, whether the patient should be an inpatient or outpatient and the type of involuntary treatment the patient should be ordered to obtain.[40] If the court finds that the patient should be an inpatient, the court will order that the patient be transported to a treatment facility where the patient will be admitted for care and treatment.[41] The court may order hospitalization for any period not to exceed 6 months, subject to the power of the CMO to discharge the patient.[42] If continued hospitalization is necessary beyond 6

---

34. *Id.*
35. O.C.G.A. § 37-3-81.
36. *Id.*
37. *Id.*
38. *Id.*
39. *Id.*
40. O.C.G.A. § 37-3-81.1.
41. *Id.*
42. *Id.*

months, the CMO must apply for an order authorizing continued hospitalization for an additional 12 months.[43]

(B)(5) Standards for Involuntary Hospitalization

To commit a person as a mentally ill person requiring involuntary inpatient treatment, the court must find that the individual

1. has a disorder of thought or mood that significantly impairs judgment, behavior, capacity to recognize reality, or ability to cope with the ordinary demands of life;[44] and

2. presents a substantial risk of imminent harm to that person or others, as manifested by either recent overt acts or recent expressed threats of violence that present a probability of physical injury to that person or others; or

3. is so unable to care for his own physical health and safety as to create an imminently life-endangering crisis.[45]

This statutory standard complies with the constitutional requirement that a mental illness alone cannot justify involuntary commitment. There must also be a finding that the person is dangerous to himself or herself, or to others.[46]

(B)(6) Discharge

Each individualized service plan must be reviewed at regular intervals to determine the patient's progress and whether the plan should be modified.[47] In addition, if the patient is able to secure the services of a private psychologist or physician, the psychologist or physician can see the patient at any reasonable time.[48] If the patient is found to no longer require involuntary inpatient treatment, the CMO may, after considering the recommendation of the treatment team

1. discharge the patient from involuntary outpatient or inpatient treatment, or both;

2. discharge the patient from involuntary inpatient treatment and require that the patient obtain outpatient treatment; or

3. transfer the patient to voluntary status at the patient's request.[49]

---

43. *Id. See* O.C.G.A. § 37-3-83 for procedures for continuing involuntary hospitalization beyond the initial period authorized by the court order.
44. O.C.G.A. § 37-3-1(11).
45. O.C.G.A. § 37-3-1(9.1).
46. O'Connor v. Donaldson, 422 U.S. 563, 95 S. Ct. 2486 (1975). *See* Remar, *supra* note 11, at 3–7.
47. O.C.G.A. § 37-3-85.
48. O.C.G.A. § 37-3-162(d).
49. O.C.G.A. § 37-3-85.

Notice of the discharge or transfer of status must be given to the patient and his representatives. If the hospitalization was court ordered, notice must be given to the court. If the patient was under criminal charges, notice must be given to the law enforcement agency originally having custody of the patient.[50]

50. *Id.*

8.5

Treatment of Alcoholics

At one time, Georgia law contained provisions relating to the treatment of alcoholics and intoxicated individuals designed to provide a continuum of treatment, rather than criminal prosecution, for alcoholic persons. The Act was never funded and never went into effect.[1] The effective date was to be originally July 1, 1983, but it was subsequently extended three times. In 1989, the effective date was extended to July 1, 1995. In its 1994 session, the General Assembly repealed the Act in its entirety.[2] (See chapter 8.6.)

---

1. O.C.G.A. § 37-7-1(15.1).
2. O.C.G.A. §§ 37-8-1 to 37-8-53.

8.6

Voluntary Admission and Involuntary Commitment of Drug-Dependent Individuals and Drug Abusers

Georgia law provides for the voluntary admission and the involuntary civil commitment of alcoholics, drug-dependent persons, and drug abusers. MHPs may be involved in the evaluation, diagnosis, treatment and discharge process. The relevant statutes,[1] Georgia Code Annotated, Chapter 7 of Title 37, mirror the statutes governing the voluntary admission[2] and involuntary commitment[3] of mentally ill adults and are virtually identical, both procedurally and substantively, except for the definitions of alcoholism, drug dependency, and drug abuse.[4]

Under Chapter 7, an individual may be subjected to involuntary treatment, either as an inpatient or outpatient, if he is an alcoholic, drug-dependent individual, or drug abuser requiring involuntary treatment. An *alcoholic* is defined as

> [a] person who habitually lacks self-control as to the use of alcoholic beverages or who uses alcoholic beverages to the extent that his health is substantially impaired or endangered or his social or economic function is substantially disrupted.[5]

A *drug dependent individual* or *drug abuser* is defined as

> [a] person who habitually lacks self-control as to the use of opium, heroin, morphine, or any derivative or synthetic drug of that group, barbiturates, other sedatives, tranquilizers, amphetamines, lysergic acid diethylamide or other hallucinogens, or

---

1. *See* O.C.G.A. §§ 37-7-1 to 37-7-8 for definitions and general provisions; §§ 37-7-20 to 37-7-24 for voluntary admission; §§ 37-7-40 to 37-7-95 for involuntary commitment.
2. *See supra* chapter 8.3, Voluntary Admission of Mentally Ill Adults.
3. *See supra* chapter 8.4, Involuntary Civil Commitment of Mentally Ill Adults.
4. *See* O.C.G.A. § 37-7-1.
5. O.C.G.A. § 37-7-1(1).

any drug, dangerous drug, narcotic drug, marijuana, or controlled substance, ... or a person who uses such drugs to the extent that his health is substantially impaired or endangered or his social or economic function is substantially disrupted; provided, however, that no person shall be deemed a drug dependent individual or abuser solely by virtue of his taking, according to directions, any such drugs pursuant to a lawful prescription issued by a physician in the course of professional treatment for legitimate medical purposes.[6]

An alcoholic, drug-dependent individual, or drug abuser may be involuntarily committed to an inpatient facility if he either (1) "presents a substantial risk of imminent harm ... as manifested by either recent overt acts or recent expressed threats of violence which present a probability of physical injury to that person or other persons" or (2) is incapacitated by alcoholic beverages, drugs, or other substances on a recurring basis. *Incapacitated by alcohol and drugs* means a person who

[a]s a result of the use of alcoholic beverages [or] drug[s], ... exhibits life-threatening levels of intoxication, withdrawal, or imminent danger thereof, or acute medical problems; or is under the influence of alcoholic beverages or drugs ... to the extent that the person is incapable of caring for himself or protecting himself due to the continued consumption or use thereof.[7]

An individual who is not in need of inpatient care may be ordered to submit to outpatient treatment if his history of drug or alcohol use establishes that outpatient treatment is required "in order to avoid predictably and imminently becoming an inpatient" and, because of his current mental state and lack of self-control, is unable to voluntarily submit to treatment.[8]

At one time, Georgia law contained provisions relating to the treatment of alcoholics and intoxicated persons designed to provide a continuum of treatment, rather than criminal prosecution, for alcoholic persons. The act was never funded and never went into effect.[9] The effective date was originally July 1, 1983 and was subsequently extended three times. In 1989, the effective date was extended to July 1, 1995. In its 1994 session, the General Assembly repealed the act in its entirety.[10]

---

6. *Id.*
7. O.C.G.A. § 37-7-1(8).
8. O.C.G.A. § 37-7-1(13).
9. O.C.G.A. § 37-7-1(15.1).
10. O.C.G.A. §§ 37-8-1 to 37-8-53.

8.7

Voluntary Admission and Court-Ordered Habilitation Services for Retarded Adults

Georgia law provides for court-ordered services for the habilitation of mentally retarded adults in mental health facilities and, to a limited extent, for voluntary admission. MHPs are involved in the entire process from evaluation, admission, and treatment to discharge.

(A) Definitions

The following terms are defined in the Georgia Mental Health Code and are central to an understanding of the law:

1. *Comprehensive evaluation team* or *comprehensive habilitation team* means and shall consist of

a group of persons with special training and experience in the assessment of needs and provision of services for mentally retarded persons, which group shall include, at a minimum, persons qualified to provide social, psychological, medical, and other services. . . .[1]

2. *Habilitation* means

the process by which program personnel help clients to acquire and maintain those life skills which will enable them to cope more effectively with the demands of their own persons and of their environment and to raise the level of their physical, mental, social, and vocational abilities.[2]

3. *Individualized program plan* means a

---

1. O.C.G.A. § 37-4-2(4).
2. O.C.G.A. § 37-4-2(8).

proposed habilitation program written in behavioral terms, developed by the comprehensive evaluation team and specifically tailored to the needs of an individual client. Each plan shall include a statement of the nature of the client's specific problems and specific needs; a description of intermediate and long-range habilitation goals and a projected timetable for their attainment; a description of the proposed habilitation program and its relation to habilitation goals; identification of the facility and types of professional personnel responsible for execution of the client's habilitation program; a statement of the least restrictive environment necessary to achieve the purposes of habilitation, based upon the needs of the client; an explanation of criteria for acceptance or rejection of alternative environments for habilitation; and proposed criteria for release of the client into less restrictive habilitation environments upon obtaining specified habilitation goals.[3]

4. *Mentally retarded person* refers to a person having a significantly subaverage general intellectual functioning existing concurrently with deficits in adaptive behavior and originating in the developmental period.[4]

5. *Mentally retarded person requiring temporary and immediate care* refers to

a person who is mentally retarded and who presents a substantial risk of imminent harm to himself or others; who is in need of immediate care, evaluation, stabilization, or treatment for certain developmental, medical, or behavioral needs; and for whom there currently exists no available, appropriate community residential setting for meeting the needs of the person.[5]

6. *Respite care* means

care and supervision . . . while the individuals with whom the person to be admitted usually resides are unavailable due to illness, absence, or needed rest. The level of treatment administered during such admission shall not exceed the level normally received . . . while such person is living in his usual environment.[6]

(B) Voluntary Admission

Although there is a more comprehensive program available for mentally retarded minors who apply for voluntary admission to a hospital setting,[7] the voluntary admission of a mentally retarded adult is limited under Georgia law to admissions for temporary or respite care[8] and for dental services.[9] The superintendent may

---

3. O.C.G.A. § 37-4-2(9).
4. O.C.G.A. § 37-4-2(12).
5. O.C.G.A. § 37-4-2(13.1).
6. O.C.G.A. § 37-4-21(a).
7. *See supra* chapter 4.19.
8. O.C.G.A. § 37-4-21.

admit any mentally retarded person for respite care if there is an available bed appropriate to the specific needs of the client.[10] The request for admission may be made by the person to be admitted if he is 18 or older; by his parents, guardian, or person standing *in loco parentis;*[11] or by his guardian if he has been declared legally incompetent.[12]

An admission for respite care can be for no longer than 2 weeks.[13] The period may be extended for additional periods of respite care, but not more than twice within any 6-month period.[14] A person who is living in a nursing home or personal care home is not eligible for respite care.[15]

A mentally retarded adult may also be voluntarily admitted to a treatment facility for dental services if the person cannot get the services elsewhere.[16] The admission may be only for the period of time necessary to receive the dental services, including a necessary recovery period.[17]

(C) Court-Ordered Services

Any person may file a petition for a court-ordered program of services for a mentally retarded person.[18] The petition must assert that the petitioner believes the person to be mentally retarded and that the petitioner is the parent, guardian, or person standing *in loco parentis* of the person and that the petitioner cannot obtain adequate services otherwise, or (2) that the petitioner believes that the parent, guardian, or person acting *in loco parentis* has failed or is unable to secure adequate services.[19]

The court will review the petition and, if it finds reasonable cause to believe that the allegations are true, will issue an order within 72 hours of the petition's filing for the client's examination by a comprehensive evaluation team.[20] Notice of the order will be provided to the client and to two representatives appointed by

---

9. O.C.G.A. § 37-4-22.
10. O.C.G.A. § 37-4-21(b).
11. *In loco parentis* means in the place of a parent. It normally refers to a person who takes the position of a lawful parent by assuming the obligations incident to the parental relation without going through the formalities necessary for legal adoption. Barron's *Law Dictionary* 233 (2d ed. 1984).
12. O.C.G.A. § 37-4-21(b).
13. O.C.G.A. § 37-4-21(c).
14. *Id.*
15. *Id.*
16. O.C.G.A. § 37-4-22.
17. *Id.*
18. O.C.G.A. § 37-4-22.
19. *Id.*
20. *Id.*

the court.[21] If the client and his representatives fail to comply with the evaluation order within 5 days after the date set by the order, the comprehensive evaluation team will notify the court, and the court may compel the attendance of the client before the comprehensive evaluation team.[22]

The comprehensive evaluation team will file a written report with the court within 10 days after examining the client.[23] If a majority of the team concludes that the client is mentally retarded and that he should receive services from the Department of Human Resources, the report submitted to the court will be in the form of an individualized program plan.[24]

The court will set a hearing on the petition and will provide notice of the hearing to the client and his representatives or guardian. The hearing must be held no sooner than 10 days and no later than 15 days, excepting weekends and holidays, after the filing of the report by the comprehensive evaluation team.[25] If, after a full and fair hearing at which the client is given all his due process rights, the court finds that the client is mentally retarded and is in need of such additional services, the department will recommend a habilitative program for the client, based on the individualized program plan submitted, which is an alternative to care in a facility.[26] If the court finds that such an alternative program is available and such program seems feasible, the court will order compliance.[27] If the court concludes that the least restrictive available alternative that would accomplish the goals of the plan is for the client to be admitted to a facility, the court will order such admission only if it specifically finds that

1. the client requires direct medical services;
2. the client needs 24-hour training in a residential care facility; and

---

21. *Id.*
22. *Id.*
23. *Id.*
24. *Id.*
25. *Id.*
26. *Id.*
27. *Id.* In S.H. v. Edwards, 860 F.2d 1045 (11th Cir. 1988), *cert. denied* 491 U.S. 905, 109 S. Ct. 3187 (1989); *rehearing en banc granted,* 880 F.2d 1203 (11th Cir. 1989) the Eleventh Circuit rejected a claim that the mentally retarded have a substantive due process right to habilitation in a community setting. Relying on the U.S. Supreme Court decision in Youngberg v. Romeo, 457 U.S. 307 (1982), the court found that Georgia's decision to keep the plaintiffs in institutions while awaiting community placement was not a deviation from accepted professional standards. The court ignored the undisputed evidence that members of the plaintiff class were not receiving the treatment recommended by the professionals in charge of their care. The court also implicitly rejected the argument that there was a state-created entitlement to treatment in the least restrictive setting by holding that the state was under no constitutional obligation to fund sufficient community placements.

3. the court has been notified that an appropriate bed is available and that the specified services can be provided.[28]

The court may order that the client be admitted to the facility for any period not to exceed 6 months, subject to earlier release by the superintendent.[29] If continued care beyond the period set by the order is deemed necessary, the person in charge of the client's habilitation shall apply for an order extending the placement for a period of up to 1 year.[30]

(D) Physician's Certification for Evaluation and Temporary Care

Any physician, psychologist, or clinical social worker may execute a certificate stating that he has personally examined a person within the preceding 48 hours and has found that the person appears to be a mentally retarded person requiring temporary and immediate care.[31] The certificate will expire after 7 days.[32] Upon receiving such a certificate, any responsible family member or representative named in the certificate may transport the client to the nearest facility.[33] A peace officer may also transport the client to a facility if the client's family member or representative is unable or unwilling to do so.[34]

A client taken to a facility under authority of such a certificate will be examined by a physician and may be given emergency care and treatment as needed.[35] The client must be discharged within 48 hours, excluding weekends and holidays, unless the superintendent files a petition for a full and fair hearing stating that the client has been personally examined by a physician or psychologist and found to be a mentally retarded person requiring temporary and immediate care.[36]

Immediately upon admission to a facility under this provision, the facility will give the client written notice of his right to petition for a writ of *habeas corpus* and to the right to legal counsel.[38] The filing of a petition authorizes continued admission

---

28. *Id.*
29. *Id.*
30. *Id.*
31. O.C.G.A. § 37-4-40.1.
32. *Id.*
33. *Id.*
34. *Id.*
35. O.C.G.A. § 37-4-40.2.
36. *Id.*
37. O.C.G.A. § 37-4-40.3.
38. O.C.G.A. § 37-4-40.4.

pending completion of a full and fair hearing.[39] Within 5 days, excluding weekends and holidays, facility staff, along with staff of the community mental retardation program, will conduct a comprehensive evaluation, develop an individualized program plan for the client, and file the plan with the court.[40]

Within 20 days of the filing of the petition, the court will hold a full and fair hearing as described and may take any action as previously described.[41]

(E) Continuation of Court-Ordered Habilitation

The superintendent of the facility in which a mentally retarded individual is being treated may seek an order authorizing an additional period of treatment for a period up to 1 year.[42] A Committee for Continued Habilitation Review may, after an evaluation of the patient's progress in accomplishing his treatment goals, make such a recommendation to the superintendent.[43] The committee will give the client and his representative notice of their right to be present at a meeting and to present an alternative individualized program plan secured at the client's expense.[44] An updated individualized program plan will be presented to the committee, and the committee will report its written recommendation to the superintendent as to whether continued habilitation in the facility is necessary.[45]

On the basis of the committee's recommendation, the superintendent may discharge the client or file a petition for an order authorizing continued habilitation, along with copies of the updated individualized program plan and the committee's report.[46] The petition will be served on the client and his representative, informing them of the right to file a request for a hearing with a hearing examiner along with their other due process rights, including the right to counsel.[47]

If a hearing is not requested, the hearing examiner will make an independent review of the petition and reports and may either order a hearing or may order continued habilitation for a period

---

39. *Id.*
40. *Id.*
41. O.C.G.A. § 37-4-42.
42. *Id.*
43. *Id.*
44. *Id.*
45. *Id.*
46. *Id.*
47. *Id.*

not to exceed 1 year.[48] If a hearing is requested or if the hearing examiner orders a hearing, the examiner will hold a full and fair hearing and may issue any order that the court is authorized to enter, except that he may issue an order for continued habilitation for a period not to exceed 1 year, subject to the power of the superintendent to discharge earlier.[49]

(F) Discharge

Upon regular, periodic reviews of the client's progress toward achieving the goals of his individualized program plan, if the client is found no longer to be in need of habilitation services, the client shall be discharged.[50] At least 14 days before discharge, notice of such action will be given to the client, his representatives, and, if the admission was court ordered, to the court.[51]

---

48. *Id.*
49. O.C.G.A. § 37-4-44.
50. *Id.*

Hospice Care

Hospice care is a program of psychological, medical, and physical support services offered to terminally ill persons and their families. The purpose of hospice care is to provide for death with dignity in a comforting environment, to increase the quality of the remaining days of life, and to assist the patient and the family to deal with issues of death and dying. Hospice care is provided by a team composed of members of the various helping professions and may include MHPs.

Georgia law specifically provides for the licensure and regulation of hospice care programs. A *hospice* is defined as a public or private agency that provides to terminally ill persons and their families, regardless of ability to pay, a centrally administered and autonomous continuum of palliative and supportive care, directed and coordinated by a hospice care team.[1] *Hospice care* is defined as

> medical, nursing, social, spiritual, volunteer, and bereavement services substantially all of which are provided to the patient and to the patient's family regardless of ability to pay under a written care plan established and periodically reviewed by the patient's attending physician, by the medical director of the hospice program, and by the hospice care team.[2]

The hospice care team is an interdisciplinary unit composed of members of the various helping professions, including physicians, nurses, social workers, clergy, or other counselors and volunteers.[3] No hospice may be operated without first obtaining a

---

1. O.C.G.A. § 31-7-172(3).
2. O.C.G.A. § 31-7-172(4).
3. O.C.G.A. § 31-7-172(5).

license from the Georgia Department of Human Resources. However, there is no requirement that the hospice obtain a certificate of need in order to provide its services.[4] Although hospice care is generally provided in the patient's home, care may also be provided by the hospice on an outpatient and short-term inpatient basis.[5]

---

4. O.C.G.A. § 31-7-179.
5. O.C.G.A. § 31-7-172(3).

Appendix

Table of Cases

References are to page numbers in this book

D

E

F

G

H

I

J

K

M

Table of Statutes

References are to page numbers in this book

Official Code of Georgia Annotated

Federal Rules of Civil Procedure

Federal Rules of Criminal Procedure

Federal Rules of Evidence

Internal Revenue Code

United States Code

Table of Rules of Court

Table of Administrative Regulations

References are to page numbers in this book

Rules of the Department of Human Resources

Rules of State Administrative Agencies

Table of References to Constitution

References are to page numbers in this book

Georgia Constitution

Article	Page
Art. 1, Sec. 1	115, 324, 348, 352
Art. 1, Sec. 2	140

Article	Page
Art. 2, Sec. 1	300
Art. 3, Sec. 6	143
Art. 4, Sec. 2	404, 405

United States Constitution

Amendment	Page
Fourth Amendment ...	115
Fifth Amendment	348
Sixth Amendment	348

Amendment	Page
Eighth Amendment ...	352
Fourteenth Amendment	244, 400

Index

References are to chapters.

Rape trauma syndrome, 6.7

About the Authors

Robert B. Remar is a partner in the Atlanta law firm of Kirwan, Parks, Chesin, and Remar. He has served as General Counsel to the Georgia Psychological Association since 1990 and represents mental health professionals in professional liability, licensing, regulatory, and business matters. He has authored a number of articles on mental health issues and is a frequent speaker on mental health law subjects. Mr. Remar also has a substantial litigation practice representing both plaintiffs and defendants in commercial and business litigation, constitutional law and civil rights, employment law, and environmental law, in addition to mental health law. He regularly handles complex litigation matters including class action lawsuits.

Mr. Remar lectures extensively to professional and civic groups in the areas of constitutional law and civil rights, mental health law, and litigation practice. He is active in professional and civic associations and has served as chair of the Individual Rights Section, the Consumer Rights and Remedies Committee, and the Death Penalty Representation Committee of the Georgia Bar, as well as serving on its Legislative Advisory Committee. He is a past president of the American Civil Liberties Union of Georgia and the Georgia Consumer Center, Inc. He currently serves on the Executive Committee of the ACLU National Board of Directors. Remar is an Adjunct Professor at the Georgia State University College of Law and serves as an administrative law judge for the Georgia Public Service Commission. He is a Master of the Bench in the Lamar Inn of Court of the American Inns of Court and is listed in *Who's Who In American Law.*

Remar is a graduate of the University of Massachusetts at Amherst (1970) and Boston College Law School (1974). He was admitted to the Georgia Bar in 1974 and the Massachusetts Bar in 1975.

Richard N. Hubert, who is a native of Atlanata, Georgia, graduated from Emory University Law School (LL.B., 1960), after attending Stetson University for one year on an athletic scholarship and Duke University. During law school, he was associate editor of the *Journal of Public Law* and a National Moot Court finalist. He is a member of the National Panel of the American Arbitration Association and a former municipal court judge. He has served as adjunct professor at Morehouse School of Medicine, where he

481

taught medical–legal courses. He has been a regular participant in Georgia Psychological Association and American Association of Psychotherapists seminars and workshops.

Mr. Hubert has practiced law in Atlanta for over 35 years and has been head of Chamberlain, Hrdlicka, White, Williams, and Martin's Atlanta litigation section since 1988.

Richard Hubert is currently serving on the executive committee of and is president-elect of the Lawyers Club of Atlanta, is active in the litigation section of the Atlanta Bar Association, and is an active participant in the life of his community and church. He performed on the stage of Atlanta theater before forsaking his career as an actor in favor of the courtroom.